The International Library of Bioethics

Volume 113

The *International Library of Bioethics* comprises international and interdisciplinary volumes on foundational and applied issues in bioethics. The series focuses on perennial topics of aging, mental health, preventive medicine, medical research issues, end of life, biolaw, and other areas of bioethics, whilst expanding into other current and future questions involving the living world. The *International Library of Bioethics* examines the role of bioethics against the background of increasing globalization and interdependency of the world's cultures and government.

The series explores meaningful ways to answer the questions of how to direct biotechnology to human and other living things' ends; how to deal with changed values in the areas of religion, society, and culture; and how to formulate a new way of thinking—that is, to create a new, practical bioethics.

The *International Library of Bioethics* welcomes book proposals representing the broad interest of the series' focus. We especially encourage proposals addressing aspects of changes in biological and medical research and clinical health care, health policy, medical and biotechnology, and other applied ethical areas involving living things, with an emphasis on those interventions and alterations that force us to re-examine foundational issues.

Matthew C. Altman · David Schwan
Editors

Ethics and Medical Technology

Essays on Artificial Intelligence, Enhancement, Privacy, and Justice

Springer

Editors
Matthew C. Altman
Central Washington University
Ellensburg, WA, USA

David Schwan
Central Washington University
Ellensburg, WA, USA

ISSN 2662-9186 ISSN 2662-9194 (electronic)
The International Library of Bioethics
ISBN 978-3-031-94689-9 ISBN 978-3-031-94690-5 (eBook)
https://doi.org/10.1007/978-3-031-94690-5

This Springer imprint is published by the registered company Springer Nature Switzerland AG
The registered company address is: Gewerbestrasse 11, 6330 Cham, Switzerland

Contents

Editors and Contributors

About the Editors

Matthew C. Altman is Chair and Professor of Philosophy at Central Washington University, USA. His research focuses on applied ethics, the history of philosophy, and the philosophy of law. Altman has published on such diverse topics as restorative justice, performance-enhancing drugs, mass incarceration, suicide, the problem of other minds, mandatory ultrasound laws, same-sex marriage, and the state of academic philosophy. He is the author, co-author, or editor of nine books, including *The Hackett Introduction to Medical Ethics* (with Cynthia D. Coe, 2025) and *A Theory of Legal Punishment* (2021).

David Schwan is a Senior Lecturer in the Department of Philosophy and Comparative Religion at Central Washington University, USA. In addition, he serves as the Director of the EthicsLab initiative at CWU. His research focuses on the intersection between applied ethics and moral psychology. He has published on empathy in medicine, the ethics of electronic health records, and medical scribes. His current research focuses on the ethics of advanced technology (AI/carebots) in medical care.

Contributors

Matthew C. Altman Central Washington University, Ellensburg, WA, USA

Lars Assen Section of Knowledge, Transformation, and Society (KiTeS), University of Twente, Enschede, The Netherlands

Rina Bliss Rutgers University, New Brunswick, NJ, USA

Bryan Cwik University of Florida, Gainesville, FL, USA

Stephen Damianos Neurorights Foundation, New York, NY, USA

Kathinka Evers Uppsala University, Uppsala, Sweden

Michele Farisco Uppsala University, Uppsala, Sweden

Luciano Floridi Yale University, New Haven, CT, USA;
Department of Legal Studies, University of Bologna, Bologna, Italy

Sharona Hoffman Case Western Reserve University School of Law, Cleveland, OH, USA

Katharine Lawrence New York University, New York, NY, USA

Christopher F. Masciari MD Anderson Cancer Center, Houston, TX, USA

Jessica Morley Yale University, New Haven, CT, USA

Lauren Nuckols Central Washington University, Ellensburg, WA, USA

Amitabha Palmer MD Anderson Cancer Center, Houston, TX, USA

David Schwan Central Washington University, Ellensburg, WA, USA

Łukasz Szoszkiewicz Adam Mickiewicz University, Poznań, Poland

Simona Tiribelli University of Macerata, Macerata, Italy

Ryan Tonkens Lakehead University, Thunder Bay, ON, Canada

Natalia Wewior Broad Institute, Cambridge, MA, USA

Chapter 1
Introduction: Technological Innovation and Moral Evolution

David Schwan and Matthew C. Altman

Abstract Advances in medical technology—from antibiotics and organ transplantation to gene editing and artificial intelligence—have transformed healthcare and raised new ethical questions about the nature of medicine. These technologies not only alter diagnostic and therapeutic practices but also mediate how humans relate to one another and understand concepts such as health, illness, death, autonomy, and care. Drawing on ethics, law, history, and sociology, this volume offers a multidisciplinary framework for understanding how technological innovation reshapes ethical norms and social practices. As medicine becomes increasingly data-driven and technologically mediated, new frameworks and practices are needed to guide its development toward appropriate human ends.

Keywords Medical technology · Bioethics · Medical ethics · Technological mediation · Clinical practice

1.1 Introduction

The invention of groundbreaking medical technologies in the twentieth century raised many ethical issues around appropriate care for patients, the role of practitioners, and how to consider risks that are hard to predict. These debates have only intensified in the twenty-first century as the pace of technological change has accelerated. New technologies are being implemented in clinical settings that would have seemed like science fiction a few decades ago. For example, recently researchers have used AI models to accurately detect cancer in a seemingly healthy pancreas approximately a year and a half before the eventual clinical diagnosis (Mayo Clinic 2023). These results represent a major medical advancement in oncology. Or consider one of the

D. Schwan (✉) · M. C. Altman
Central Washington University, Ellensburg, WA, USA
e-mail: david.schwan@cwu.edu

M. C. Altman
e-mail: matthew.altman@cwu.edu

M. C. Altman and D. Schwan (eds.), *Ethics and Medical Technology*, The International Library of Bioethics 113, https://doi.org/10.1007/978-3-031-94690-5_1

many gene-based therapies that have recently been approved by the US Food and Drug Administration (FDA). Researchers used CRISPR to harvest a patient's blood-forming stem cells, edit their genes, and then reinsert them to encourage hemoglobin production. Clinical trials found that 93.5% of the patients with sickle cell disease experienced no pain crises for at least a year post-treatment (Klein 2024).

Such cases highlight the potential of new technologies to improve health and well-being. At the same time, they are transforming care delivery and raising urgent ethical and legal questions. The chapters in this volume explore these issues from philosophical, sociological, legal, and historical perspectives. Our goal is to provide students, ethicists, researchers, and medical professionals with an overview of the present state of new and emerging medical technologies as well as the attendant ethical issues that must be addressed.

1.2 What Is Technology?

Scholarship on the philosophy of technology is extensive and interdisciplinary, and there are many proposed definitions of technology in the literature. To take only a few examples, technology has been defined as human-made artifacts (material or immaterial), devices, infrastructure, systems, human labor, an activity, a skill, an instance of volition, an idea (realized or not), or even a way of seeing the world (Coeckelbergh 2020). Given the diversity of candidates, we treat "technology" as denoting a complex network of conceptual family resemblances. Such an approach encourages careful observation and analysis of concrete applications of technology (and technological concepts) in ordinary human experience without ignoring commonalities among different accounts.

Taking a functional approach, Peter-Paul Verbeek (2005) describes three ways that technology pertains to human activities and interests:

1. Instrumentalism: Technology is a neutral means or tool to achieve our goals.
2. Substantivism: Technology is not neutral; it determines parts of society or culture.
3. Mediation theory: Technology mediates human relations with other individuals, the world, and technology itself.

Following Verbeek (2005) and Don Idhe (1990), we adopt a broadly mediative account. Technology is not a neutral tool, but it goes beyond structuring specific aspects of society. Instead, it "shape[s] human existence" itself (Verbeek 2015, 28), transforming our experiences in three distinct ways:

1. embodiment relations, where the technology indirectly "becomes" a part or extension of the physical body (e.g., stethoscopes);
2. hermeneutic relations, where we "read" features of the world through a technology, translating the representation into clinically relevant information (e.g., CT scans); and

3. alterity relations, where we confront technology as an other that may resist or remain opaque to us (e.g., stubborn electronic health record systems) (Idhe 1990, 107).

Although resolving disputes about the ideal philosophical account of technology would go beyond the scope of this Introduction, the mediative approach is especially useful for understanding medical technologies because they frame and shift our basic perceptions of each other and the world.

1.3 The Social Value of Bioethics

People often say that our ethical, legal, and policy frameworks struggle to keep pace with technological change. There is some truth to this claim. After all, laws and regulations are usually implemented after the development of new tools or processes. It is sometimes easier to invent something than it is to sort out its ethical implications. In addition, academics and policymakers typically lack the technical and subject matter expertise to craft detailed policies.

However, it is important to distinguish the academic discussion of new technology from the public policies related to it. In our view, bioethics has generally kept pace with technological advances in medicine. Sometimes ethical discussion began contemporaneously with the relevant scientific or medical research programs. For example, the Human Genome Project, which was launched in 1990, included proactive programs at the outset to address the ethical, social, and legal implications of research related to human cloning (National Human Genome Research Institute 2012).

There is also ample evidence of ethically anticipatory work in contemporary bioethics. For example, the cloning of Dolly the sheep in the mid-1990s received wide media coverage, with many commentators expressing concerns about the ethics of cloning. However, such concerns had been discussed in detail several decades earlier in the bioethical literature (Orentlicher 1999). Or consider the fact that ethical debates about modifying human embryos or germline editing emerged in the 1980s, decades before the technology itself was feasible (Baumann 2016). Finally, while the field of neuroethics was not formalized until 2002, research on the social ramifications of neuroscientific discoveries was already being published in the mid-1990s (Leefmann et al. 2016). Although fine-grained issues often become clear only when a new practice emerges, academics have a history of delineating the ethical implications of potential new technologies in advance.

Presently, those working on the ethics of medical technology find themselves at a challenging and exciting juncture. Emerging technologies will fundamentally reshape healthcare practices in the next few decades. As a result, academic research in this area will likely involve speculation about the future while also acknowledging the limitations inherent in this kind of prediction. For students, researchers, clinicians, and patients, technology will continue to raise profound philosophical questions about the purpose of medicine, the components of well-being, and what it means to be human.

1.4 A Brief (and Selective) History of Twentieth-Century Medical Technology and Ethics

The origins of medical technology extend to human prehistory. For example, archaeologists have found evidence of Neolithic forms of trepanation, a process where stone tools were used to drill holes in the skull for surgical purposes. Some patients seem to have survived the process (Gross 2012). Finding early evidence of pharmacology is more challenging given the nature of the physical evidence, but one recent study found carbonized traces of *Ephedra* (a plant utilized in traditional medicine) in a Moroccan burial site dated to the late Pleistocene period, about fifteen thousand years ago (Morales et al. 2024). Archeologists have also discovered clay tablets from the Sumerian period (3500–2000 BCE) that describe the use of willow leaves for pain and inflammation (Mahdi et al. 2006).

Our aim in this section is to illustrate the complex relationship between ethics and contemporary medical technology, so we set aside earlier milestones such as the invention of the microscope, the initial development of vaccines, the discovery and application of germ theory, and the use of anesthesia for surgery (see Porter 1997, 2006). Instead, we discuss four technological advancements in the twentieth century that both redefined medical practice and raised distinct ethical concerns: (1) penicillin, (2) hemodialysis, (3) the mechanical respirator and electroencephalography (EEG), and (4) organ transplantation.

1.4.1 Penicillin

The invention of penicillin in 1928 was the result of a laboratory accident. Alexander Fleming, a Scottish bacteriologist working at St. Mary's Hospital in London, returned from a holiday to find that a fungus had invaded one of his agar plates (Gaynes 2017). Noticing that bacteria did not grow around the mold colony, he isolated the mold and identified it as belonging to the *Penicillium* genus. In a 1929 article, Fleming showed that this "penicillin" fungus could inhibit bacterial growth in vitro (Lobanovska and Pilla 2017). About a decade later, Ernst Chain, Howard Florey, and a team of researchers at Oxford University successfully isolated, purified, and chemically characterized penicillin, which led to several initial human trials (Gaynes 2017). Later, mass production was made possible by combining a potent strain of penicillin with a waste product from corn, which was available in large quantities in the United States. As the US entered World War II, it took over the production of penicillin.

Once penicillin was produced at scale, it revolutionized the treatment of infections and transformed the world of pharmaceutical medicine. However, it also raised significant ethical questions. Because the initial production of penicillin (even at scale) was relatively limited, one question that arose was how to allocate it. A seriously wounded solider with a severe infection might require a substantial dose of the scarce antibiotic to survive and potentially return to service. But, instead of giving a large amount of the drug to one patient, a field physician might decide (based on a kind of utilitarian calculus) to give smaller doses to more patients struggling with minor infections so they could return to combat more quickly. In some cases, soldiers with less serious injuries were treated first, a form of "reverse triage" (Hurst and Ray 2024). In other cases, "the drug was given to soldiers with gonorrhea rather than used on wound infections" (Mitchell 2008, S5). This raises questions about the just distribution of scarce medical resources as well as whether fundamental principles of triage apply differently in civilian contexts than in war. In the United States, the Committee on Chemotherapeutic and Other Agents (COC) established guidelines that largely prioritized the military effort overseas, though allowances were made for urgent civilian cases where its use would be "of value" (Adams 1989, 200).

The appearance of penicillin-resistant bacteria also raised ethical challenges around how to balance short-term benefits against long-term risks. While penicillin was praised as a miracle drug, Fleming himself expressed concern about antibiotic resistance in his Nobel Prize lecture: "The time may come when … the ignorant man may easily underdose himself and by exposing his microbes to non-lethal quantities of the drug make them resistant" (1945, 93). Fleming's remarks underscored the importance of educating providers to consider not only the immediate clinical benefits of antibiotics but also potential harms to public health that may result from their misuse.

1.4.2 Hemodialysis

In the early twentieth century, John Abel, Leonard Rowntree, and Benjamin Turner invented an experimental artificial kidney that could be used for dialysis in animals. While dialysis was being developed concurrently worldwide, the crucial breakthrough occurred in 1942, when Dutch physician Willem Kolff created a form of hemodialysis that could be used in a clinic. A limitation of Kolff's machine was that it could not treat long-term kidney disease, since patients had to be surgically attached to it, and the procedure could only be performed a limited number of times. This constraint was overcome in 1960 when Seattle physician Belding Scribner and engineer Wayne Quinton invented the "Quinton-Scribner shunt," which connected a cannula (tube) in the patient's radial artery to a cannula in the cephalic vein. This allowed patients to receive dialysis repeatedly because clinicians could temporarily replace the shunt with the blood circuit of the mechanical kidney. Before the shunt, nine of out ten patients died; this new technology reversed those odds (Baker 2014, 2).

Although this breakthrough offered life-saving treatment for patients with long-term kidney disease, it also raised new ethical issues. The main challenge for the Seattle Artificial Kidney Center was deciding how to allocate this scarce and expensive treatment. Potential patients were screened for medical necessity, psychiatric conditions, and ability to pay. The Kidney Center also assembled an anonymous, seven-member panel of peers (a lawyer, clergyman, housewife, banker, labor leader, state official, and surgeon) as an Admissions Advisory Committee—nicknamed the "God Committee"—to determine who would receive dialysis.

The God Committee's approach generated a flurry of popular and academic critiques and raised broader questions about the allocation of scarce resources (Alexander 1962; Ross 2012). Critics noted that the multi-staged selection criteria hid several ethical assumptions. For example, patients without additional co-morbidities were favored over those with co-morbidities. Age was also a factor, with patients over fifty less likely to receive treatment. The most controversial selection criterion was the "Social Worth Evaluation," which seemed to yield ad hoc, bourgeois evaluations of patients based on their expected contributions to society. One critic caustically concluded: "The Pacific Northwest is no place for a Henry David Thoreau with bad kidneys" (Sanders and Dukeminier 1968, 378).

This marked a turning point in medical ethics. As Albert Jonsen notes, the selection process "was a dramatic instance of the new medicine meeting traditional medical ethics," which involved the "shocking" process of physicians ceding moral authority to an independent group of laypeople (2003, 214). Although "European medical societies never abandoned their jurisdiction over medical ethics" (Baker 2014, 279), in the US, the moral ambiguity generated by new technologies empowered a diverse group of "ex-theologians, lawyers, philosophers, social scientists … nurses, physicians, and researchers" to create new discourses and conceptual frameworks to address the problems they raised (279). Some scholars suggest that this was the beginning of American bioethics as a distinct discipline.

1.4.3 The Mechanical Respirator and Electroencephalography

Many of the advances we have described were a boon for the treatment of disease and extending human life. But other technological innovations challenged our collective understanding of life and death itself. For several centuries, a person was "declared dead when her heart stopped beating and her lungs ceased to function" (Whetstine 2008, 65). While this definition of death was relatively uncontroversial, it was often more challenging to determine when or whether a person had died. Until the early twentieth century, the medical establishment lacked the understanding of physiology to "accurately test for death" (65). Typically, physicians relied on observable processes such as the lack of a pulse, unresponsiveness to stimuli, or the absence of breathing. Although these tests were not infallible, in most cases they aligned with common intuitions about when death occurred.

The development and refinement of two technologies in the twentieth century complicated this picture and sparked debates in medicine, public policy, and academia around the metaphysics of death and the ethics of end-of-life care. First, the mechanical respirator (also known as a ventilator or breathing machine) provided artificial assistance so that otherwise incapacitated patients could continue breathing, sustaining their vital functions even when natural respiration had ceased or was no longer possible. Second, electroencephalography measured electrical activity in the brain with sensors on the scalp, giving physicians diagnostic information that was previously unavailable.

Techniques for assisting respiration began in the late nineteenth century. An early form of technological ventilation—the so-called iron lung—used negative pressure, placing the patient in a sealed chamber (except for their head) and mechanically regulating their breathing by adjusting air pressure. An alternate technique involved positive pressure ventilation, where (for example) a mask and bag could be used to circulate air into a patient's lungs. While this technique was often effective, it was typically employed only for intermittent conditions.

Invasive mechanical ventilators became available in the 1940s and 50s. This form of ventilator delivered oxygen into the lungs with positive pressure via an endotracheal tube. For the first time, it was possible to provide sustained respiration for patients with severe respiratory failure. Unlike the iron lung, which was bulky and gave clinicians only limited access to the patient's body through portholes, even early versions of positive pressure invasive ventilators were smaller and more portable, allowed direct access to the body, and delivered oxygen more consistently and efficiently (Young and Sykes 1990).

These assisted breathing technologies called into question the very meaning of life and death. On the traditional cardiopulmonary model of death, death occurred when heart and lung function ceased. However, artificial respiration made it possible to sustain a patient (even without apparent consciousness) so that they were breathing and alive according to the traditional definition but were not what most people would consider a living person. Was a patient in this state really alive? And if they were, when (if ever) was it permissible to withdraw these kinds of technological supports?

These questions were further complicated by the development of electroencephalography (EEG) in the late nineteenth and early twentieth centuries. By 1929, German neuropsychiatrist Hans Berger had successfully recorded EEG activity in human subjects using electrodes, and he had discovered that differences in mental states and cognitive activity were reflected in EEG patterns. By the mid-twentieth century, EEGs had become widely used to assess a variety of neurological conditions, including monitoring patients who were in comas or persistent vegetative states (Collura 1993). This led to a growing recognition that, in some cases, a patient could maintain cardiopulmonary activity (with or without ventilator support) yet have little brain activity. People's intuitions about the boundary between life and death became unsettled. Was a person alive if their heart and lungs functioned through artificial means? Was it different if a person was in a persistent vegetative state, with a functioning brain stem that naturally supported their animal functions, but with no higher brain activity?

The widespread use of the ventilator for critically ill patients also raised concerns for transplant surgeons. By the 1960s, new surgical techniques and immunosuppressant drugs made it possible to successfully transplant life-saving organs. However, the criteria for determining death remained unclear since even patients with severe brain injuries could have beating hearts. This confluence of new technologies and the growing potential for organ transplantation led to a reexamination of the traditional, cardiopulmonary definition of death.

A committee at Harvard Medical School was formed to develop a revised definition, which became known as the Harvard Brain Death Criteria. In 1968, they proposed that a patient in an "irreversible coma" who was "unresponsive," lacked "movements or breathing," with "no reflexes" and a "flat … EEG" should be considered dead (Ad Hoc Committee 1968, 337–338). The report provided clear guidance to medical professionals and courts, and it "became authoritative soon after its publication" (Jonsen 2003, 240). Starting in 1970, several US states enacted legislation that included the new definition. Yet there were substantial problems with it. Critics called attention to its rationale, which was stated at the beginning of the article: "Obsolete criteria for the definition of death can lead to controversy in obtaining organs for transplantation" (Ad Hoc Committee 1968, 337). This comment suggested that part of the reason for this new definition was to obtain healthy organs for transplantation, which seemed to prioritize the interests of transplant surgeons and their patients over independent, theoretical issues of how to understand life and death.

The President's Commission for the Study of Ethical Problems in Medicine and Biomedical and Behavioral Research was formed in 1978 with a mandate to develop a "uniform definition of death" (President's Commission 1981, 1). After much discussion, research, and review of existing arguments, the Commission issued a report that included the following statute, intended to replace previous legal definitions of death:

> Uniform Determination of Death Act (UDDA): An individual who has sustained either (1) irreversible cessation of circulatory and respiratory functions, or (2) irreversible cessation of all functions of the entire brain, including the brain stem, is dead. A determination of death must be made in accordance with accepted medical standards. (President's Commission 1981, 2)

According to this proposal, death is determined using traditional criteria, either cardiopulmonary or neurological. The Commission did not substantially revise clinical practice or change the ordinary understanding of death. It provided a clear justification for removing life support from individuals who had lost full brain function but could be kept breathing through mechanical respiration. Since such individuals were considered dead, their organs could be permissibly harvested (if they were donors) and used to save other people's lives.

1.4.4 Organ Transplantation

The earliest documented transplant in the modern era was a successful skin graft that occurred in 1869. New techniques for surgical skin grafts were used to treat injuries during World War I and World War II, but there was "a general consensus that transplantation of anything other than skin was not feasible due to rejection" (Nordham and Ninokawa 2021, 125).

The first successful kidney transplant occurred in 1954 with two identical twins. The organ recipient survived the surgical procedure and lived an additional eight years. Further transplant cases followed, also typically involving twins. The challenge for transplant surgeons and patients was finding potential donor organs that would not be rejected. This led to growing interest in research related to immunosuppressive drugs.

The key breakthrough occurred in 1962, when British surgeon Roy Calne discovered that using chemical suppressive agents such as azathioprine prolonged survival after renal transplants in dogs. This led to the first renal transplant from a deceased donor between non-genetically related human patients. In the next few years, the general shortage of viable organs also led to attempted transplants from nonhuman species (xenotransplantation). American transplant surgeon Keith Reemtasma attempted thirteen transplantations of chimpanzee kidneys to human recipients. Most of the transplants failed within four to eight weeks (Cooper 2012).

The first lung transplant was performed in 1963, and the first heart transplant in 1964. In both cases, patients survived the procedure but died eighteen days later (Nordham and Ninokawa 2021, 126). Subsequent transplants were more successful, with one patient living almost two years. While surgeons worldwide continued to perform organ transplants, "the results were not encouraging" and the practice raised a variety of ethical and legal issues (Jonsen 2003, 201).

One set of problems was mentioned in the previous section. According to the cardiopulmonary account of death, a potential donor was only considered dead when the heart and lungs had ceased to function. This left medical teams little time to remove, transport, and transplant viable organs that would have any chance of not being rejected. However, the growing use of the mechanical ventilator allowed clinicians to sustain respiration (and potentially a beating heart) when a patient would have otherwise died. This posed the questions mentioned earlier: Were such patients actually dead? Was it permissible to remove some of their organs when their circulatory system was still functioning?

Additional issues emerged even in transplant cases that were more likely to be successful. For example, was removing the organ of a consenting family member a violation of the traditional medical maxim to "do no harm"? It may be easier to answer this question in cases involving competent adults who could consent to the procedure, but it is more difficult with minors or the cognitively disabled. In one case, Jerry Strunk, a twenty-seven-year-old with cognitive disability, was proposed as a kidney donor for his brother Tommy. Their mother, serving as Jerry's guardian, petitioned the court to allow the transplant in part because Jerry's mental well-being depended on Tommy's survival. The court permitted the procedure (*Strunk v. Strunk*, 445 S.W.2d 145 [1969]). Cases involving minors raised novel issues about how to understand consent. Judicial review of several cases allowed surgeries only under specific conditions, including parental permission and assent of the minor, medical necessity, and psychological stability of the organ recipient.

While some of these issues were being resolved in the courts, they also revealed disagreements over who should have the authority to make ethical judgments in such cases. For some physicians, "the very idea of incorporating ethics experts, *nonresearchers*, into the review of research was rejected as insulting" (Baker 2014, 286). For example, Owen Wangensteen, professor and mentor to many transplant surgeons at the time, claimed that clinicians had not only technical but also ethical authority: "The fellow who holds the apple can peel it best. ... If you are thinking of theologians, lawyers, and philosophers and others ... I cannot see how they could help. I would leave these decisions to responsible people doing the work" (286).

These tensions reached a turning point when it was revealed that the US Public Health Service had, over a forty-year period, deceived 399 African Americans into participating in a study of untreated syphilis—even though doctors knew that penicillin was an effective cure. In response to the Tuskegee Syphilis Study and other scandals, the National Research Act was signed into law in 1974, requiring all federally funded research involving human participants to be reviewed by institutional review boards (IRB). It also led to the creation of the National Commission for the Protection of Human Subjects of Biomedical and Behavioral Research, which identified three basic ethical principles that should govern such research: respect for persons, beneficence, and justice.

1.4.5 Summing Up

Although we have not given a comprehensive account of ethics and medical technology, even this brief history illustrates how important technological disruptions in the twentieth century reshaped settled ways of thinking about human life and death, and raised ethical issues that required additional analysis, new frameworks, and novel applications. This gave rise to medical ethics as a distinct subfield of philosophy. We continue to ask the questions that were posed decades ago, and we still appeal to and debate many of the moral principles that were articulated by those who initially confronted such radical technological change.

1.5 Emerging Issues in the Twenty-First Century

Today, advances in medical technology are again poised to reshape healthcare and pose new ethical challenges. Innovations in genomics and precision medicine have made it possible to target treatments to individual genetic profiles. The rapid expansion of electronic health records (EHRs) in the last two decades and the more recent growth of telemedicine have altered both the accessibility of medicine and central features of the patient-clinician experience. Further, as artificial intelligence is integrated into medicine, it raises concerns about privacy, equity, and the nature of healthcare.

1.5.1 The Human Genome, Precision Medicine, and Gene Editing

The discovery of the structure of DNA in the mid-twentieth century was a watershed moment in science, transforming genetics, molecular biology, and our understanding of heredity. Within the decade, Marshall Nirenberg had "cracked the genetic code," showing how the information contained in DNA was used to construct proteins (Genomics Education Programme 2016).

From this discovery, three technological advances ushered in the modern era of precision, gene-based medicine. First, researchers in the 1970s produced recombinant DNA molecules by splicing, joining, and inserting hybrid DNA into host cells (National Human Genome Research Institute 2013). Scientists could now engage in direct and relatively controlled genetic engineering, which led to subsequent breakthroughs in synthetic insulin development, vaccines, and a variety of gene therapies. Second, researchers developed a complete roadmap of the human genome. In 1990, the Human Genome Project began to sequence the complete set of genetic instructions found in human DNA. This project was largely completed in 2003, with the remaining gaps finished by 2022 (National Institutes of Health 2022). Third, while what is now known as CRISPR (Clustered Regularly Interspaced Short Palindromic Repeats) was discovered in 1987, it was not until 2012 that a landmark paper by Emmanuelle Charpentier and Jennifer Doudna (Jinek et al. 2012) showed that genetic "scissors" could be used to "cut specific sites in isolated DNA," essentially creating a "programmable gene-editing system" (Ishino et al. 2018).

As our ability to map, edit, and engineer the human genome has advanced, questions have been raised about how these technologies should be used, who should benefit, and what limits should be placed on their applications. Broadly, there are three types of ethical concerns that have emerged in the literature: the distinction between genetic enhancements and genetic therapies, issues of genetic discrimination and inequity, and worries about privacy and consent related to genomic data.

First, ethicists examine whether and how to distinguish genetic therapies from genetic enhancements: therapies prevent and treat disease, while enhancements augment traits beyond what is medically necessary. In some cases, the distinction seems relatively straightforward. For example, using gene editing to treat sickle cell disease, blindness, or cancer all seem to be therapeutic in nature. But the possibility of manipulating genes to enhance intelligence, physical performance, or aesthetic appearance have generated debates about whether we ought to artificially improve naturally occurring human traits, particularly if those enhancements are heritable (i.e., germline gene editing). Some philosophers have claimed that genetic enhancement is a moral imperative: liberal eugenicists argue that we have an obligation to improve future children's well-being and support their autonomy (Savulescu 2007), and transhumanists see it as a collective goal to deliberately improve humanity beyond what natural evolution can achieve (Bostrom 2003). Still others have argued that the distinction between therapy and enhancement is porous (Juengst 1997). By narrowly focusing on these issues, however, we may overlook broader ethical challenges, such as the risk of introducing novel and heritable genetic information into the future human gene pool, with unpredictable consequences (Cwik 2019).

A second set of ethical problems concerns the unjust distribution of benefits. While precision medicine offers increasingly targeted and life-saving interventions, people do not have equal access to either genetic testing or the therapies themselves. Furthermore, some existing genomic datasets are incomplete because they fail to represent certain marginalized populations, and some are ambiguous because they inconsistently label or categorize specific populations. This complicates attempts to apply research findings in clinical settings (Ory et al. 2023). A growing area of discussion is the use of genetic information outside of direct clinical care. Existing laws such as the US Genetic Information Nondiscrimination Act (GINA) (2008) aim to ensure that genetic data can be used only in clinical and forensic contexts, although careful analyses find that such legal protections "fall short in many ways" (Chapman et al. 2019).

Finally, the growth of large genomic databases has intensified concerns about patient consent, data security, and privacy. Laws such as the Health Insurance Portability and Accountability Act (HIPAA) in the US protect personal health information and aim to balance the use of patient data for research with respect for patient privacy. However, unlike other aspects of a patient's health record, each individual's DNA profile is unique. Sharing this information, even for research purposes, poses risks to privacy, especially since study participants can be reidentified using this genomic data along with publicly available databases (Gymrek et al. 2013). Because of this, the US National Institutes of Health (NIH) "controls access to sensitive or potentially identifiable information in these databases" (National Human Genome Research Institute 2023). While better privacy protections have been developed in clinical and research contexts, the last two decades have seen substantial growth in direct-to-consumer genetic testing for both health and ancestry information. These at-home kits carry more privacy risks than most consumers realize. Genetic information revealed by these tests is not fully protected under GINA, which applies only to health insurance and employer discrimination. Additionally, most direct-to-consumer genetic testing companies are not bound by HIPAA, meaning that consumer data can be shared with or sold to third parties, including researchers, insurance companies, and law enforcement.

1.5.2 Electronic Health Records

In addition to medical techniques, new technologies have also been created to capture, store, and transmit enormous amounts of sensitive medical data. While the practice of keeping written medical records extends into the ancient world, the foundations of the modern electronic health record (EHR) or electronic medical record (EMR) systems do not appear until the 1960s, when academic medical centers developed "clinical information systems" to organize and standardize patient charts (Evans 2016). The US government followed suit in the 1970s, when they began using EHRs in the Department of Veterans Affairs. While practical and storage limitations hampered early systems in the 1980s, a consensus emerged in the 1990s that computerized systems would help reduce medical errors (Atherton 2011).

Even though the hardware was becoming increasingly affordable and powerful, the widespread use of EHRs was still "delayed by high costs, data entry errors, poor initial physicians' acceptance, and lack of any real incentive" (Evans 2016, S49). In the United States, a series of federal interventions in the 2000s played a critical role in changing that. First, President George W. Bush created the Office of the National Coordinator for Health Information Technology (ONC), which was tasked with developing a national health IT infrastructure and encouraging the adoption of EHRs by providers (Wells 2025). Second, the Certification Commission for Healthcare Information Technology (CCHIT) was established to ensure that EHR systems met basic requirements related to interoperability and security. Nonetheless, adoption rates of EHRs in the early 2000s were still low, since providers had few financial incentives to incorporate new and complex software into their practices. A 2008 study found that only 1.5% of surveyed hospitals and clinics had implemented an EHR system in all clinical units (Jha et al. 2009).

The turning point occurred when the Health Information Technology for Economic and Clinical Health (HITECH) Act was signed into law by President Barack Obama in 2009. Among other things, HITECH allocated billions of dollars to incentivize hospitals and clinics to adopt and demonstrate meaningful use of EHR tools. It also strengthened HIPAA privacy and security regulations and required that hospitals and clinics enact better data-sharing standards to improve connectivity. The impact of this law was substantial. In 2004, the percentage of office-based physicians using any form of EHR system was 20.8%. By 2015, EHR use had jumped to 86.9%. As of 2021, 88% of US office-based physicians used some form of EHR, with a growing number (78%) using a government-certified EHR system (Office of the National Coordinator, n.d.).

EHRs make patient information more shareable within a healthcare team, which increases communication among clinicians and makes possible better continuity of care. But it also changes our sense of what confidentiality means. A patient's healthcare record is accessible to numerous people: various physicians (primary care physician, surgeon, etc.), house officers (surgical and ICU staff, etc.), nurses (on multiple shifts), pharmacists, nutritionists, chart reviewers (quality and risk management officers, financial officers, insurance auditors, etc.), and more. EHR use coupled with team-based care models means that "the confidentiality principle is compromised systematically in the course of routine medical care" (Siegler 1982, 1518).

EHR use also impacts the kind of work that clinicians do. Ideally, EHRs enable them to reliably and safely store medical records and to streamline their workflow, freeing them to focus on patient care. However, the impact of EHR use on the practice of medicine has been mixed, arguably generating as many problems as it purports to solve. One regular complaint from clinicians is that these virtual paperwork burdens intrude on their personal time outside clinical consultations. These tasks involve documenting appointments (including coding conditions for insurance reimbursement), charting progress notes, ordering medications, submitting preauthorization requests, and keeping up with internal emails and other communications. A recent study found that physicians "spend nearly six hours on [the EHR] for every eight hours of patient scheduled time" (Robeznieks 2024).

The time commitments required for EHR documentation are problematic for several reasons. First, excessive time on data entry reduces direct engagement with and care for patients. While many physicians see genuine value in EHR use, a poll of primary care physicians found that 49% agreed that it "detracts from their clinical effectiveness" (Stanford Medicine 2018). Given that clinicians regularly have to include additional billing and compliance information (as well as clinical data) in EHRs, it is not surprising that the length of clinical notes has doubled since the HITECH Act was passed (Budd 2023).

In other cases, problems of usability and design hamper clinicians in their medical practice. For example, EHRs may have confusing or cumbersome menu systems (e.g., long, unorganized dropdowns). One researcher noted that it took thirty-two clicks to "order and record having given a flu shot" (Robeznieks 2024). In another case, physicians were required to manually log in to a system up to 140 times during a workday (Budd 2023). For many clinicians, modern medicine increasingly feels like it is more about data entry than caring for patients.

In addition to being inefficient, poor user interface (UI) design also imposes cognitive demands on clinicians. Relevant health data may be fragmented in a digital record system, making it difficult to review and synthesize during interactions with patients. Often, clinicians are faced with unmanageable numbers of EHR alerts: for example, in some systems, one in four medication orders leads to an alert. This can lead to "alert fatigue," where overburdened clinicians no longer distinguish trivial alerts from serious alerts, which increases the risk of medical errors and patient harm (McGreevey et al. 2020).

Providers regularly identify EHR use as one of the most significant stressors in their medical practice, and it is a "prominent contributor" to clinician burnout (Jha et al. 2018; Budd 2023). Some promising practical and technological advances have been developed to mitigate these problems, such as the use of scribes or AI "assistants" for nonessential medical data entry. In these technological transitions, the risk of medical error and professional loss (as physicians leave practices due to burnout) remain pressing areas of concern in clinical practice and public health.

1.5.3 Telemedicine

Another fundamental shift in patient care has been the rapid expansion of telemedicine and telehealth. The former can be broadly understood as "the exchange of medical information from one site to another through electronic communication," and the latter as any "two-way, real-time interactive communication between a patient and a physician or practitioner at a distant site through telecommunications equipment that includes, at a minimum, audio and visual equipment" (American Medical Association, n.d.). Telemedicine in its modern form has existed for decades. In one early case, heart rhythms were transmitted over the telephone, and by the 1940s physicians were sharing radiologic images by the same medium using an early form of line-by-line fax technology. As technological capabilities grew, so did the scale of telemedicine. By 1960, it was possible for NASA to engage in (almost) real-time monitoring of astronauts in flight by medical teams. Applications of telehealth continued to grow slowly in the following decades. Often this was for specialized consultation (e.g., radiology) or to provide necessary services at a distance (e.g., to rural populations) when local care was unavailable.

The growth of the internet in the 1990s had a substantial impact on telehealth, as did the introduction of broadband internet in the early 2000s. Clinicians could now reliably engage in video consultations and transmit larger amounts of data in less time. By 2016, 76% of hospital systems in the US utilized some form of telemedicine, with radiology, psychiatry, and cardiology being the most frequent applications (Hyder and Razzak 2020). However, its general integration into medical practice "remained low, and the logistics were complex" (Shaver 2022, 518).

This changed rapidly with the outbreak of the SAR-CoV-2 virus in 2019. As the virus spread in 2020, Congress relaxed regulations on interstate medical practice, privacy, and insurance coverage for telemedicine. Visits could now be made from home (for clinicians and patients), use easily accessible video platforms (e.g., Zoom), and be reimbursed as though the appointment was in person (Shaver 2022). These changes led to an explosion in the practice of telehealth. One nationwide study showed that telehealth encounters increased 766% in the first few months of the pandemic (Weiner et al. 2021). In some hospital systems, they surged 8,729% compared to the previous, pre-COVID year (Ramaswamy et al. 2020).

While use of telehealth has "quieted significantly" since the COVID-19 pandemic, it is still above pre-pandemic levels (Brouillette 2024). A survey by the US Department of Health and Human Services (HHS) found that between 2021 and 2022, telehealth usage rates fluctuated between 20.5% and 24.2% (Lee et al. 2023). A more recent national study found higher utilization, with 43% of adults reporting telehealth use in 2022 (Chang et al. 2024). And while many patients (approximately

40%) stated that they would continue to use it going forward, most preferred in-person care when it is available (Bestsennyy et al. 2021; Predmore et al. 2021).

Access to telehealth during the COVID-19 pandemic was important to maintain medical care while mitigating the risk of transmission. And the fact that telehealth applications have not fallen to pre-pandemic levels suggests that clinicians and patients see value in this new modality. However, its continued integration into clinical practice is worth ongoing ethical investigation. First, while telehealth offers clear benefits in terms of accessibility, it raises concerns about the comparative quality of (virtual) care and how it affects the clinician-patient relationship. The available evidence on quality of care is fairly promising. For example, one recent review of meta-analyses found that "telehealth can be equivalent or more clinically effective" than typical in-person care (Snoswell et al. 2023).

Although these outcomes are impressive, clinical effectiveness varies across medical disciplines and practices. For example, while current data suggests that most primary care physicians (76.7%) and medical specialists (73.1%) were "able to provide a similar quality of care during telemedicine visits," the average falls to 50.6% for surgical specialists (Myrick et al. 2024, 1). This suggests that the nature of some clinical interactions and "hands on" examinations are difficult to replicate virtually, particularly when the condition is more directly physically embodied.

A related worry is that the virtually mediated nature of telehealth will negatively impact the clinician-patient relationship. Here the evidence is more mixed. Recent qualitative data suggests that, despite important benefits, telehealth patients have a reduced sense of connection with their providers and that it is more challenging to establish relationships with new providers. Clinicians expressed concern about the lack of physical presence (and touch), and both clinicians and patients noted challenges with communication and shared decision-making (Andreadis et al. 2023). This has led some researchers to propose clearer telehealth competencies for medical education that emphasize both technical care (e.g., physical exams and tests) and virtual communication skills (e.g., eye contact and body language) (Cruz-Panesso et al. 2023).

A second ethical concern relates to medical data and privacy. In a traditional clinical context, a medical exam takes place in a private setting, and personal health information (PHI) from the consultation is securely transmitted and stored in a clinic or hospital system. With telehealth, it is sometimes difficult for patients and clinicians to find suitably private spaces, even in their homes. In addition, many common video chat apps (such as FaceTime) are not HIPAA compliant, so patients must locate and learn to use alternative platforms, which creates barriers to access, particularly for those with less technological proficiency.

Finally, the virtual expansion of the clinic with telehealth poses new risks to patient medical data. As medical information is increasingly distributed across multiple platforms and accessed by clinicians, IT teams, and patients through patient portals and apps, the potential for security and surveillance vulnerabilities grows. There are two areas of particular concern. First, telehealth visits have become a critical means of providing access to medication abortion services, especially in countries or regions with restrictive laws. While this form of virtual abortion care has increased accessibility, it also introduces new legal challenges related to government surveillance. Another worry is related to the security of health information. This kind of personal data is highly valued by criminals, so the added complexities of telehealth pose increased risk of authorized access. Between 2009 and 2024, over 6,759 data breaches were reported to HHS, representing nearly 850 million healthcare records (Adler 2025). The frequency and severity of these kinds of breaches are growing rapidly, so there is an urgent need for robust security measures and strict oversight.

1.5.4 Artificial Intelligence

Artificial intelligence has its roots in the early twentieth century, though the concept of simulated intelligence was not formalized until the Dartmouth Summer Research Project on Artificial Intelligence in 1956 (McCarthy et al. 1955). In the following decades, AI research advanced through expert systems in the 1970s, statistical learning methods in the 1990s, and deep learning techniques in the 2010s. These developments paved the way for modern applications of AI such as machine learning, which improves system performance without explicit instructions; deep learning, which uses models built on neural networks to detect patterns; and natural language processing, which trains machines to understand, interpret, and generate ordinary language (Alowais et al. 2023).

AI applications in healthcare are rapidly expanding and now serve an important role in drug discovery, clinical decision support, imaging analysis and diagnostics, predictive analytics, personalized medicine, and surgery. While these technologies are already delivering improved accuracy, efficiency, and accessibility, they raise concerns about bias and the inequitable distribution of benefits. They are also reshaping the role of clinicians, the nature of the clinical encounter, and the clinician-patient relationship.

Before addressing specific applications, it is important to acknowledge a structural limitation of AI: algorithmic bias. This kind of bias can emerge in complex ways: in selecting the problems to solve, in the datasets themselves (both reflecting existing biases and introducing new biases), in modeling and evaluation, and in how the algorithm is applied in practice. For example, imagine that a particular group has been historically underserved or excluded and so has lower healthcare costs relative to the wider population. If an AI model is trained on this dataset, it may mistakenly infer that the group has low healthcare needs when the opposite is true (Obermeyer et al. 2019). Or a predictive model that is largely trained on data from male patients will be less accurate in predicting heart attacks in females. A growing literature has developed to identify and mitigate algorithmic bias.

As noted earlier, the widespread use of EHR systems has been a mixed blessing. Many clinicians complain that they spend more time on EHR navigation and data entry than they devote to patients themselves. Newer AI-powered, "smart" EHRs may lessen or remove some of these barriers. For example, smart EHRs can help clinicians prepare for appointments by summarizing notes, autocompleting medical terminology, and combined with "ambient" AI scribes, can take notes during appointments. Recent research suggests that this reduces both paperwork fatigue and burnout more generally (Waldren and Billings 2024).

Some of the most impressive results of medical AI have occurred in diagnosis and testing. While AI-driven clinical decision-support systems currently only exist as prototypes, initial results are promising. In one case, an AI system trained on a large EHR dataset was able to accurately predict patient responses to antidepressants (Sheu et al. 2023). AI systems have been developed to detect and monitor a variety of health conditions such as cancer, heart disease, retinopathy, strokes, and depression. Some AI tools now regularly outperform skilled diagnosticians, particularly in radiology (Kim et al. 2020). These kinds of advances may detect diseases earlier and reduce human error.

AI is also revolutionizing the process of drug discovery. Traditional drug discovery is expensive, and it is time-consuming to bring a drug to market. Using AI, researchers can now make better predictions about disease-associated targets and drug toxicities, and can optimize the design of clinical trials. For example, the development of AlphaFold 2 allowed researchers to predict the three-dimensional structure of nearly all two hundred million known proteins based on their amino acid sequence, something it would have taken "a billion years of PhD time to complete at the rate of five years per protein" (Ranger 2025). These kinds of advances significantly shorten the time to develop new drugs, which reduces costs, indirectly benefiting patients.

For all these advantages, applying AI technologies to medicine introduces new risks and ethical challenges. One major risk is that, as clinicians outsource more cognitive tasks to machines, they will become less adept at their work. For example, potential overreliance on machine-generated summaries or suggestions can lead to automation bias, where users become overly reliant on machine outputs and fail to verify results. As AI tools and smart EHR systems become better at diagnosis, clinicians may lose opportunities to practice their diagnostic skills, which can atrophy over time. High case volumes are critical for developing diagnostic proficiency, and removing these cases from early-career physicians may result in long-term deskilling in crucial areas such as visual perception tasks in radiology (Povyakalo et al. 2013).

Another ongoing challenge is the "black box problem." In many cases, it is not possible in principle to determine how an AI algorithm arrived at a conclusion or prediction. This is particularly troubling when the judgments of the clinician and the machine are in tension. Will clinicians feel pressured to justify any deviation from the findings of medical AI, even when their training and intuition suggest otherwise? And who is liable in cases where a faulty judgment results in patient harm? Research suggests that physicians already defer to AI-generated outputs, even when those outputs introduce systematic biases, raising concerns about the erosion of independent clinical judgment (Jabbour et al. 2023).

Finally, AI tools affect the clinician-patient relationship. While many of the benefits of AI technologies will help patients (such as improved outcomes and new medications), the growing automation of the clinical setting may reduce the personal side of medical practice. As AI tools grow in clinical prominence, humanistic medical virtues such as empathy, moral attention, and a holistic understanding of the patient's experience may be sidelined. As patient interactions are increasingly mediated, clinicians may struggle to maintain the meaningful relationships required to build trust with patients and provide effective care.

1.6 Summary of Chapters

New technologies reshape social practices. Medical technologies mediate relationships between patients and clinicians, and they challenge us to rethink basic aspects of health, life, and death. The chapters in this volume explore how these technologies are transforming healthcare and, in the process, raising novel ethical, legal, and philosophical questions that must be addressed.

Part I examines how new technologies are altering the nature of the clinical encounter, shifting the clinician-patient relationship in substantial and subtle ways. In Chap. 2, Jessica Morley and Luciano Floridi assess the state of AI ethics, categorizing the risks of AI and mapping its effects at individual, institutional, and societal levels. In Chap. 3, Simona Tiribelli challenges a common idea that AI bias is merely a technical flaw, arguing that these biases expose deeper inequities in healthcare that can be leveraged to design fairer medical systems. In Chap. 4, Amitabha Palmer and David Schwan show how AI-driven clinical tools, if they are adopted uncritically, may deskill physicians, reshape medical knowledge, and diminish their moral character. Amitabha Palmer and Christopher Masciari extend this discussion to telemedicine in Chap. 5. Although telemedicine can expand access, it also risks reducing care to mere technical transactions, displacing central humanistic values. Finally, in Chap. 6, Kathinka Evers and Michele Farisco examine the rise of robotic caregivers and explore how the reliance on machines to provide care for children may impact the children's development and influence social and ethical norms.

As medicine moves beyond treating disease and toward enhancing human well-being, difficult questions arise regarding the nature of humanity, our obligations to future generations, and the role of clinicians. Part II considers the ethical implications of regenerative medicine and enhancement technologies. The first three chapters focus on genetic therapies and enhancements: Natalia Wewior argues that a full ethical evaluation of somatic gene therapies should consider not only risks but also substantial benefits that may accrue if we institute the proper institutional safeguards (Chap. 7); Bryan Cwik examines the "targets problem," arguing that the distinction between therapy and enhancement is often blurred by the social values embedded in genomic science (Chap. 8); and Ryan Tonkens warns that, without careful regulation, genetic enhancements may deepen social divisions and create new forms of biological privilege (Chap. 9). In Chap. 10, Lars Assen uses the case of stem cell research to argue that researchers should play a more active role in anticipating ethical challenges. Chapters 11 and 12 consider how society and the law will both shape and be shaped by neurotechnology. Rina Bliss questions how AI-assisted cognitive enhancements might redefine agency and stratify cognitive ability along socioeconomic lines, while Łukasz Szoszkiewicz and Stephen Damianos argue that, in the absence of formal regulation, medical providers can use existing human rights law to guide the ethical use of neurotechnology in ways that benefit persons with disabilities and children.

As healthcare systems become increasingly reliant on big data and AI-driven analytics, new questions also emerge regarding privacy, autonomy, and fairness—issues that are addressed in Part III. In Chap. 13, Katharine Lawrence describes the various ways that electronic health records can encode biases and reinforce disparities in diagnosis and treatment. In Chap. 14, Sharona Hoffman explores the growing vulnerabilities in medical data privacy, particularly the health information gathered through wearables, online searches, and social media. In Chap. 15, Lauren Nuckols develops these concerns with regard to big data, noting that the commodification of health data by insurers and corporations threatens patient autonomy and reinforces biases. Finally, in Chap. 16, Matthew Altman explores how technology and data can be used to influence behavior through digital nudging, arguing that, when designed transparently, these interventions can improve public health without undermining autonomy. Each of these discussions emphasizes the ongoing need for safeguards to ensure that we protect patient privacy and respect autonomy in ways that avoid exacerbating existing injustices.

1.7 Conclusion

Taken together, the contributions in this volume illustrate how emerging medical technologies do more than attempt to improve health outcomes or reduce inefficiencies. They also alter fundamental features of modern medicine. In clinical settings, smart EHR systems, telehealth, and carebots are shifting the nature of the clinician-patient relationship. Gene editing is challenging the distinction between therapy and enhancement. And as big data and algorithmic decision-making become fully integrated into healthcare, new forms of bias are emerging. Technological innovation must be accompanied by ongoing ethical attention, different approaches to medical education, and new legal and regulatory frameworks. Change need not occur in any particular way; it is a function of our collective interests and priorities. If we aspire to maintain access to healthcare technology that is just and equitable, we must actively shape its development and align it with those ideals. This book is part of that effort.

References

Adams, David P. 1989. "Wartime Bureaucracy and Penicillin Allocation: The Committee on Chemotherapeutic and Other Agents, 1942–44." *Journal of the History of Medicine and Allied Sciences* 44 (2) (April): 196–217. https://doi.org/10.1093/jhmas/44.2.196.

Ad Hoc Committee of the Harvard Medical School to Examine the Definition of Brain Death. 1968. "A Definition of Irreversible Coma: Report of the Ad Hoc Committee of the Harvard Medical

School to Examine the Definition of Brain Death." *JAMA: Journal of the American Medical Association* 205 (6) (August 5): 337–340. https://doi.org/10.1001/jama.1968.03140320031009.

Adler, Steve. 2025. "Healthcare Data Breach Statistics." *HIPAA Journal.* Last modified March 20, 2025. https://www.hipaajournal.com/healthcare-data-breach-statistics/.

Alexander, Shana. 1962. "They Decide Who Lives, Who Dies: Medical Miracle Puts Moral Burden on Small Committee." *Life* 53 (19) (November 9): 102–125.

Alowais, Shuroug A., Sahar S. Alghamdi, Nada Alsuhebany, Tariq Alqahtani, Abdulrahman I. Alshaya, Sumaya N. Almohareb, et al. 2023. "Revolutionizing Healthcare: The Role of Artificial Intelligence in Clinical Practice." *BMC Medical Education* 23: article no. 689. https://doi.org/10.1186/s12909-023-04698-z.

American Medical Association. n.d. "Telehealth Resource Center: Definitions." Accessed March 26, 2025. https://www.ama-assn.org/practice-management/digital/telehealth-resource-center-definitions.

Andreadis, Katerina, Kimberly Muellers, Jessica S. Ancker, Carol Horowitz, Rainu Kaushal, and Jenny J. Lin. 2023. "Telemedicine Impact on the Patient-Provider Relationship in Primary Care During the COVID-19 Pandemic." *Medical Care* 61 (4) (April): S83–S88. https://doi.org/10.1097/MLR.0000000000001808.

Atherton, Jim. 2011. "Development of the Electronic Health Record." *Virtual Mentor* 13 (3) (March): 186–189. https://doi.org/10.1001/virtualmentor.2011.13.3.mhst1-1103.

Baker, Robert. 2014. *Before Bioethics: A History of American Medical Ethics from the Colonial Period to the Bioethics Revolution.* New York: Oxford University Press.

Baumann, Martina. 2016. "CRISPR/Cas9 Genome Editing—New and Old Ethical Issues Arising from a Revolutionary Technology." *NanoEthics* 10 (2) (August): 139–159. https://doi.org/10.1007/s11569-016-0259-0.

Bestsennyy, Oleg, Greg Gilbert, Alex Harris, and Jennifer Rost. 2021. "Telehealth: A Quarter-Trillion-Dollar Post-COVID-19 Reality?" McKinsey & Company. July 9. https://www.mckinsey.com/industries/healthcare/our-insights/telehealth-a-quarter-trillion-dollar-post-covid-19-reality.

Bostrom, Nick. 2003. "Human Genetic Enhancements: A Transhumanist Perspective." *Journal of Value Inquiry* 37 (4) (December): 493–506. https://doi.org/10.1023/b:inqu.0000019037.67783.d5.

Brouillette, Monique. 2024. "In a Postpandemic Era, Is Telehealth Still a Vital Tool?" *Annals of Emergency Medicine* 83 (3) (March): A11–A14. https://www.annemergmed.com/article/S0196-0644(24)00034-9/fulltext.

Budd, Jeffrey. 2023. "Burnout Related to Electronic Health Record Use in Primary Care." *Journal of Primary Care & Community Health* 14. https://doi.org/10.1177/21501319231166921.

Chang, Eva, Robert B. Penfold, and Nancy D. Berkman. 2024. "Patient Characteristics and Telemedicine Use in the US, 2022." *JAMA Network Open* 7 (3) (March 22): e243354. https://doi.org/10.1001/jamanetworkopen.2024.3354.

Chapman, Carolyn Riley, Kripa Sanjay Mehta, Brendan Parent, and Arthur L. Caplan. 2019. "Genetic Discrimination: Emerging Ethical Challenges in the Context of Advancing Technology." *Journal of Law and the Biosciences* 7 (1) (January–June): lsz016. https://doi.org/10.1093/jlb/lsz016.

Coeckelbergh, Mark. 2020. *Introduction to Philosophy of Technology.* New York: Oxford University Press.

Collura, Thomas F. 1993. "History and Evolution of Electroencephalographic Instruments and Techniques." *Journal of Clinical Neurophysiology* 10 (4) (October): 476–504. https://doi.org/10.1097/00004691-199310000-00007.

Cooper, David K. C. 2012. "A Brief History of Cross-Species Organ Transplantation." *Baylor University Medical Center Proceedings* 25 (1): 49–57. https://doi.org/10.1080/08998280.2012.11928783.

Cruz-Panesso, Ilian, Issam Tanoubi, and Pierre Drolet. 2023. "Telehealth Competencies: Training Physicians for a New Reality?" *Healthcare* 12 (1) (January 1): article no. 93. https://doi.org/10.3390/healthcare12010093.

Cwik, Bryan. 2019. "Moving Beyond 'Therapy' and 'Enhancement' in the Ethics of Gene Editing." *Cambridge Quarterly of Healthcare Ethics* 28 (4) (October): 695–707. https://doi.org/10.1017/S0963180119000641.

Evans, R. S. 2016. "Electronic Health Records: Then, Now, and in the Future." *Yearbook of Medical Informatics* 25 (S1): S48–S61. https://doi.org/10.15265/IYS-2016-s006.

Fleming, Alexander. 1945. "Penicillin: Nobel Lecture, December 11, 1945." NobelPrize.org. https://www.nobelprize.org/uploads/2018/06/fleming-lecture.pdf.

Gaynes, Robert. 2017. "The Discovery of Penicillin—New Insights after More Than 75 Years of Clinical Use." *Emerging Infectious Diseases* 23 (5) (May): 849–853. https://doi.org/10.3201/eid2305.161556.

Genomics Education Programme. 2016. "Cracking the Genetic Code." December 20. https://www.genomicseducation.hee.nhs.uk/blog/cracking-the-genetic-code/.

Gross, Charles G. 2012. *A Hole in the Head: More Tales in the History of Neuroscience.* Cambridge, MA: MIT Press.

Gymrek, Melissa, Amy L. McGuire, David Dolan, Eran Halperin, and Yaniv Erlich. 2013. "Identifying Personal Genomes by Surname Inference." *Science* 339 (6117) (January 18): 321–324. https://doi.org/10.1126/science.1229566.

Hurst, Daniel J., and T. L. Ray. 2024. "Reassessing Reverse Triage in Future Conflict." *BMJ Military Health.* https://doi.org/10.1136/military-2024-002774.

Hyder, Maryam A., and Junaid Razzak. 2020. "Telemedicine in the United States: An Introduction for Students and Residents." *Journal of Medical Internet Research* 22 (11) (November): e20839. https://doi.org/10.2196/20839.

Idhe, Don. 1990. *Technology and the Lifeworld: From Garden to Earth.* Bloomington: Indiana University Press.

Ishino, Yoshizumi, Mart Krupovic, and Patrick Forterre. 2018. "History of CRISPR-Cas from Encounter with a Mysterious Repeated Sequence to Genome Editing Technology." *Journal of Bacteriology* 200 (7) (April). https://doi.org/10.1128/jb.00580-17. https://doi.org/10.1128/JB.00580-17.

Jabbour, Sarah, David Fouhey, Stephanie Shepard, Thomas S. Valley, Ella A. Kazerooni, Nikola Banovic, Jenna Wiens, and Michael W. Sjoding. 2023. "Measuring the Impact of AI in the Diagnosis of Hospitalized Patients: A Randomized Clinical Vignette Survey Study." *JAMA: Journal of the American Medical Association* 330 (23) (December 19): 2275–2284. https://doi.org/10.1001/jama.2023.22295.

Jha, Ashish K., Andrew R. Iliff, Alain A. Chaoui, Steven Defossez, Maryanne C. Bombaugh, and Yael R. Miller. 2018. *A Crisis in Health Care: A Call to Action on Physician Burnout.* Massachusetts Medical Society, Massachusetts Health and Hospital Association, Harvard T. H. Chan School of Public Health, and Harvard Global Health Institute. https://www.massmed.org/Publications/Research,-Studies,-and-Reports/Physician-Burnout-Report-2018/.

Jha, Ashish K., Catherine M. DesRoches, Eric G. Campbell, Karen Donelan, Sowmya R. Rao, Timothy G. Ferris, Alexandra Shields, Sara Rosenbaum, and David Blumenthal. 2009. "Use of Electronic Health Records in U.S. Hospitals." *New England Journal of Medicine* 360 (16) (April 16): 1628–1638. https://doi.org/10.1056/NEJMsa0900592.

Jinek, Martin, Krzysztof Chylinski, Ines Fonfara, Michael Hauer, Jennifer A. Doudna, and Emmanuelle Charpentier. 2012. "A Programmable Dual-RNA-Guided DNA Endonuclease in Adaptive Bacterial Immunity." *Science* 337 (6096) (August 17): 816–821. https://doi.org/10.1126/science.1225829.

Jonsen, Albert R. 2003. *The Birth of Bioethics.* New York: Oxford University Press.

Juengst, Eric T. 1997. "Can Enhancement Be Distinguished from Prevention in Genetic Medicine?" *Journal of Medicine and Philosophy* 22 (2) (April): 125–142. https://doi.org/10.1093/jmp/22.2.125.

Kim, Hyo-Eun, Hak Hee Kim, Boo-Kyung Han, Ki Hwan Kim, Kyunghwa Han, Hyeonseob Nam, Eun Hye Lee, and Eun-Kyung Kim. 2020. "Changes in Cancer Detection and False-Positive Recall in Mammography Using Artificial Intelligence: A Retrospective, Multireader Study." *Lancet Digital Health* 2 (3) (March): e138–e148. https://doi.org/10.1016/S2589-7500(20)30003-0.

Klein, Jessica. 2024. "Cutting Edge Gene Therapy: Vertex Pharmaceuticals and CRISPR Therapeutics Casgevy." *Time*. October 30. https://time.com/7094725/vertex-pharmaceuticals-and-crispr-therapeutics-casgevy/.

Lee, Euny C., Violanda Grigorescu, Idia Enogieru, Scott R. Smith, Lok Wong Samson, Ann B. Conmy, and Nancy De Lew. 2023. "Updated National Survey Trends in Telehealth Utilization and Modality (2021–2022)." HP-2023-09. US Department of Health and Human Services, Office of the Assistant Secretary for Planning and Evaluation. April 19. https://aspe.hhs.gov/sites/default/files/documents/7d6b4989431f4c70144f209622975116/household-pulse-survey-telehealth-covid-ib.pdf.

Leefmann, Jon, Clement Levallois, and Elisabeth Hildt. 2016. "Neuroethics 1995–2012: A Bibliometric Analysis of the Guiding Themes of an Emerging Research Field." *Frontiers in Human Neuroscience* 10: article no. 336. https://doi.org/10.3389/fnhum.2016.00336.

Lobanovska, Mariya, and Giulia Pilla. 2017. "Penicillin's Discovery and Antibiotic Resistance: Lessons for the Future?" *Yale Journal of Biology and Medicine* 90 (1) (March): 135–145. https://pmc.ncbi.nlm.nih.gov/articles/PMC5369031/.

Mahdi, J. G., A. J. Mahdi, A. J. Mahdi, and I. D. Bowen. 2006. "The Historical Analysis of Aspirin Discovery, Its Relation to the Willow Tree and Antiproliferative and Anticancer Potential." *Cell Proliferation* 39 (2) (April): 147–155. https://doi.org/10.1111/j.1365-2184.2006.00377.x.

Mayo Clinic. 2023. "From Challenge to Change: AI's Leap in Early Pancreatic Cancer Identification." November 30. https://www.mayoclinic.org/medical-professionals/cancer/news/from-challenge-to-change-ais-leap-in-early-pancreatic-cancer-identification/mac-20558901.

McCarthy, J., M. L. Minsky, N. Rochester, and C. E. Shannon. 1955. "A Proposal for the Dartmouth Summer Research Project on Artificial Intelligence." August 31. https://www-formal.stanford.edu/jmc/history/dartmouth/dartmouth.html.

McGreevey, John D. III, Colleen P. Mallozzi, Randa M. Perkins, Eric Shelov, and Richard Schreiber. 2020. "Reducing Alert Burden in Electronic Health Records: State of the Art Recommendations from Four Health Systems." *Applied Clinical Informatics* 11 (1) (January): 1–12. https://doi.org/10.1055/s-0039-3402715.

Mitchell, Glenn W. 2008. "A Brief History of Triage." *Disaster Medicine and Public Health Preparedness* 2 (S1) (September): S4–S7. https://doi.org/10.1097/DMP.0b013e3181844d43.

Morales, Jacob, Yolanda Carrión Marco, Joanne H. Cooper, Elaine Turner, Alison Freyne, Joshua Hogue, Ismail Ziani, R. Nicholas E. Barton, Abdeljalil Bouzouggar, and Louise T. Humphrey. 2024. "Late Pleistocene Exploitation of *Ephedra* in a Funerary Context in Morocco." *Scientific Reports* 14: article no. 26443. https://doi.org/10.1038/s41598-024-77785-w.

Myrick, Kelly L., Mohsin Mahar, and Carol J. DeFrances. 2024. "Telemedicine Use among Physicians by Physician Specialty: United States, 2021." *NCHS Data Brief*. No. 493 (February). https://doi.org/10.15620/cdc:141934.

National Human Genome Research Institute. 2012. "Review of the Ethical, Legal and Social Implications Research Program and Related Activities (1990–1995)." Last modified October 1, 2012. https://www.genome.gov/10001747/elsi-program-review-19901995.

National Human Genome Research Institute. 2013. "1972: First Recombinant DNA." Last modified April 26, 2013. https://www.genome.gov/25520302/online-education-kit-1972-first-recombinant-dna.

National Human Genome Research Institute. 2023. "Direct-to-Consumer Genetic Testing FAQ for Healthcare Professionals." Last modified June 14, 2023. https://www.genome.gov/For-Health-Professionals/Provider-Genomics-Education-Resources/Healthcare-Provider-Direct-to-Consumer-Genetic-Testing-FAQ.

National Institutes of Health. 2022. “First Complete Sequence of a Human Genome.” *NIH Research Matters*. April 12. https://www.nih.gov/news-events/nih-research-matters/first-complete-sequence-human-genome.

Nordham, Kristen D., and Scott Ninokawa. 2021. “The History of Organ Transplantation.” *Baylor University Medical Center Proceedings* 35 (1): 124–128. https://doi.org/10.1080/08998280.2021.1985889.

Obermeyer, Ziad, Brian Powers, Christine Vogeli, and Sendhil Mullainathan. 2019. “Dissecting Racial Bias in an Algorithm Used to Manage the Health of Populations.” *Science* 366 (6464) (October 25): 447–453. https://doi.org/10.1126/science.aax2342.

Office of the National Coordinator for Health Information Technology. n.d. “Office-Based Physician Electronic Health Record Adoption. Health IT Quick-Stat #50.” Accessed March 26, 2025. https://www.healthit.gov/data/quickstats/office-based-physician-electronic-health-record-adoption.

Orentlicher, David. 1999. “The Misperception That Bioethics and the Law Lag behind Advances in Biotechnology: A Response to Michael H. Shapiro.” *Indiana Law Review* 33 (1): 163–172. https://mckinneylaw.iu.edu/practice/law-reviews/ilr/pdf/vol33p163.pdf.

Ory, Marcia G., Omolola E. Adepoju, Kenneth S. Ramos, Patrick S. Silva, and Deborah Vollmer Dahlke. 2023. “Health Equity Innovation in Precision Medicine: Current Challenges and Future Directions.” *Frontiers in Public Health* 11: 1119736. https://doi.org/10.3389/fpubh.2023.1119736.

Porter, Roy. 1997. *The Greatest Benefit to Mankind: A Medical History of Humanity*. New York: Norton.

Porter, Roy, ed. 2006. *The Cambridge History of Medicine*. Cambridge: Cambridge University Press.

Povyakalo, Andrey A., Eugenio Alberdi, Lorenzo Strigini, and Peter Ayton. 2013. “How to Discriminate between Computer-Aided and Computer-Hindered Decisions: A Case Study in Mammography.” *Medical Decision Making* 33 (1) (January): 98–107. https://doi.org/10.1177/0272989X12465490.

Predmore, Zachary S., Elizabeth Roth, Joshua Breslau, Shira H. Fischer, and Lori Uscher-Pines. 2021. “Assessment of Patient Preferences for Telehealth in Post-COVID-19 Pandemic Health Care.” *JAMA Network Open* 4 (12) (December 1): e2136405. https://doi.org/10.1001/jamanetworkopen.2021.36405.

President’s Commission for the Study of Ethical Problems in Medicine and Biomedical and Behavioral Research. 1981. *Defining Death: A Report on the Medical, Legal and Ethical Issues in the Determination of Death*. Washington, DC: US Government Printing Office.

Ramaswamy, Ashwin, Miko Yu, Siri Drangsholt, Eric Ng, Patrick J. Culligan, Peter N. Schlegel, and Jim C. Hu. 2020. “Patient Satisfaction with Telemedicine During the COVID-19 Pandemic: Retrospective Cohort Study.” *Journal of Medical Internet Research* 22 (9) (September): e20786. https://doi.org/10.2196/20786.

Ranger, Steve. 2025. “AI Designed Drugs in Trials This Year, Says Google DeepMind Chief.” *SCI*. January 23. https://www.soci.org/news/2025/1/ai-designed-drugs-in-trials-this-year-says-google-deepmind-chief.

Robeznieks, Andis. 2024. “Five Physician Specialties That Spend the Most Time in the EHR.” American Medical Association. September 11. https://www.ama-assn.org/practice-management/digital/five-physician-specialties-spend-most-time-ehr.

Ross, Will. 2012. “God Panels and the History of Hemodialysis in America: A Cautionary Tale.” *Virtual Mentor* 14 (11) (November): 890–896. https://journalofethics.ama-assn.org/article/god-panels-and-history-hemodialysis-america-cautionary-tale/2012-11.

Sanders, David, and Jesse Dukeminier Jr. 1968. “Medical Advance and Legal Lag: Hemodialysis and Kidney Transplantation.” *UCLA Law Review* 15 (2): 357–413.

Savulescu, Julian. 2007. “Genetic Interventions and the Ethics of Enhancement of Human Beings.” In *The Oxford Handbook of Bioethics*, ed. Bonnie Steinbock, 516–535. Oxford: Oxford University Press. https://doi.org/10.1093/oxfordhb/9780199562411.003.0023.

Shaver, Julia. 2022. "The State of Telehealth before and after the COVID-19 Pandemic." *Primary Care* 49 (4) (December): 517–530. https://doi.org/10.1016/j.pop.2022.04.002.

Sheu, Yi-Han, Colin Magdamo, Matthew Miller, Sudeshna Das, Deborah Blacker, and Jordan W. Smoller. 2023. "AI-Assisted Prediction of Differential Response to Antidepressant Classes Using Electronic Health Records." *NPJ Digital Medicine* 6: article no. 73. https://doi.org/10.1038/s41746-023-00817-8.

Siegler, Mark. 1982. "Confidentiality in Medicine—A Decrepit Concept." *New England Journal of Medicine* 307 (24) (December 9): 1518–1521. https://doi.org/10.1056/NEJM198212093072411.

Snoswell, Centaine L., Georgina Chelberg, Keisha R. De Guzman, Helen M. Haydon, Emma E. Thomas, Liam J. Caffery, and Anthony C. Smith. 2023. "The Clinical Effectiveness of Telehealth: A Systematic Review of Meta-analyses from 2010 to 2019." *Journal of Telemedicine and Telecare* 29 (9) (October): 669–684. https://doi.org/10.1177/1357633X211022907.

Stanford Medicine. 2018. *White Paper: The Future of Electronic Health Records.* September. https://med.stanford.edu/content/dam/sm/ehr/documents/EHR-White-Paper.pdf.

Verbeek, Peter-Paul. 2005. *What Things Do: Philosophical Reflections on Technology, Agency, and Design.* University Park, PA: Penn State University Press.

Verbeek, Peter-Paul. 2015. "Beyond Interaction: A Short Introduction to Mediation Theory." *Interactions* 22 (3) (May–June): 26–31. https://doi.org/10.1145/2751314.

Waldren, Steven E., and Edmund Billings. 2024. *AI Assistant for Clinical Review and Value-Based Care.* American Academy of Family Physicians. January. https://www.aafp.org/dam/AAFP/documents/practice_management/innovation_lab/report-navina-ai-clinical-review-phase2.pdf.

Weiner, Jonathan P., Stephen Bandeian, Elham Hatef, Daniel Lans, Angela Liu, and Klaus W. Lemke. 2021. "In-Person and Telehealth Ambulatory Contacts and Costs in a Large US Insured Cohort before and during the COVID-19 Pandemic." *JAMA Network Open* 4 (3) (March 23): e212618. https://doi.org/10.1001/jamanetworkopen.2021.2618.

Wells, Nora. 2025. "Assistant Secretary for Technology Policy/Office of the National Coordinator for Health Information Technology (ASTP/ONC)." *In Focus.* No. 12352. Congressional Research Service. Updated March 21, 2025. https://www.congress.gov/crs-product/IF12352.

Whetstine, Leslie M. 2008. "The History of the Definition(s) of Death: From the 18th Century to the 20th Century." In *End-of-Life Communication in the ICU: A Global Perspective*, ed. David W. Crippen, 65–78. New York: Springer. https://doi.org/10.1007/978-0-387-72966-4_4.

Young, J. D., and M. K. Sykes. 1990. "Artificial Ventilation: History, Equipment and Techniques." *Thorax* 45 (10) (October): 753–758. https://doi.org/10.1136/thx.45.10.753.

David Schwan is a Senior Lecturer in the Department of Philosophy and Comparative Religion at Central Washington University, USA. In addition, he serves as the Director of the EthicsLab initiative at CWU. His research focuses on the intersection between applied ethics and moral psychology. He has published on empathy in medicine, the ethics of electronic health records, and medical scribes. His current research focuses on the ethics of advanced technology (AI/carebots) in medical care.

Matthew C. Altman is Chair and Professor of Philosophy at Central Washington University, USA. His research focuses on applied ethics, the history of philosophy, and the philosophy of law. Altman has published on such diverse topics as restorative justice, performance-enhancing drugs, mass incarceration, suicide, the problem of other minds, mandatory ultrasound laws, same-sex marriage, and the state of academic philosophy. He is the author, co-author, or editor of nine books, including *The Hackett Introduction to Medical Ethics* (with Cynthia D. Coe, 2025) and *A Theory of Legal Punishment* (2021).

Part I
The Patient Experience

Chapter 2
The Ethics of AI in Healthcare: An Updated Mapping Review

Jessica Morley and Luciano Floridi

Abstract Artificial intelligence's impact on healthcare is undeniable. What is less clear is whether it will be ethically justifiable. Just as we know that AI can be used to diagnose disease, predict risk, develop personalized treatment plans, monitor patients remotely, or automate triage, we also know that it can pose significant threats to patient safety and the reliability (or trustworthiness) of the healthcare sector as a whole. These ethical risks arise from (a) flaws in the evidence base of healthcare AI (epistemic concerns); (b) the potential of AI to transform fundamentally the meaning of health, the nature of healthcare, and the practice of medicine (normative concerns); and (c) the "black box" nature of the AI development pipeline, which undermines the effectiveness of existing accountability mechanisms (traceability concerns). In this chapter, we systematically map (a)–(c) to six different levels of abstraction: individual, interpersonal, group, institutional, sectoral, and societal. The aim is to help policymakers, regulators, and other high-level stakeholders delineate the scope of regulation and other "softer" governing measures for AI in healthcare. We hope that by doing so, we may enable global healthcare systems to capitalize safely and reliably on the many benefits of healthcare AI.

Keywords Artificial intelligence · Ethics · Healthcare · Health policy · Machine learning

J. Morley (✉) · L. Floridi
Yale University, New Haven, CT, USA
e-mail: jessica.morley@yale.edu

L. Floridi
e-mail: luciano.floridi@yale.edu

L. Floridi
Department of Legal Studies, University of Bologna, Bologna, Italy

M. C. Altman and D. Schwan (eds.), *Ethics and Medical Technology*, The International Library of Bioethics 113, https://doi.org/10.1007/978-3-031-94690-5_2

2.1 Introduction

That artificial intelligence (AI) will have an impact on healthcare is, at this point, undeniable. In the US alone, healthcare AI startups have raised over $60 billion in the last ten years (Desai and Rubin 2024). AI is prominently featured in the healthcare strategies of nations such as Estonia, Israel, South Korea, and the United Kingdom. What is less clear is whether the inevitable impact of AI on healthcare will be ethically justifiable. Just because we now know that AI *could* be used to diagnose disease, predict risk, develop personalized treatment plans, monitor patients remotely, or automate triage, it is not apparent that it *should* be used for these purposes. AI is not merely a new type of medical device or drug. It is a new form of agency capable of coupling, re-coupling, and de-coupling different parts of the healthcare system (e.g., patients and their data, research and practice, and the presence of the healthcare provider and the location of the patient) in ways that may fundamentally transform the meaning of health, the nature of healthcare, and the practice of medicine. The negative consequences of this fundamentally transformative (that is, re-ontologizing) process for patient safety and the reliability or trustworthiness of the healthcare sector could be significant if they are not anticipated and proactively mitigated.

With this need for proactive mitigation of ethical harms in mind, in 2019, we mapped the patient safety and trustworthiness issues raised exclusively[1] by the use of AI in healthcare (Morley et al. 2020). We found that the causes of these ethical issues could be epistemic (related to misguided, inconclusive, or inscrutable evidence), normative (related to unfair outcomes and transformative effects), or related to traceability, and that these issues could arise at six levels of abstraction[2] (LoA): individual, interpersonal, group, institutional, societal, or sectoral. We then used these findings (summarized in Table 2.1), to elaborate eleven key questions for policymakers, regulators, and developers, aimed at helping them to achieve this proactive mitigation. We hoped that by encouraging policymakers and others to think in terms of our proposed ethical framework, we could help delineate the scope of emerging regulation and other "softer" governing measures for AI in healthcare.

The intervening five years have seen some progress in this regard. In 2019, the Royal Australian and New Zealand College of Radiologists produced ethical principles for AI in medicine, the EU High-Level Ethics Group on AI Ethics produced its guidelines for trustworthy AI, and the American Medical Association published its augmented intelligence in healthcare policy. Similarly, in 2021, the US Food and Drug Administration published its AI/ML-based software as a medical device action plan, and the World Health Organization published its guidance on the ethics and governance of AI.

---

[1] Ethical issues related to data sharing, data access, data privacy, general surveillance/nudging, consent, and ownership of health data were excluded, as they apply to all digital health technologies, not just AI.

[2] An LoA can be imagined as an interface that enables one to observe some aspects of a system analyzed while making other aspects opaque or indeed invisible (Floridi 2008).

Table 2.1 Summary of the epistemic, normative, and traceability concerns associated with healthcare AI at the six different LoAs identified by the literature in 2019 adapted from Morley et al. (2020)

	Ethical concern	Explanation	Example impact on patient safety or system trustworthiness	Presentation at different levels of abstraction
Epistemic concerns	Inconclusive evidence	Algorithmic outcomes (e.g., classification) are probabilistic and not infallible. They are rarely sufficient to posit the existence of a causal relationship	EKG readers in smartwatches may "diagnose" a patient as suffering from arrhythmia when it may be due to a fault with the watch not being able to accurately read that user's heartbeat (for example, due to the color of their skin) or the norm is inappropriately calibrated for that individual	**Individual**: Misdiagnosis or missed diagnosis **Interpersonal**: Loss of trust in provider-patient relationships, de-personalization of care **Group**: Misdiagnosis or missed diagnosis at scale—some groups are more affected than others **Institutional**: Waste of funds and resources not directed to areas of greater need **Sectoral**: Excessively broad data sharing between public and private entities **Societal**: Poorer public healthcare provision and worsening health outcomes for society
	Inscrutable evidence	Recipients of an algorithmic decisions very rarely have complete oversight of the data used to train or test an algorithm, or the data points used to reach a specific decision	A clinical decision support system deployed in a hospital may make a treatment recommendation, but it may not be clear on what basis it has made that decision, raising the risk that it has used data that are inappropriate for the individual in question or that there is a bug in the system leading to issues with over- or under-prescribing	
	Misguided evidence	Algorithmic outcomes can only be as reliable (or as neutral) as the data they are based on	Watson for Oncology was widely used in China for diagnosis via image recognition but was primarily trained on a Western dataset, leading to issues with concordance and poorer results for Chinese patients than their Western counterparts	

(continued)

Table 2.1 (continued)

	Ethical concern	Explanation	Example impact on patient safety or system trustworthiness	Presentation at different levels of abstraction
Normative concerns	Unfair outcomes	An action can be found to have more of an impact (positive or negative) on one group of people	An algorithm learns to prioritize patients it predicts to have better outcomes for a particular disease. This turns out to have a discriminatory effect on people within the Black and minority ethnic communities	**Individual**: Surveillance and undermining of autonomy and integrity of self **Interpersonal**: Deskilling of healthcare providers, overreliance on AI tools, undermining of consent practices, and redefining roles in the healthcare system **Group**: Profiling and discrimination against certain groups seen as being less healthy or higher risk **Institutional**: Transformation of care pathways and imposing of specific values at scale, redefining good care **Sectoral**: Siloing of new AI tool development within the private sector **Societal**: Inequalities in outcomes
	Transformative effects	Algorithmic activities, like profiling, re-conceptualize reality in unexpected ways	An individual using a personal health app has limited oversight over what passive data it is collecting and how that is being transformed into a recommendation to improve, limiting their ability to challenge any recommendations made and a loss of personal autonomy and data privacy	
Traceability		The harm caused by algorithmic activity is hard to debug (to detect the harm and find its cause), and it is hard to identify who should be held responsible for the harm caused	If a decision made by clinical decision support software leads to a negative outcome for the individual, it is unclear who to assign the responsibility and/or liability to and, therefore, to prevent it from happening again	**Individual**: "Bad users" could come to be blamed for their own ill health **Interpersonal**: See Institutional **Group**: Specific groups framed as being more morally irresponsible with regard to their health than others **Institutional**: Lack of clarity over liability with regard to issues with safety and effectiveness could halt adoption or result in certain groups being blamed more often than others **Sectoral**: See Institutional **Societal**: Society must decide through regulation preferable answers to the question regarding liability and risk allocation in healthcare provision. However, all groups in society may not be given an equal say in this process

Although such developments are promising and worthy of recognition, the overall pace of progress has been slow and has lagged considerably behind technological development. As a consequence, policymakers and regulators at national, international, and supranational levels find themselves having to simultaneously (a) develop governance mechanisms designed to mitigate the known ethical risks associated with the AI of five years ago; and (b) scope the unknown or emerging ethical risks associated with contemporary generative AI (for example, large language models) or ambient AI[3] (Martinez-Martin et al. 2021). This is problematic because, as long as the lag between ethical governance and technological development persists, the safety of patients continues to be at risk, and the reliability (or trustworthiness) of the healthcare sector continues to be under threat. Thus, over the following pages, we hope to shorten the lag by: (i) assessing whether the previously identified (or known) ethical risks have changed or been exacerbated over the past five years; (ii) identifying any new (or unknown) ethical risks that have been introduced by the arrival of generative and ambient AI; and (iii) anticipating ethical risks that may potentially arise in the future if the current trajectory of rapidly developing technology and slowly progressing policy is allowed to continue. Specifically, Sect. 2.2 provides a detailed description of the methodology; Sect. 2.3 presents the findings, outlining in detail the epistemic, normative, and traceability ethical considerations that arise at the individual, interpersonal, group, institutional, sectoral, and societal LoAs; Sect. 2.4 discusses what is missing from the reviewed literature in order to identify the guiding questions that still need to be answered by policymakers and regulators; and Sect. 2.5 concludes the chapter.

2.2 Methodology

A mapping review methodology was used to find literature from across disciplinary boundaries, highlighting the ethical issues associated with patient safety and healthcare sector trustworthiness unique to the use of AI. The literature searches were conducted in September 2024. Scopus and PubMed[4] were searched systematically using the terms in Table 2.2.

Initial results were screened by the title. After duplicates were removed, the inclusion and exclusion criteria (Table 2.3) were used to reduce the 682 selected articles to 108. Figure 2.1 shows the entire selection process according to the PRISMA 2020 reporting guideline.

The included articles were first reviewed to identify any new epistemic, normative, or traceability-related patient safety or trustworthiness ethical concerns. Next, each article was examined more thoroughly for any new or emerging ethical concerns

[3] Ambient AI works in the background without direct interaction with the user—for example, AI that transcribes clinical notes from a consultation.

[4] In 2019, five databases were searched. This time, as the baseline had already been established, we decided to focus on the databases that produced the greatest volume of literature in 2019.

Table 2.2 Terms used to search Scopus and PubMed, and results

Search terms	Scopus number of search results	Scopus number of articles selected on title	PubMed number of search results	PubMed number of articles selected on title
Ethics AND algorithm AND health	709	117	2164	324
Ethics AND "Artificial Intelligence" OR AI AND health	1409	307	2330	300
Moral AND "Artificial Intelligence" OR AI AND health	169	53	333	99
Fair AND "Artificial Intelligence" OR AI AND health	221	41	349	30
Moral OR ethics AND "Machine Learning" OR ML AND health	101	28	173	48
Fair AND "Machine Learning" OR ML AND health	275	29	290	11

Table 2.3 Inclusion and Exclusion criteria used to screen the identified literature

Inclusion criteria	Exclusion criteria
Published between 2019–2024 Written in English Written in article format Focused on the ethics of AI Providing a normative discussion of AI ethics Focused on the use of AI in human healthcare High-quality article Generalizable conclusions	Not in English Not in an article format Insufficiently focused on the ethics of AI Providing a quantitative solution or other non-normative argument Insufficiently focused on AI Poor quality Non-generalizable conclusions

not included in the original map. Particular attention was paid to concerns exclusive to generative or ambient AI. Finally, the included articles were combined with those used to inform the original map and analyzed, not from the "what is present?" perspective, but rather from the perspective of "what is missing?" Or, what are the potential future patient safety or reliability issues that may arise that have not yet been identified by the literature? An anticipatory ethics approach was adopted to do this. The results from these analyses will now be discussed.

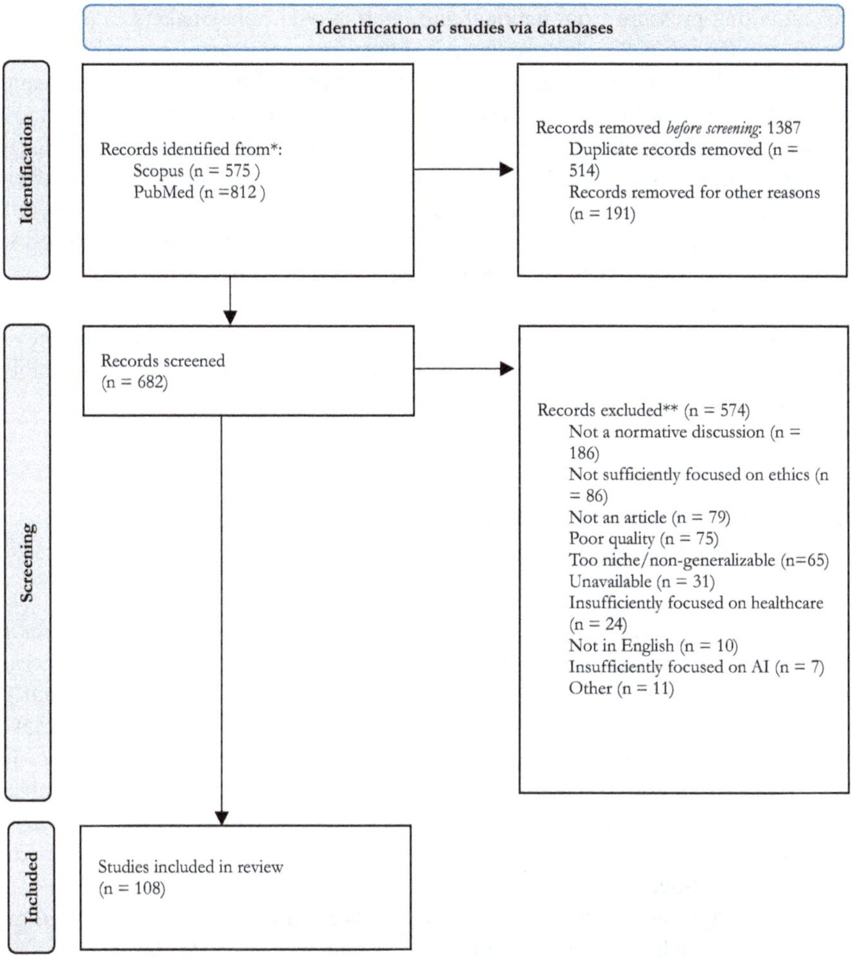

Fig. 2.1 PRISMA flow diagram of the literature search

2.3 Findings

Repeating the 2019 literature searches in 2024 revealed a nearly threefold increase in published literature on the ethics of artificial intelligence in healthcare. PubMed searches for "ethics AND Artificial Intelligence" returned 34,193 results for 2014–2019 compared to 127,923 for 2019–2024. Scopus searches for "ethics AND Artificial Intelligence AND health" yielded 239 results in 2019 and 1409 in 2024.

This increase reflects (i) growing awareness of, and interest in, the ethical issues raised by the use of AI in healthcare from philosophers, social scientists, digital ethicists, clinicians, and other science and technology scholars; (ii) significant investment in ethics-related scholarship separate to investment in technical AI development; and

(iii) mounting pressure from national and international policymakers to pay more attention to the safety threats posed by AI. However, despite this surge in the volume of AI ethics literature, the *range* of ethical issues explored by the literature remains relatively narrow, with limited focus on generative or ambient AI. Although most (67/108) included articles were published after the launch of ChatGPT (a particularly prominent large language model), only six highlighted ethical issues related to generative AI ethics, and just one addressed ethical issues related to ambient AI. Overall, the reviewed literature revealed just three additional considerations not included in the original framework: negative environmental impact (which is not included as it is an ethical risk for all uses of AI); deception and dignity (Sætra 2022); and decisional privacy (Mühlhoff 2023). Otherwise, the included articles focused on previously highlighted ethical concerns, emphasizing their persistence and vulnerability to exacerbation by contemporary AI.

2.3.1 Epistemic Concerns: Inconclusive, Inscrutable, and Misguided Evidence

By focusing on the flaws in the quality, accuracy, and validity of the evidence upon which AI models base their clinical "decisions," epistemic and ethical concerns make clear the fallibility of AI outputs and the consequences of this fallibility. Just because an AI model can recognize a pattern does not automatically make the pattern meaningful nor the action it informs clinically efficacious or safe. In brief, AI models trained on poor-quality data can produce inaccurate or discriminatory outputs that may lead to patient fatalities (Alowais et al. 2023; Bartlett 2023); models that are initially well-trained and properly validated may introduce patient safety risks post-deployment due to the negative effects of dataset drift or even data poisoning (Chen and Esmaeilzadeh 2024); and large language models may regurgitate or hallucinate harmful misinformation (De Angelis et al. 2023; Jayakumar et al. 2023; Moodley 2023; Toma et al. 2023; Wang et al. 2023; Stevens and Beaulieu 2024). The consequences of these issues may arise at any of the LoAs included in the original framework, each of which will now be discussed.

At the individual LoA, there is a considerable risk of misdiagnosis. In 2019, we highlighted that this could happen in at least two ways: either by an individual using a wearable device that has a bug or is inappropriately calibrated for them (e.g., they could be told that they are suffering from a health condition when they are not, or vice versa), or a healthcare provider relying on clinical decision support software (Ruckenstein and Schüll 2017) could be given an inaccurate diagnosis or recommendation which they do not question due to a tendency to accept the decisions of automated systems uncritically (Challen et al. 2019). In 2024, it is still possible that misdiagnosis may occur because of either of these epistemic failures. However, large language models (LLMs) have also introduced several new ways in which AI-based misdiagnosis may occur. LLMs are stochastic (i.e., based on probabilities and randomness), meaning they can produce different (realistic and convincing) outputs for a given input (Choudhury 2022; Alowais et al. 2023). Consequently, unless very mindfully prompted, LLMs may output different diagnoses for the same input set of symptoms (Harrer 2023) or, as briefly mentioned above, they may hallucinate (or fabricate) entirely new diagnoses (Abhari et al. 2024). LLMs may also attempt to personalize their outputs to best suit, what they predict to be, the user's expectations—potentially perpetuating beliefs in misinformed diagnoses (Arnold 2021; Yu et al. 2024).

Not only do these potential causes of AI-derived misdiagnosis pose a risk to individuals, but they also reverse the advantage of healthcare AI solutions being able to operate at scale by introducing the group LoA ethical concern of misdiagnosis or missed diagnosis happening repeatedly. While a healthcare provider might give one person the wrong diagnosis and then be corrected, a faulty AI model, based on misguided, inscrutable, or inconclusive evidence, could provide the same wrong diagnosis to thousands of people at a time (Topol 2019). This risk is especially pronounced for LLMs, given how widely and publicly they are available. Yet, this scale does not mean that the risk of AI-based misdiagnosis is the same for all groups within the population (or all users of healthcare AI solutions). There are multiple sources of bias throughout the AI development pipeline, from conceptualization (due to historical inequal access), through development (due to non-representative datasets), validation, and all the way to access and marketing (Abràmoff et al. 2023; Flores et al. 2023). These biases make it more likely that AI models will draw incorrect, and potentially harmful inferences about specific population subgroups (most likely marginalized groups). An AI model trained to predict cervical cancer risk on a nonrepresentative dataset might, for example, infer that a particular subgroup of the population (e.g., a specific ethnic group) is at lower risk simply because people from that subgroup are underrepresented in the training dataset. Alternatively, an AI model trained on a dataset with no social data included (e.g., data on socioeconomic status or other social determinants of health) may incorrectly infer that a particular subgroup is at higher risk of developing a specific condition for biological or genomic reasons, when the actual cause of the increased relative risk is social[5] (Aquino et al. 2023). Repeated at scale, these epistemic mistakes can exacerbate inequalities in healthcare outcomes (Baumgartner et al. 2023).

AI model ignorance of the social determinants of health also raises several ethical considerations at the interpersonal LoA. Healthcare provider-patient relationships are primarily based on trust and empathy, and while AI models can take over tasks that are more routine and standardized, they cannot reproduce the emotional virtues of which human healthcare providers are capable (Ngiam and Khor 2019). This is because empathetic care requires the combination of *techne* (collecting, analyzing, and deploying information) and *phrenos* (knowledge and judgment based on experience to achieve a good outcome) (Arnold 2021). AI models only replicate *techne*: they have no semantic understanding of how life experience or cultural context alters

[5] The WHO estimates that 30–55% of all health outcomes are related to the social determinants of health.

health outcomes, nor can they factor in a patient's values, beliefs, or lifestyle preferences. Consequently, a growing reliance on AI, and the quantitative and objective evidence that fuels clinical algorithms (Cabitza et al. 2017), could result in the discreditation of other forms of diagnosis and treatment (Rosenfeld et al. 2019). This could lead to the dehumanization or depersonalization of care provision (Juengst et al. 2016) from a service based on *listening* and *theory* to one based purely on *categorization*. For this reason, Thomas Grote and Philipp Berens (2020) believe that calls to defer diagnostic decisions to algorithms lack epistemic justification.

Far from being lone voices in a crowd, Grote and Berens's (2020) view that AI may currently be overpromising and under-delivering in the field of healthcare has grown in popularity over the last five years as the scarcity of clinically validated and successfully implemented AI solutions has become more obvious (Abràmoff et al. 2023; Bürger et al. 2024). As LLMs are proving more popular among clinicians than other forms of AI (Blease et al. 2024), fewer people may question them. However, as it remains entirely unclear how to benchmark and evaluate the performance of LLMs in healthcare (Choudhury and Chaudhry 2024; Ong et al. 2024) (i.e., the epistemic justification remains unclear), it is equally possible that rapid abandonment will occur. This would cause the same voices to grow louder instead. Thus, at the institutional, sectoral, and societal LoAs, there is considerable risk that over-investment in non-validated AI solutions could significantly waste public funds. Like any other sector, healthcare is resource-constrained. If too much money is "wasted" on AI, there may not be sufficient money to pay for other more effective, more reliable, or more human solutions. Over time, this may lead to poorer quality, less reliable, public healthcare provision (Holzmeyer 2021; Bak et al. 2022).

2.3.2 Normative Concerns: Unfair Outcomes and Transformative Effects

While epistemic and ethical implications primarily focus on the impact of poor-quality evidence on the performance of individual AI models, and how these aggregate to create interpersonal, group, institutional, sectoral, and societal harms, normative ethical concerns focus on how the integration of AI into healthcare systems may fundamentally alter the nature of care delivery. Specifically, by focusing on how the implementation of AI may reconfigure relationships between different parts of the healthcare ecosystem, normative ethical implications stress AI's potential to (a) change how health and illness are conceptualized, categorized, and managed (De Togni et al. 2021); (b) reshape the embodied and affective experiences of both patients and clinicians; (c) reinforce social inequalities (d'Elia et al. 2022); and (d) erode trust in human healthcare professionals (Fournier-Tombs and McHardy 2023). How these issues arise at each of the LoA will now be discussed.

At the individual LoA, the increased uptake of AI-based diagnostic and therapeutic interventions poses a considerable risk to the concept of integrity of self (the ability of an individual to understand the forces acting on them) (Cheney-Lippold 2019; Mathiesen and Broekman 2022). First, individuals are being encouraged to share more and more personal data about themselves (Racine et al. 2019) both for the purpose of training AI models and as the input for AI models. These data can be used in opaque, potentially harmful ways over which individuals have minimal control (Sterckx et al. 2016). Second, for an individual to exert agency over an AI-derived clinical decision, they would need to understand the underlying data, processes, and technical possibilities involved in it being reached (DuFault and Schouten 2020). They would also need to ensure their values are considered by the decision-making algorithm (McDougall 2019). This is not only a new responsibility that patients have never previously been expected to shoulder (de Boer and Kudina 2021), but one that requires a level of eHealth literacy that the vast majority of the population does not have (Kim and Xie 2017). Thus, the increasing use of algorithmic decision-making in clinical settings can negatively affect individual autonomy. This loss of autonomy may undermine the ability for individuals to be involved in shared decision-making, to give meaningful informed consent, refuse treatment, contest their diagnosis (Ploug and Holm 2022), or act on their right not to know (Armitage 2024).

Amplifying this loss of autonomy is the fact that AI models can be "hypersausive," as they are capable of strongly influencing behavior in nontransparent ways (Floridi 2024). Such "digital nudges" are not value-free and may, especially with the advent of generative AI, be difficult to detect (Capasso and Umbrello 2022): a patient engaging with a "medical agent" may not know that they are not communicating with a human. This potential for deception adds a threat to human dignity to the existing threat to the integrity of the self (Sætra 2022; Rudschies and Schneider 2024). Ultimately, given that damage to a person's psychological integrity can be perceived as harm, not accounting for these potentialities poses the risk of creating a healthcare system that violates the first principle of medical ethics: *primum non nocere* ("first, do no harm") (Morley and Floridi 2020).

Although, as evidenced by the preceding paragraphs, much of the reviewed literature focuses on AI's potential to undermine *patient* autonomy by harming psychological integrity, AI models can also undermine *clinician* autonomy by threatening epistemic authority (Arnold 2021). Rather than being seen as a simple tool or medical device (e.g., a blood pressure cuff) that clinicians (or other healthcare providers) can use as a decision aid, AI is increasingly being positioned as a decision-making agent that may diminish the clinician's role in the decision-making process (Bélisle-Pipon et al. 2021; Kasperbauer 2021). This is an ethical risk that emerges at the interpersonal LoA, fundamentally changing the nature of the therapeutic relationship between patients and clinicians. If clinicians feel excluded from the clinical decision-making loop, they may feel unable to exert their own agency over the decision-making capacity of AI models (i.e., they may defer the epistemic authority to the algorithm), which may, in turn, undermine the reliability of (or patient trust in) clinicians (De Togni et al. 2021; Rudschies and Schneider 2024). However, more than this, making the clinician one part of a decision-making triad between patient, clinician, and algorithm also changes the nature of the clinician's fiduciary responsibility (Habli et al. 2020). While the introduction of the algorithm decision-making partner may *lessen the control* a clinician has over the decision-making process, especially in light of automation bias and algorithmic opacity (Ciliberti et al. 2023; Dalton-Brown 2020; DeCamp and Lindvall 2020; Habli et al. 2020), this may not lessen their legal responsibility. Clinicians may still be held liable for negative outcomes even if they feel uninvolved in (or are physically removed from) the relevant decision (Quinn et al. 2021; Iqbal et al. 2022; Bartlett 2023; Ennis-O'Connor and O'Connor 2024). At the same time, adding algorithms into the decision-making mix may *increase* other clinician responsibilities. For example, the predictive element of AI might extend the clinician's duty to warn beyond communicable diseases; the data-intensive nature of AI might require clinicians to take on additional "data work"; and the requirement to ensure AI is "explainable" may exacerbate anxiety and pressure to justify medical choices and ensure informed consent (de Boer and Kudina 2021). Consequently, AI may add to the cognitive burden faced by clinicians rather than lessen it, and weaken the connection between clinician and patient rather than strengthen it.

These and other consequences of algorithmically mediated clinical decision-making will probably not be equally distributed (Pot et al. 2021). This becomes apparent at the group LoA. AI models, including generative AI models, are notoriously better able to identify illnesses and injuries that have well-established and fairly set (and therefore automatable) diagnostic criteria and treatment protocols (Morley et al. 2020). Models that tackle these problems are also far easier to verify, validate, and evaluate for accuracy, efficacy, and safety. When used to diagnose or treat maladies that meet these conditions, the impact of the displacement of the human clinician from the decision-making loop on the clinical outcome of the patient in question might be minimal. However, easily learnable patterns of this nature are far more likely to exist for afflictions most commonly suffered by white men, as there is a greater volume of health and medical trials data for this group than there is for almost any other potential patient group. Models trained to recognize these conditions on biased or nonrepresentative datasets can make considerably poorer decisions for the patients excluded from the data—for example, younger black women. Similarly, AI models are far less likely to perform well (at least in a verifiable way) when faced with illnesses and injuries that affect smaller, more marginalized population groups, and are likely to perform especially poorly when dealing with patient edge cases that may be treated as statistical outliers and removed from training datasets (Dalton-Brown 2020; Grote and Keeling 2022). In these circumstances, the displacement of the clinician from the decision-making loop could exacerbate existing inequalities between the "haves" and the "have-nots" of the digital healthcare ecosystem, i.e., those that generate data on themselves to ensure accurately trained AI models and those that do not (Topol 2019; Bærøe et al. 2022; Abràmoff et al. 2023).

Overcoming this bias inequality problem is challenging. Creating statistically representative or fair datasets is a necessary but insufficient step or, as Elle Lett and William La Cava state, "equilibrating model performance across groups does not guarantee equitable health outcomes" (2023, 476). This is because equality, which typically underpins fairness metrics, and equity are different normative concepts. Equality is focused only on the existence of difference, i.e., there are different outcomes between groups A and B, and all difference is perceived negatively. This is problematic in healthcare, where insisting on, for example, equality in treatment regardless of patients' age, sex, or ethnicity, might neglect critical dimensions of medical practice, including dignity preservation and quality of life optimization (Liu et al. 2023). Put simply, different people have different healthcare needs, even *if* they have the same condition and wish to achieve the same outcome. Everybody might have the same life expectancy goal, but different individuals will need different interventions to achieve that goal. Equity focuses on this difference in need, and it seeks to identify where the difference (or inequality) exists because of some form of injustice, such as the unfair distribution of healthcare resources (Pot et al. 2021; Pruski 2024; Rueda et al. 2024). Statistically fair datasets, or equally accurate AI models, will not mitigate these biases or inequities—especially as they may not be immediately apparent but appear long after model deployment (latent bias) (DeCamp and Lindvall 2020). Since, as the COVID-19 pandemic made clear, a person's health and well-being are inherently tied to the well-being of others given the interconnected nature of public health, unless more comprehensively tackled, this issue of inequitable outcomes will become a societal LoA risk, and the health outcomes of the overall population may worsen (De Togni et al. 2021; Weissglass 2022; Amugongo et al. 2023).

If solutions to the group and societal LoA normative harms associated with biased AI models cannot be found in technical fixes for individual datasets or individual algorithms, then it is necessary to look at a higher LoA. Specifically, it is essential to look at the institutional and sectoral LoA. Once at the institutional and sectoral LoA, it becomes clear that one of the reasons AI for healthcare is both struggling to deliver on its promised benefits and posing difficult-to-mitigate ethical risks is an imbalance of power between public healthcare systems and private technology companies (Graham 2023; Freitas 2024). While public healthcare systems may know how clinical care is organized and managed, technological innovation and knowledge of AI are concentrated in big private tech companies (Murdoch 2021). This is making healthcare systems increasingly reliant on the proprietary products of these private companies, for example, specific generative AI models. This is not simply a problem because proprietary products can be modified or taken offline without notice, but because it represents ceding control of medicine and healthcare to opaque corporate interests (Toma et al. 2023). In essence, by handing over epistemic authority for clinical decisions to AI models, public healthcare systems are also handing over epistemic authority for planning and strategic decisions related to what care *is* and what constitutes *good* care to private third-party companies that may be motivated to optimize profit rather than patient safety. This shift in power makes it difficult for the healthcare sector as a whole to dictate what problems it would like AI to solve (i.e., what types of decision it would like to delegate to AI). Thus, to effectively mitigate the potential negative normative consequences of AI implementation, it is essential to tackle this power imbalance a priori. Otherwise, this process of transforming the provision of care risks over-fitting healthcare systems to a specific set of values that may not represent those of society at large (Morley et al. 2020) and may significantly damage system reliability.

2.3.3 Concerns Related to Traceability

The preceding discussion of the normative ethical risks associated with the increasing use of AI in healthcare highlighted how AI has the potential to transform the delivery of healthcare fundamentally. At the core of this transformation process is the development of a far more complex network consisting of humans and nonhuman agents. The complexity of this resultant network makes responsibility attribution difficult because a fault, which may result in a patient safety issue, may have multiple causes that are hard to trace (Chen et al. 2023). This is concerning because, according to Ryan Felder (2021), the transparent organization of responsibility in a healthcare system serves at least two purposes: (a) to incentivize healthcare providers to act ethically in all circumstances, and (b) to ensure the foundation of patient trust in the reliability of healthcare providers is sufficiently solid for healthcare to flourish. The ethical consequences of this will now be discussed at the different LoAs.

AI developers and healthcare policymakers hope that AI will be the key that unlocks P4 medicine at the individual LoA: making healthcare more personalized, predictive, participatory, and preventative. The central idea is that by encouraging individuals to provide more personal health and well-being data to private third parties for the purpose of algorithmic monitoring (participation), AI models can (i) predict when, how, and why individuals will become unwell; and (ii) provide a personalized preventative plan that—if followed correctly—should alleviate this risk of future illness. The concern is that if this process fails, in the sense that it does not result in an individual taking appropriate action to improve their health, this process of algorithmic surveillance risks creating an elaborate mechanism for victim-blaming (Morley et al. 2020). The individual may be perceived as a "bad patient" for failing to act upon the allegedly objective and evidence-based advice of the algorithm, and may, therefore, be framed as being morally responsible for their poor health and not deserving of state-provided healthcare. Yet, due to the lack of transparency over the complex development pipeline, there can be no certainty that the poor outcome was due to the lack of action by the individual: it could be a faulty device, buggy code, or the result of biased datasets (Topol 2019). Alternatively, the algorithmic advice could be uninterpretable by the individual (Jongepier and Keymolen 2022), ignorant of the individual's values and their wider social determinants (Birch et al. 2022; Huang et al. 2022), or manipulated to achieve a goal more related to private profit than individual health. Not only does this process represent a new form of paternalism, which Anto Čartolovni et al. (2022) refer to as "computernalism," but also a new form of infringement on "decisional privacy": a manipulation of individual deliberative agency over highly personal health-related decisions (Fairfield and Reynolds 2022; Jongepier and Keymolen 2022). This invasion highlights why this process is a matter of ethical concern, even if a negative outcome resulted purely from an individual's disregarding the guidance of a predictive algorithm.

Individuals do not always come into contact with these kinds of algorithmic predictions through their own independent actions. Instead, individuals might be presented with the outputs of algorithmic predictions in their clinician's office or via an app that a clinician has recommended that they use. In these instances, the lack of traceability undermines the trustworthiness and reliability of the clinician-patient decision-making process, which hinges on informed consent and information sharing (Murphy et al. 2021; Banja et al. 2022; Ahmad and Eckert 2023; Elendu et al. 2023; Upadhyay et al. 2023; Bekbolatova et al. 2024; Shaw et al. 2024). Thus, there are also ethical consequences of the overarching "black box" nature of algorithmic outputs at the interpersonal LoA. Indeed, the consequences scale still further, to the group LoA, when it is considered that persistent bias might mean that some groups come to be seen as being more morally irresponsible about their healthcare than others. As mentioned above, weaker healthcare provision for some ultimately weakens health outcomes for all, rendering this problem a societal issue as well.

Finally, at the institutional and sectoral LoAs, a lack of traceability translates into a lack of auditability and consequential reliability (Char et al. 2020). Individual healthcare institutions, and the healthcare sector as a whole, are increasingly being incentivized and put under pressure to adopt AI solutions to improve efficiency and productivity. This is even though there is no internationally agreed standard for validating the efficacy, accuracy, or safety of AI systems, nor for calibrating potential harm. Additionally, most AI systems are proprietary, and no regulations or standards insist on transparent reporting of how the system was developed or by whom. Institutions are, therefore, at risk of procuring systems about which they do not know how the problem the algorithm is solving was selected, how the data the algorithm is trained on was collected, how the outcome was defined and why, how the algorithm was developed, how the safety and efficacy of the algorithm was verified, what infrastructure is required to ensure the successful implementation of the AI system, nor what aspects of performance need to be monitored post-deployment (Chen et al. 2021). All these issues, magnified in the context of generative AI, undermine healthcare institutions' evaluative and decisional autonomy (Char et al. 2020). Ultimately, if this lack of auditability results in the procurement and deployment of even *one* AI system that causes significant patient harm, the likely outcome will be a chilling of enthusiasm for the potential of AI to save lives and an undermining of the trustworthiness and reliability of the healthcare sector (Zhang and Zhang 2023).

2.4 Discussion

As stated at the outset, by repeating the mapping process we followed in 2019, we sought to (i) assess whether the previously identified (or known) ethical risks have changed or been exacerbated over the past five years; (ii) identify any new (or unknown) ethical risks that have been introduced by the arrival of generative and ambient AI. Having surveyed the newly included literature, it is now clear that (a) all the ethical risks identified in 2019 have endured (see Table 2.4), and while it is possible that ethical harms not discussed in the literature have been addressed, few of these literature-based ethical risks have yet been effectively mitigated through technological or regulatory innovation; (b) several of the known ethical risks have been exacerbated through the introduction of generative and ambient AI, with the threats to epistemic certainty, epistemic authority, and autonomy at all levels from individual to institutional, being particularly affected (see italicized text in Table 2.4); and (c) generative and ambient AI have introduced new risks related to decisional privacy and dignity as well as introduced new causes of existing risks such as hallucinated or misinformed diagnoses (see italicized and bold text in Table 2.4).

Combined, these ethical concerns make clear that the implementation of AI into healthcare systems represents a far more significant change than simply replacing paper with data. It heralds a new era of healthcare, founded on an algorithm-based, data-centric, and networked model of care delivered through a multi-agent system comprised of human agents (e.g., clinicians, tech developers) and artificial agents (e.g., clinical decision support, health apps). Compared to the previous late twentieth century evidence-based, patient-centric, and 1:1 relationship model of care, the developing algorithmically-enhanced twenty-first-century model of care may be more standardized, but less caring; prioritize evidence availability over accuracy; be more transactional than relational (Launer 2024); and, overall, be insufficiently concerned about the potential patient harm—including psychological harm and manipulation—that may arise from a mismatch between the advice of an algorithm and the real life of a patient (Bouaud et al. 2015; Grote and Berens 2020). Yet, the literature seems reluctant to engage with the macro or *systemic* level consequences of this paradigmatic shift in healthcare brought about by a collision of technology, neoliberalism, capitalism, and everyday medicalization (Gaeta, 2023, 2). This reluctance may be why an underestimation and oversimplification of the ethical considerations is currently acting as an impediment to healthcare AI achieving a justifiable return on investment (Karpathakis et al. 2024). If this oversimplification is not corrected, and the development of associated policy and regulation struggles to pick up pace, then there are at least two systemic level consequences for patient safety and system reliability that can be anticipated: personalized unwellness and the inverse data quality law.

2.4.1 Personalized Unwellness

Rather than bringing in a new era of personalized medicine, the implementation of healthcare AI may usher in an era of personalized unwellness. First, by expanding into the realms of social media, direct-to-consumer wearables and apps, and the recording of lifestyle and fitness data, the algorithmication of healthcare may make the concepts of health and illness more fluid (Rubeis 2023). A diagnosis of Autism Spectrum Disorder, Anxiety, Borderline Personality Disorder, or ADHD may no longer require an examination of clinical symptoms by a doctor but the viewing of a targeted advert on Instagram or the watching of a "for you" video on TikTok. Second, by emphasizing prediction and prevention, the increased reliance on healthcare AI may redefine the concept of health itself. Health may no longer be viewed merely as the absence of disease but as a holistic state of emotional, physical, and spiritual wellness (Baker 2022) that is always endangered from future developments, can

Table 2.4 Summary of the updated epistemic, normative, and traceability ethical concerns of healthcare AI at the six different LoA

	Individual	Interpersonal	Group	Institutional	Sectoral	Societal
Epistemic concerns	Misdiagnosis, missed diagnosis, ***hallucinated diagnosis, misinformed diagnosis*** *undermining epistemic certainty*	*Loss of trust, empathy and* phrenos *in clinician-patient relationships, dehumanization and depersonalization of care*	Misdiagnosis, missed diagnosis, *hallucinated diagnosis, misinformed diagnosis* at scale—some groups are more affected than others	Waste of funds and resources not directed to areas of greater need	See Institutional	Poor public healthcare provision and worsening health outcomes for society
Normative concerns	Surveillance, undermining of autonomy and integrity of self, *increased personal responsibility, hypersuasion* ***deception & loss of dignity***	*Loss of epistemic authority, weakening of clinician-patient therapeutic relationship*	Profiling and discrimination, *exclusion of outliers and data "have-nots," worsening inequities in healthcare outcomes*	Transformation of care pathways & imposing of specific values at scale- redefining "good care"	*Power imbalance between public healthcare systems and private, for-profit providers of proprietary systems*	Poor public healthcare provision and worsening health outcomes for society
Traceability concerns	"Bad patients" could come to be blamed for their own ill health, ***infringement of decisional privacy***	*Undermining of informed consent and shared decision-making*	Specific groups are framed as being more morally irresponsible with regard to their health than others	*Lack of auditability undermines institutional decisional autonomy and creates an accountability gap*	*See Institutional*	Poor public healthcare provision and worsening health outcomes for society

always be improved, and requires constant digital monitoring (Rubeis 2023). Good patient norms may shift, so that people will not only be expected to strive to maintain their health, but also to see themselves as incomplete or permanently unwell, needing continuous improvement, de-aging, slimming, beautifying, and more (Dionne 2020; Roetman 2020). This may render good but permanently unwell patients in a scenario where they must submit passively to the advice of many potentially manipulative and poorly evidenced algorithms, lest they wish to be perceived as a threat to public health.

2.4.2 The Inverse Data Quality Law

Devised by Julian Tudor Hart in 1971, the inverse care law states that "the availability of good medical care tends to vary inversely with the need for it in the population served" and that this law "operates more completely where medical care is most exposed to market forces" (Tudor Hart 1971, 405). The insufficiently governed use of healthcare AI may result in a new inverse data quality law where "the availability of high-quality healthcare data varies inversely with need for healthcare in the population served." More than just a consequence of the digital divide and unequal access to smartphones and wearables at an individual consumer level, this is a systemic-level consequence that may arise from inequities across the entire AI development pipeline, including variations in (i) access to twenty-first-century digital infrastructure inside healthcare institutions; (ii) digital health literacy, leaving some individuals more vulnerable to manipulation by online misinformation than others; (iii) awareness of algorithms, boosting the confidence of some individuals, and undermining the confidence of others, in the use of online triage systems or symptom checkers; (iv) attitudes toward privacy and system trustworthiness, and increasing the willingness of some, and decreasing the willingness of others, to "donate" their data to research or service planning; (v) the design of electronic health records and the availability of clinical codes for recording the specific diagnosis or treatment, influencing the ability of a care provider to accurately record, in detail, an individual's symptoms or diagnosis; and many more factors. Ultimately, the growing risk is that those who generate high-quality data about themselves and their "wellness" will be more likely to have access to higher-quality healthcare, even if they are less likely to *need* access to healthcare, resulting in the creation of a two-tiered global healthcare system between the "worried well" and the "ignored sick."

To avoid these and other systemic consequences of healthcare AI implementation, policymakers, regulators, and other relevant stakeholders must begin to pay more attention to the enduring, exacerbated, and emerging ethical risks highlighted in this review. Guided by the questions in Table 2.5 (new questions in italics), they must move beyond the constant production and reproduction of simplistic, high-level guidelines that do little to protect against the risks of ethics washing, ethics shopping, and ethics dumping (Floridi 2019), and focus instead on the creation of an appropriate, enforceable, and reliable regulatory infrastructure that ensures all the concerns highlighted are accounted for and appropriately redressed (Kerasidou et al. 2022). It is only by developing this regulatory infrastructure and operationalizing it through a combination of best practices for ethical inclusivity, software development, implementation and regulatory science, and human–computer interaction (Alowais et al. 2023) that healthcare systems will be able to avoid the greatest potential ethical risk safely: opportunity cost (Floridi et al. 2018).

2.5 Limitations

All research has limitations, and this mapping review is no exception. First, the articles selected were restricted to those written in English. This means that, as in 2019, some ethical issues will have been overlooked, and the overview of ethical issues provided almost certainly suffers from a Western bias. Second, academic literature, much like regulation, struggles to keep pace with technological development. This review did not include literature published on pre-print servers (e.g., SSRN or arXiv) or grey literature. It is entirely possible that, given the relatively short timeframe since the arrival of generative and ambient AI, much of the discussion regarding the ethical implications has not yet been formally published and may, therefore, have been excluded. We do not believe that these limitations detract from the comprehensiveness of the final ethical map, but we do encourage readers to view it as a living rather than a final product.

2.6 Conclusion

By updating this mapping review of the literature on the ethics of healthcare AI, we have sought to highlight how the ethical implications of healthcare AI have endured and changed over the last five years following the arrival of generative and ambient AI. As the literature on this topic is extensive, we have endeavored to make this overview more useful by organizing the findings into three core themes (epistemic, normative, and traceability) and six different levels of abstraction (individual, interpersonal, group, institutional, sectoral, and societal). The comprehensiveness of the resultant analysis may appear overly negative or Luddite-like. It is possible that having reached the end of this chapter, the impression given is that efforts to implement healthcare AI are too risky and should be abandoned. This is not our intention—far from it. Since all humans have the right to benefit from the outputs of science (Vayena and Tasioulas 2016), and other rights can be suspended or superseded in the name of public health, it would be highly unethical to suggest that global efforts to implement healthcare AI—with such clear capacity to save and improve lives—should be abandoned. Instead, we intend to stress the importance of being mindful of the re-ontologizing effects of algorithmically enhanced healthcare and encourage policymakers, developers, clinicians, and patients to pause and assess (a)

Table 2.5 Eighteen key questions to guide policymakers, regulators, and other high-level stakeholders in the design of a comprehensive regulatory infrastructure for healthcare AI

Key question	Relevant ethical issue & LoA
What skills will the professional healthcare workforce require in order to make safe and effective use of AI-Health solutions in the future?	Epistemic (individual, interpersonal, group, societal) Normative (interpersonal, group, institutional, sectoral) Traceability (individual, group)
Which tasks should be delegated to AI-Health solutions, and which should not?	Epistemic (individual, interpersonal, group, institutional, societal) Normative (interpersonal, group, institutional, societal) Traceability (individual, group, institutional)
What evidence is needed to prove the clinical effectiveness of an AI-Health solution?	Epistemic (individual, interpersonal, group, sectoral, societal) Normative (sectoral) Traceability (individual, group, institutional, societal)
What mechanisms should be put in place to enable people to report and seek redress for AI-Health associated harms?	Epistemic (individual, group, sectoral, societal) Normative (individual, group, sectoral, societal) Traceability (individual, group, institutional)
What mechanisms should be put in place to ensure all relevant stakeholder views are included in the development of AI-Health solutions?	Epistemic (group, sectoral, societal) Traceability (individual, group, institutional, societal)
How can the explainability of AI-Health solutions be guaranteed?	Epistemic (individual, group) Normative (individual, group, sectoral) Traceability (individual, institutional)
What mechanisms can be implemented to ensure the reliability, replicability, and safety of AI-Health solutions?	Epistemic (individual, group, sectoral) Normative (group, sectoral, societal) Traceability (individual, group, institutional)
How can transparency over how algorithmic tools are integrated into the healthcare workflow, how it shapes decisions, and how it affects process optimization within medical services, be guaranteed?	Epistemic (individual, interpersonal, group, institutional, sectoral, societal) Normative (group, interpersonal, institutional, societal) Traceability (individual, institutional, societal)
How can traditional and nontraditional sources of health data be incorporated into AI-Health decision-making? And how can it be appropriately protected and how can it be harmonized?	Epistemic (individual, group, institutional, sectoral, societal) Normative (individual, group, institutional, sectoral, societal) Traceability (individual, group, institutional, sectoral)
How are bioethical concepts (beneficence, nonmaleficence, autonomy, and justice) challenged by AI-Health?	Epistemic (interpersonal, societal) Normative (individual, group, institutional, societal) Traceability (individual, societal)

(continued)

Table 2.5 (continued)

Key question	Relevant ethical issue & LoA
How can concepts such as fairness, accountability, and transparency be maintained at scale?	Epistemic (group, institutional, sectoral, societal) Normative (institutional, sectoral, societal) Traceability (societal)
How can the epistemic authority of clinicians be maintained, protected, and (if necessary) enhanced?	*Epistemic (interpersonal)* *Normative (interpersonal)*
How can the processes of informed consent and shared decision-making be adapted to ensure patients are protected from deception and their dignity is upheld?	*Epistemic (individual, interpersonal, societal)* *Normative (individual, interpersonal, societal)* *Traceability (individual)*
What mechanisms must be implemented to redress the power imbalance between public healthcare institutions and private big tech companies?	*Traceability (institutional, sectoral, societal)*
To what extent should healthcare regulators be held responsible for hallucinated, misinformed, or disinformed content produced by generative AI? How could such responsibility be operationalized?	*Epistemic (individual, interpersonal, group, institutional, sectoral, societal)* *Traceability (individual, sectoral, societal)*
How can liability be clarified for harms caused by AI products marketed directly to consumers, e.g., AI-based triaging or diagnostic apps?	*Epistemic (individual, interpersonal, sectoral, societal)* *Normative (individual, interpersonal, sectoral, societal)* *Traceability (interpersonal, sectoral)*
How might the use of ambient AI in clinical consultations undermine the concept of patient-clinician confidentiality? How might confidentiality be protected? Might the use of ambient AI for consultations relating to particularly sensitive conditions be deemed inappropriate?	*Normative (individual, interpersonal, institutional)* *Traceability (institutional)*
What education should be provided to patients and the public better to protect them from hypersuasive manipulation by AI systems?	*Epistemic (individual)*

whether the benefits of the intended consequences outweigh the risks of the unintended consequences, (b) what success *should* look like (and why it should look like that), and (c) how the overarching system might be designed to maximize the chances of success. We hope that by encouraging this more mindful (and necessarily slower) approach to the implementation of healthcare AI, policymakers and other high-level decision-makers can help capitalize on opportunities while avoiding (potentially chilling) risks. Ultimately, as we said in 2019, we hope that this reflection will encourage the development of a system of transparent and distributed responsibility, where (a) all those involved in the clinical algorithm supply chain can be held proportionately and appropriately accountable for the safety and well-being of patients and healthcare practitioners alike, and (b) the medical community at large feel willing and able to safely adopt lifesaving, life-changing, and life-enhancing AI technologies.

References

Abhari, Shahabeddin, Somayeh Fatahi, Ashish Saragadam, Dmytro Chumachenko, and Plinio Pelegrini Morita. 2024. "A Road Map of Prompt Engineering for ChatGPT in Healthcare: A Perspective Study." In *Studies in Health Technology and Informatics*, eds. John Mantas, Arie Hasman, George Demiris, Kaija Saranto, Michael Marschollek, Theodoros N. Arvanitis, et al., 998–1002. Amsterdam: IOS Press. https://doi.org/10.3233/SHTI240578.

Abràmoff, Michael D., Michelle E. Tarver, Nilsa Loyo-Berrios, Sylvia Trujillo, Danton Char, Ziad Obermeyer, Malvina B. Eydelman, and William H. Maisel. 2023. "Considerations for Addressing Bias in Artificial Intelligence for Health Equity." *NPJ Digital Medicine* 6 (1) (September 12): article no. 170. https://doi.org/10.1038/s41746-023-00913-9.

Ahmad, M. A., and C. M. Eckert. 2023. "Show Your Work: Responsible Model Reporting in Health Care Artificial Intelligence." *Surgical Clinics of North America* 103 (2S) (June): e1–e11. https://doi.org/10.1016/j.suc.2023.03.002.

Alowais, Shuroug A., Sahar S. Alghamdi, Nada Alsuhebany, Tariq Alqahtani, Abdulrahman I. Alshaya, Sumaya N. Almohareb, et al. 2023. "Revolutionizing Healthcare: The Role of Artificial Intelligence in Clinical Practice." *BMC Medical Education* 23 (1) (September 22): article no. 689. https://doi.org/10.1186/s12909-023-04698-z.

Amugongo, Lameck Mbangula, Nicola J. Bidwell, and Caitlin C. Corrigan. 2023. "Invigorating Ubuntu Ethics in AI for Healthcare: Enabling Equitable Care." In *FAccT '23: Proceedings of the 2023 ACM Conference on Fairness, Accountability, and Transparency*, 583–592. New York: Association for Computing Machinery. https://doi.org/10.1145/3593013.3594024.

Aquino, Yves Saint James, Stacy M. Carter, Nehmat Houssami, Annette Braunack-Mayer, Khin Than Win, Chris Degeling, Lei Wang, and Wendy A Rogers. 2023. "Practical, Epistemic and Normative Implications of Algorithmic Bias in Healthcare Artificial Intelligence: A Qualitative Study of Multidisciplinary Expert Perspectives." *Journal of Medical Ethics*. https://doi.org/10.1136/jme-2022-108850.

Armitage, Richard C. 2024. "Digital Health Technologies: Compounding the Existing Ethical Challenges of the 'Right' Not to Know." *Journal of Evaluation in Clinical Practice* 30 (5) (August): 774–779. https://doi.org/10.1111/jep.13980.

Arnold, Mark Henderson. 2021. "Teasing Out Artificial Intelligence in Medicine: An Ethical Critique of Artificial Intelligence and Machine Learning in Medicine." *Journal of Bioethical Inquiry* 18 (1) (March): 121–139. https://doi.org/10.1007/s11673-020-10080-1.

Bærøe, Kristine, Torbjørn Gundersen, Edmund Henden, and Kjetil Rommetveit. 2022. "Can Medical Algorithms Be Fair? Three Ethical Quandaries and One Dilemma." *BMJ Health and Care Informatics* 29 (1) (April): e100445. https://doi.org/10.1136/bmjhci-2021-100445.

Bak, Marieke, Vince Istvan Madai, Marie-Christine Fritzsche, Michaela Th. Mayrhofer, and Stuart McLennan. 2022. "You Can't Have AI Both Ways: Balancing Health Data Privacy and Access Fairly." *Frontiers in Genetics* 13 (June 13): 929453. https://doi.org/10.3389/fgene.2022.929453.

Baker, Stephanie Alice. 2022. "Alt. Health Influencers: How Wellness Culture and Web Culture Have Been Weaponised to Promote Conspiracy Theories and Far-Right Extremism during the COVID-19 Pandemic." *European Journal of Cultural Studies* 25 (1) (February): 3–24. https://doi.org/10.1177/13675494211062623.

Banja, John D., Rolf Dieter Hollstein, and Michael A. Bruno. 2022. "When Artificial Intelligence Models Surpass Physician Performance: Medical Malpractice Liability in an Era of Advanced

Artificial Intelligence." *Journal of the American College of Radiology* 19 (7) (July): 816–820. https://doi.org/10.1016/j.jacr.2021.11.014.

Bartlett, Benjamin. 2023. "The Possibility of AI-Induced Medical Manslaughter: Unexplainable Decisions, Epistemic Vices, and a New Dimension of Moral Luck." *Medical Law International* 23 (3) (September): 241–270. https://doi.org/10.1177/09685332231193944.

Baumgartner, Renate, Payal Arora, Corinna Bath, Darja Burljaev, Kinga Ciereszko, Bart Custers, et al. 2023. "Fair and Equitable AI in Biomedical Research and Healthcare: Social Science Perspectives." *Artificial Intelligence in Medicine* 144 (October): 102658. https://doi.org/10.1016/j.artmed.2023.102658.

Bekbolatova, Molly, Jonathan Mayer, Chi Wei Ong, and Milan Toma. 2024. "Transformative Potential of AI in Healthcare: Definitions, Applications, and Navigating the Ethical Landscape and Public Perspectives." *Healthcare* 12 (2) (January-2): 125. https://doi.org/10.3390/healthcare12020125.

Bélisle-Pipon, Jean-Christophe, Vincent Couture, Marie-Christine Roy, Isabelle Ganache, Mireille Goetghebeur, and I. Glenn Cohen. 2021. "What Makes Artificial Intelligence Exceptional in Health Technology Assessment?" *Frontiers in Artificial Intelligence* 4 (November): 736697. https://doi.org/10.3389/frai.2021.736697.

Birch, Jonathan, Kathleen A. Creel, Abhinav K. Jha, and Anya Plutynski. 2022. "Clinical Decisions Using AI Must Consider Patient Values." *Nature Medicine* 28 (2) (February): 229–232. https://doi.org/10.1038/s41591-021-01624-y.

Blease, Charlotte R., Cosima Locher, Jens Gaab, Maria Hägglund, and Kenneth D. Mandl. 2024. "Generative Artificial Intelligence in Primary Care: An Online Survey of UK General Practitioners." *BMJ Health & Care Informatics* 31 (1). https://doi.org/10.1136/bmjhci-2024-101102.

Boer, Bas de, and Olya Kudina. 2021. "What Is Morally at Stake When Using Algorithms to Make Medical Diagnoses? Expanding the Discussion beyond Risks and Harms." *Theoretical Medicine and Bioethics* 42 (5–6) (December): 245–266. https://doi.org/10.1007/s11017-021-09553-0.

Bouaud, Jacques, Jean-Philippe Spano, Jean-Pierre Lefranc, Isabelle Cojean-Zelek, Brigitte Blaszka-Jaulerry, Laurent Zelek, et al. 2015. "Physicians' Attitudes Towards the Advice of a Guideline-Based Decision Support System: A Case Study with OncoDoc2 in the Management of Breast Cancer Patients." *MEDINFO 2015: eHealth-Enabled Health*: 264–269. https://doi.org/10.3233/978-1-61499-564-7-264.

Bürger, Valerie K., Julia Amann, Cathrine K. T. Bui, Jana Fehr, and Vince I. Madai. 2024. "The Unmet Promise of Trustworthy AI in Healthcare: Why We Fail at Clinical Translation." *Frontiers in Digital Health* 6. https://doi.org/10.3389/fdgth.2024.1279629.

Cabitza, Federico, Raffaele Rasoini, and Gian Franco Gensini. 2017. "Unintended Consequences of Machine Learning in Medicine." *JAMA: Journal of the American Medical Association* 318 (6) (August 8): 517–518. https://doi.org/10.1001/jama.2017.7797.

Capasso, Marrianna, and Steven Umbrello. 2022. "Responsible Nudging for Social Good: New Healthcare Skills for AI-Driven Digital Personal Assistants." *Medicine, Health Care and Philosophy* 25 (1) (March): 11–22. https://doi.org/10.1007/s11019-021-10062-z.

Čartolovni, Anto, Ana Tomičić, and Elvira Lazić Mosler. 2022. "Ethical, Legal, and Social Considerations of AI-Based Medical Decision-Support Tools: A Scoping Review." *International Journal of Medical Informatics* 161 (May): 104738. https://doi.org/10.1016/j.ijmedinf.2022.104738.

Challen, Robert, Joshua Denny, Martin Pitt, Luke Gompels, Tom Edwards, and Krasimira Tsaneva-Atanasova. 2019. "Artificial Intelligence, Bias and Clinical Safety." *BMJ Quality & Safety* 28 (3) (March): 231–237. https://doi.org/10.1136/bmjqs-2018-008370.

Char, Danton S., Michael D. Abràmoff, and Chris Feudtner. 2020. "Identifying Ethical Considerations for Machine Learning Healthcare Applications." *American Journal of Bioethics* 20 (11): 7–17. https://doi.org/10.1080/15265161.2020.1819469.

Chen, Yan, and Pouyan Esmaeilzadeh. 2024. "Generative AI in Medical Practice: In-Depth Exploration of Privacy and Security Challenges." *Journal of Medical Internet Research* 26 (March): e53008. https://doi.org/10.2196/53008.

Chen, Irene Y., Emma Pierson, Sherri Rose, Shalmali Joshi, Kadija Ferryman, and Marzyeh Ghassemi. 2021. "Ethical Machine Learning in Healthcare." *Annual Review of Biomedical Data Science* 4: 123–144. https://doi.org/10.1146/annurev-biodatasci-092820-114757.

Chen, Antian, Chenyu Wang, and Xinqing Zhang. 2023. "Reflection on the Equitable Attribution of Responsibility for Artificial Intelligence-Assisted Diagnosis and Treatment Decisions." *Intelligent Medicine* 3 (2) (May): 139–143. https://doi.org/10.1016/j.imed.2022.04.002.

Cheney-Lippold, John. 2019. *We Are Data: Algorithms and the Making of Our Digital Selves*. New York: New York University Press.

Choudhury, Avishek. 2022. "Factors Influencing Clinicians' Willingness to Use an AI-Based Clinical Decision Support System." *Frontiers in Digital Health* 4 (August): 920662. https://doi.org/10.3389/fdgth.2022.920662.

Choudhury, Avishek, and Zaira Chaudhry. 2024. "Large Language Models and User Trust: Consequence of Self-Referential Learning Loop and the Deskilling of Health Care Professionals." *Journal of Medical Internet Research* 26 (April 25): e56764. https://doi.org/10.2196/56764.

Ciliberti, R., V. Schiavone, and L. Alfano. 2023. "Artificial Intelligence and the Caring Relationship: Ethical Profiles." *Medicina Historica* 7: article no. e2023016. https://www.scopus.com/inward/record.uri?eid=2-s2.0-85162142171&partnerID=40&md5=fb67dfb27da5a1c62fe59541fd2aee68.

Dalton-Brown, Sally. 2020. "The Ethics of Medical AI and the Physician-Patient Relationship." *Cambridge Quarterly of Healthcare Ethics* 29 (1) (January): 115–121. https://doi.org/10.1017/S0963180119000847.

De Angelis, Luigi, Francesco Baglivo, Guglielmo Arzilli, Gaetano Pierpaolo Privitera, Paolo Ferragina, Alberto Eugenio Tozzi, and Caterina Rizzo. 2023. "ChatGPT and the Rise of Large Language Models: The New AI-Driven Infodemic Threat in Public Health." *Frontiers in Public Health* 11 (April): 1166120. https://doi.org/10.3389/fpubh.2023.1166120.

DeCamp, Matthew, and Charlotta Lindvall. 2020. "Latent Bias and the Implementation of Artificial Intelligence in Medicine." *Journal of the American Medical Informatics Association* 27 (12) (December): 2020–2023. https://doi.org/10.1093/jamia/ocaa094.

Desai, Parth, and Jake Rubin. 2024. "Where Do Healthcare Budgets Match AI Hype? A 10-Year Lookback of Funding Data." *Medium* (blog). September 9. https://flarecapitalpartners.medium.com/where-do-healthcare-budgets-match-ai-hype-a-10-year-lookback-of-funding-data-783d52010e29.

De Togni, Giulia, Sonja Erikainen, Sarah Chan, and Sarah Cunningham-Burley. 2021. "What Makes AI 'Intelligent' and 'Caring'? Exploring Affect and Relationality across Three Sites of Intelligence and Care." *Social Science and Medicine* 277 (May): 113874. https://doi.org/10.1016/j.socscimed.2021.113874.

Dionne, Émilie. 2020. "Algorithmic Mediation, the Digital Era, and Healthcare Practices: A Feminist New Materialist Analysis." *Global Media Journal: Canadian Edition* 12 (1): 49–65. http://gmj-canadianedition.ca/wp-content/uploads/2020/06/05_Dionne-Volume-11-issue-2-Final-.pdf.

DuFault, Beth Leavenworth, and John W. Schouten. 2020. "Self-Quantification and the Datapreneurial Consumer Identity." *Consumption Markets & Culture* 23 (3): 290–316. https://doi.org/10.1080/10253866.2018.1519489.

Elendu, Chukwuka, Dependable C. Amaechi, Tochi C. Elendu, Klein A. Jingwa, Osinachi K. Okoye, Minichimso John Okah, John A. Ladele, Abdirahman H. Farah, and Hameed A. Alimi. 2023. "Ethical Implications of AI and Robotics in Healthcare: A Review." *Medicine* 102 (50) (December 15): e36671. https://doi.org/10.1097/MD.0000000000036671.

d'Elia, Alexander , Mark Gabbay, Sarah Rodgers, Ciara Kierans, Elisa Jones, Irum Durrani, Adele Thomas, and Lucy Frith. 2022. "Artificial Intelligence and Health Inequities in Primary Care: A Systematic Scoping Review and Framework." *Family Medicine and Community Health* 10 (suppl. 1) (October): e001670. https://doi.org/10.1136/fmch-2022-001670.

Ennis-O'Connor, Marie, and William T. O'Connor. 2024. "Charting the Future of Patient Care: A Strategic Leadership Guide to Harnessing the Potential of Artificial Intelligence." *Healthcare Management Forum* 37 (4) (July): 290–295. https://doi.org/10.1177/08404704241235893.

Fairfield, Joshua, and Nathaniel Reynolds. 2022. "Griswold for Google: Algorithmic Determinism and Decisional Privacy." *Southern Journal of Philosophy* 60 (1) (March): 5–37. https://doi.org/10.1111/sjp.12454.

Felder, Ryan Marchall. 2021. "Coming to Terms with the Black Box Problem: How to Justify AI Systems in Health Care." *Hastings Center Report* 51 (4) (July–August): 38–45. https://doi.org/10.1002/hast.1248.

Flores, Lidia, Seungjun Kim, and Sean D. Young. 2023. "Addressing Bias in Artificial Intelligence for Public Health Surveillance." *Journal of Medical Ethics* 50 (3) (March): 190–194. https://doi.org/10.1136/jme-2022-108875.

Floridi, Luciano. 2008. "The Method of Levels of Abstraction." *Minds and Machines* 18: 303–329. https://doi.org/10.1007/s11023-008-9113-7.

Floridi, Luciano. 2019. "Translating Principles into Practices of Digital Ethics: Five Risks of Being Unethical." *Philosophy & Technology* 32: 185–193. https://doi.org/10.1007/s13347-019-00354-x.

Floridi, Luciano. 2024. "*Hypersuasion*—on AI's Persuasive Power and How to Deal with It." *Philosophy & Technology* 37 (2): article no. 64. https://doi.org/10.1007/s13347-024-00756-6.

Floridi, Luciano, Josh Cowls, Monica Beltrametti, Raja Chatila, Patrice Chazerand, Virginia Dignum, et al. 2018. "AI4People—An Ethical Framework for a Good AI Society: Opportunities, Risks, Principles, and Recommendations." *Minds and Machines* 28: 689–707. https://doi.org/10.1007/s11023-018-9482-5.

Fournier-Tombs, Eleonore, and Juliette McHardy. 2023. "A Medical Ethics Framework for Conversational Artificial Intelligence." *Journal of Medical Internet Research* 25 (July): e43068. https://doi.org/10.2196/43068.

Freitas, Ana Teresa. 2024. "Data-Driven Approaches in Healthcare: Challenges and Emerging Trends." In *Multidisciplinary Perspectives on Artificial Intelligence and the Law*, eds. Henrique Sousa Antunes, Pedro Miguel Freitas, Arlindo L. Oliveira, Clara Martins Pereira, Elsa Vaz De Sequeira, and Luís Barreto Xavier, 65–80. Cham: Springer. https://doi.org/10.1007/978-3-031-41264-6_4.

Gaeta, Amy. 2023. "Diagnostic Advertisements: The Phantom Disabilities Created by Social Media Surveillance." *First Monday* 28 (1–2) (January). https://doi.org/10.5210/fm.v28i1.12913.

Graham, Mackenzie. 2023. "Data for Sale: Trust, Confidence and Sharing Health Data with Commercial Companies." *Journal of Medical Ethics* 49 (7) (July): 515–522. https://doi.org/10.1136/medethics-2021-107464.

Grote, Thomas, and Philipp Berens. 2020. "On the Ethics of Algorithmic Decision-Making in Healthcare." *Journal of Medical Ethics* 46 (3) (March): 205–211. https://doi.org/10.1136/medethics-2019-105586.

Grote, Thomas, and Geoff Keeling. 2022. "On Algorithmic Fairness in Medical Practice." *Cambridge Quarterly of Healthcare Ethics* 31 (1) (January): 83–94. https://doi.org/10.1017/S0963180121000839.

Habli, Ibrahim, Tom Lawton, and Zoe Porter. 2020. "Artificial Intelligence in Health Care: Accountability and Safety." *Bulletin of the World Health Organization* 98 (4) (April 1): 251–256. https://doi.org/10.2471/BLT.19.237487.

Harrer, Stefan. 2023. "Attention Is Not All You Need: The Complicated Case of Ethically Using Large Language Models in Healthcare and Medicine." *eBioMedicine* 90 (April): 104512. https://doi.org/10.1016/j.ebiom.2023.104512.

Holzmeyer, Cheryl. 2021. "Beyond 'AI for Social Good' (AI4SG): Social Transformations—Not Tech-Fixes—For Health Equity." *Interdisciplinary Science Reviews* 46 (1–2): 94–125. https://doi.org/10.1080/03080188.2020.1840221.

Huang, Pei-Hua, Ki-hun Kim, and Maartje Schermer. 2022. "Ethical Issues of Digital Twins for Personalized Health Care Service: Preliminary Mapping Study." *Journal of Medical Internet Research* 24 (1) (January): e33081. https://doi.org/10.2196/33081.

Iqbal, Jeffrey David, Michael Krauthammer, and Nikola Biller-Andorno. 2022. "The Use and Ethics of Digital Twins in Medicine." *Journal of Law, Medicine & Ethics* 50 (3) (Fall): 583–596. https://doi.org/10.1017/jme.2022.97.

Jayakumar, Prakash, Koen D. Oude Nijhuis, Jacobien H. F. Oosterhoff, and Kevin J. Bozic. 2023. "Value-Based Healthcare: Can Generative Artificial Intelligence and Large Language Models Be a Catalyst for Value-Based Healthcare?" *Clinical Orthopaedics and Related Research* 481 (10) (October): 1890–1894. https://doi.org/10.1097/CORR.0000000000002854.

Jongepier, F., and E. Keymolen. 2022. "Explanation and Agency: Exploring the Normative-Epistemic Landscape of the 'Right to Explanation.'" *Ethics and Information Technology* 24: article no. 49. https://doi.org/10.1007/s10676-022-09654-x.

Juengst, Eric, Michelle L. McGowan, Jennifer R. Fishman, and Richard A. Settersten Jr. 2016. "From 'Personalized' to 'Precision' Medicine: The Ethical and Social Implications of Rhetorical Reform in Genomic Medicine." *Hastings Center Report* 46 (5) (September–October): 21–33. https://doi.org/10.1002/hast.614.

Karpathakis, Kassandra, Jessica Morley, and Luciano Floridi. 2024. "A Justifiable Investment in AI for Healthcare: Aligning Ambition with Reality." *Minds and Machines* 34 (4) (December): article no. 38. https://doi.org/10.1007/s11023-024-09692-y.

Kasperbauer, T. J. 2021. "Conflicting Roles for Humans in Learning Health Systems and AI-Enabled Healthcare." *Journal of Evaluation of Clinical Practice* 27 (3) (June): 537–542. https://doi.org/10.1111/jep.13510.

Kerasidou, Charalampia (Xaroula), Angeliki Kerasidou, Monika Buscher, and Stephen Wilkinson. 2022. "Before and beyond Trust: Reliance in Medical AI." *Journal of Medical Ethics* 48 (11) (November): 852–856. https://doi.org/10.1136/medethics-2020-107095.

Kim, Henna, and Bo Xie. 2017. "Health Literacy in the eHealth Era: A Systematic Review of the Literature." *Patient Education and Counseling* 100 (6) (June): 1073–1082. https://doi.org/10.1016/j.pec.2017.01.015.

Launer, John. 2024. "Faces or Candlesticks? Why We Need Continuity in Teams." *BMJ* 385: q1323. https://doi.org/10.1136/bmj.q1323.

Lett, Elle, and William G. La Cava. 2023. "Translating Intersectionality to Fair Machine Learning in Health Sciences." *Nature Machine Intelligence* 5 (5) (May): 476–479. https://doi.org/10.1038/s42256-023-00651-3.

Liu, Mingxuan, Yilin Ning, Salinelat Teixayavong, Mayli Mertens, Jie Xu, Daniel Shu Wei Ting, et al. 2023. "A Translational Perspective towards Clinical AI Fairness." *Npj Digital Medicine* 6 (1): article no. 172. https://doi.org/10.1038/s41746-023-00918-4.

Martinez-Martin, Nicole, Zelun Luo, Amit Kaushal, Ehsan Adeli, Albert Haque, Sara S. Kelly, et al. 2021. "Ethical Issues in Using Ambient Intelligence in Health-Care Settings." *The Lancet Digital Health* 3 (2) (February): e115–e123. https://doi.org/10.1016/S2589-7500(20)30275-2.

Mathiesen, Tiit, and Marike Broekman. 2022. "Machine Learning and Ethics." In *Machine Learning in Clinical Neuroscience*, eds. Victor E. Staartjes, Luca Regli, and Carlo Serra, 251–256. Cham: Springer. https://doi.org/10.1007/978-3-030-85292-4_28.

McDougall, Rosalind J. 2019. "Computer Knows Best? The Need for Value-Flexibility in Medical AI." *Journal of Medical Ethics* 45 (3) (March): 156–160. https://doi.org/10.1136/medethics-2018-105118.

Moodley, K. 2023. "Artificial Intelligence (AI) or Augmented Intelligence? How Big Data and AI Are Transforming Healthcare: Challenges and Opportunities." *South African Medical Journal* 114 (1): 22–26. https://doi.org/10.7196/SAMJ.2024.v114i1.1631.

Morley, Jessica, and Luciano Floridi. 2020. "The Limits of Empowerment: How to Reframe the Role of mHealth Tools in the Healthcare Ecosystem." *Science and Engineering Ethics* 26: 1159–1183. https://doi.org/10.1007/s11948-019-00115-1.

Morley, Jessica, Caio C. V. Machado, Christopher Burr, Josh Cowls, Indra Joshi, Mariarosaria Taddeo, and Luciano Floridi. 2020. "The Ethics of AI in Health Care: A Mapping Review." *Social Science & Medicine* 260 (September): 113172. https://doi.org/10.1016/j.socscimed.2020.113172.

Mühlhoff, Rainer. 2023. "Predictive Privacy: Collective Data Protection in the Context of Artificial Intelligence and Big Data." *Big Data and Society* 10 (1). https://doi.org/10.1177/20539517231166886.

Murdoch, Blake. 2021. "Privacy and Artificial Intelligence: Challenges for Protecting Health Information in a New Era." *BMC Medical Ethics* 22: article no. 122. https://doi.org/10.1186/s12910-021-00687-3.

Murphy, Kathleen, Erica Di Ruggiero, Ross Upshur, Donald J. Willison, Neha Malhotra, Jia Ce Cai, Nakul Malhotra, Vincci Lui, and Jennifer Gibson. 2021. "Artificial Intelligence for Good Health: A Scoping Review of the Ethics Literature." *BMC Medical Ethics* 22: article no. 14. https://doi.org/10.1186/s12910-021-00577-8.

Ngiam, Kee Yuan, and Ing Wei Khor. 2019. "Big Data and Machine Learning Algorithms for Health-Care Delivery." *Lancet Oncology* 20 (5) (May): e262–e273. https://doi.org/10.1016/S1470-2045(19)30149-4.

Ong, Jasmine Chiat Ling, Shelley Yin-Hsi Chang, Wasswa William, Atul J Butte, Nigam H Shah, Lita Sui Tjien Chew, Nan Liu, et al. 2024. "Ethical and Regulatory Challenges of Large Language Models in Medicine." *Lancet Digital Health* 6 (6) (June): e428–e432. https://doi.org/10.1016/S2589-7500(24)00061-X.

Ploug, Thomas, and Søren Holm. 2022. "Right to Contest AI Diagnostics: Defining Transparency and Explainability Requirements from a Patient's Perspective." In *Artificial Intelligence in Medicine*, eds. Niklas Lidströmer and Hutan Ashrafian, 227–238. Cham: Springer. https://doi.org/10.1007/978-3-030-64573-1_267.

Pot, Mirjam, Nathalie Kieusseyan, and Barbara Prainsack. 2021. "Not All Biases Are Bad: Equitable and Inequitable Biases in Machine Learning and Radiology." *Insights into Imaging* 12: article no. 13. https://doi.org/10.1186/s13244-020-00955-7.

Pruski, Michal. 2024. "What Does It Mean for a Clinical AI to Be Just: Conflicts between Local Fairness and Being Fit-for-Purpose?" *Journal of Medical Ethics*. https://doi.org/10.1136/jme-2023-109675.

Quinn, Thomas P., Manisha Senadeera, Stephan Jacobs, Simon Coghlan, and Vuong Le. 2021. "Trust and Medical AI: The Challenges We Face and the Expertise Needed to Overcome Them." *Journal of the American Medical Informatics Association* 28 (4) (April): 890–894. https://doi.org/10.1093/jamia/ocaa268.

Racine, Eric, Wren Boehlen, and Matthew Sample. 2019. "Healthcare Uses of Artificial Intelligence: Challenges and Opportunities for Growth." *Healthcare Management Forum* 32 (5) (September): 272–275. https://doi.org/10.1177/0840470419843831.

Roetman, Sara. 2020. "Self-Tracking 'Femtech': Commodifying & Disciplining the Fertile Female Body." *AoIR Selected Papers of Internet Research*. https://doi.org/10.5210/spir.v2020i0.11320.

Rosenfeld, Ariel, David Benrimoh, Caitrin Armstrong, Nykan Mirchi, Timothe Langlois-Therrien, Colleen Rollins, Myriam Tanguay-Sela, et al. 2019. "Big Data Analytics and AI in Mental Healthcare." *arXiv*: 1903.12071. https://doi.org/10.48550/arXiv.1903.12071.

Rubeis, Giovanni. 2023. "Liquid Health: Medicine in the Age of Surveillance Capitalism." *Social Science & Medicine* 322 (April): 115810. https://doi.org/10.1016/j.socscimed.2023.115810.

Ruckenstein, Minna, and Natasha Dow Schüll. 2017. "The Datafication of Health." *Annual Review of Anthropology* 46: 261–278. https://doi.org/10.1146/annurev-anthro-102116-041244.

Rudschies, Catharina, and Ingrid Schneider. 2024. "Ethical, Legal, and Social Implications (ELSI) of Virtual Agents and Virtual Reality in Healthcare." *Social Science & Medicine* 340 (January): 116483. https://doi.org/10.1016/j.socscimed.2023.116483.

Rueda, Jon, Janet Delgado Rodríguez, Iris Parra Jounou, Joaquín Hortal-Carmona, Txetxu Ausín, and David Rodríguez-Arias. 2024. "'Just' Accuracy? Procedural Fairness Demands Explainability in AI-Based Medical Resource Allocations." *AI & Society* 39 (3) (June): 1411–1422. https://doi.org/10.1007/s00146-022-01614-9.

Sætra, Henrik Skaug. 2022. "First, They Came for the Old and Demented: Care and Relations in the Age of Artificial Intelligence and Social Robots." *Human Arenas* 5 (1) (March): 25–43. https://doi.org/10.1007/s42087-020-00125-7.

Shaw, James, Joseph Ali, Caesar A. Atuire, Phaik Yeong Cheah, Armando Guio Español, Judy Wawira Gichoya, et al. 2024. "Research Ethics and Artificial Intelligence for Global Health: Perspectives from the Global Forum on Bioethics in Research." *BMC Medical Ethics* 25: article no. 46. https://doi.org/10.1186/s12910-024-01044-w.

Sterckx, Sigrid, Vojin Rakic, Julian Cockbain, and Pascal Borry. 2016. "'You Hoped We Would Sleep Walk into Accepting the Collection of Our Data': Controversies Surrounding the UK Care.Data Scheme and Their Wider Relevance for Biomedical Research." *Medicine, Health Care and Philosophy* 19 (2) (June): 177–190. https://doi.org/10.1007/s11019-015-9661-6.

Stevens, M., and A. Beaulieu. 2024. "A Careful Approach to Artificial Intelligence: The Struggles with Epistemic Responsibility of Healthcare Professionals." *Information, Communication & Society* 27 (4): 719–734. https://doi.org/10.1080/1369118X.2023.2289971.

Toma, Augustin, Senthujan Senkaiahliyan, Patrick R. Lawler, Barry Rubin, and Bo Wang. 2023. "Generative AI Could Revolutionize Health Care—But Not If Control Is Ceded to Big Tech." *Nature* 624 (7990) (November 30): 36–38. https://doi.org/10.1038/d41586-023-03803-y.

Topol, Eric J. 2019. "High-Performance Medicine: The Convergence of Human and Artificial Intelligence." *Nature Medicine* 25 (1) (January): 44–56. https://doi.org/10.1038/s41591-018-0300-7.

Tudor Hart, Julian. 1971. "The Inverse Care Law." *Lancet* 297 (7696) (February 27): 405–412. https://doi.org/10.1016/S0140-6736(71)92410-X.

Upadhyay, Umashankar, Anton Gradisek, Usman Iqbal, Eshita Dhar, Yu-Chuan Li, and Shabbir Syed-Abdul. 2023. "Call for the Responsible Artificial Intelligence in the Healthcare." *BMJ Health & Care Informatics* 30 (1) (December): e100920. https://doi.org/10.1136/bmjhci-2023-100920.

Vayena, Effy, and John Tasioulas. 2016. "The Dynamics of Big Data and Human Rights: The Case of Scientific Research." *Philosophical Transactions of the Royal Society A: Mathematical, Physical and Engineering Sciences* 374 (2083) (December 28): 20160129. https://doi.org/10.1098/rsta.2016.0129.

Wang, Changyu, Siru Liu, Hao Yang, Jiulin Guo, Yuxuan Wu, and Jialin Liu. 2023. "Ethical Considerations of Using ChatGPT in Health Care." *Journal of Medical Internet Research* 25: e48009. https://doi.org/10.2196/48009.

Weissglass, Daniel E. 2022. "Contextual Bias, the Democratization of Healthcare, and Medical Artificial Intelligence in Low- and Middle-Income Countries." *Bioethics* 36 (2) (February): 201–209. https://doi.org/10.1111/bioe.12927.

Yu, Kun-Hsing, Elizabeth Healey, Tze-Yun Leong, Isaac S. Kohane, and Arjun K. Manrai. 2024. "Medical Artificial Intelligence and Human Values." *New England Journal of Medicine* 390 (20) (May 30): 1895–1904. https://doi.org/10.1056/NEJMra2214183.

Zhang, Jie, and Zong-ming Zhang. 2023. "Ethics and Governance of Trustworthy Medical Artificial Intelligence." *BMC Medical Informatics and Decision Making* 23: article no. 7. https://doi.org/10.1186/s12911-023-02103-9.

Jessica Morley is a postdoctoral research associate at the Digital Ethics Center, Yale University, USA. She holds a BA, MSc, and PhD from the University of Oxford, where she previously served as the director of policy research at the Bennett Institute for Applied Data Science. Morley's research focuses on ensuring the secondary use of health data is technically feasible, socially acceptable, ethically justifiable, and legally compliant. She continues to contribute her expertise as a member of the National Data Guardian Panel and the NHS England AI Advisory Board, bridging the gap between academic research and practical healthcare policy implementation.

Luciano Floridi is the founding director of the Digital Ethics Center at Yale University, USA, where he is also a professor in the cognitive science program. Educated at La Sapienza University of Rome and the University of Warwick, he previously held the position of OII Professor of Philosophy and Ethics of Information at the University of Oxford. Floridi's expertise spans digital ethics, AI ethics, philosophy of information, and philosophy of technology. His research focuses on understanding the impact of emerging technologies on society and the digital transformation of human experience. Floridi's interdisciplinary approach bridges philosophy, computer science, and ethics, contributing to critical discussions on technology's impact on human potential and society.

Chapter 3
Toward Healthcare (Social) Justice: On the Value of Biases in Healthcare AI

Simona Tiribelli

Abstract Prominent debates in AI ethics contend that biases are one of the main problems to be eradicated to design fair AI systems, leading the community to develop many technical and non-technical methods mainly focused on eliminating them to create fairer AI tools in healthcare. However, such methods are shown to be often inadequate for the design of fairer healthcare AI. As I argue in this chapter, the problem is a passive understanding of biases as mere errors and technical bugs in AI systems, and of the related solutions mainly aimed at their simple removal. Instead, we should value them as proactive signals of those socio-relational determinants that intangibly and often unfairly shape healthcare access and outcomes in societies over time. This chapter focuses on gender and ethnic biases in healthcare AI and argues for their value in developing AI-based systems and services as drivers of fairer and more just healthcare ecosystems. Also, drawing on ethical theories of affirmative action, the chapter shows how this understanding of biases enables us to generate novel compensatory design actions for the development of truly fair healthcare AI systems, capable of addressing longstanding unfair inequalities in healthcare, therefore promoting better and more just healthcare ecosystems.

Keywords AI ethics · Healthcare social justice · Bias · Fairness · Affirmative action

3.1 Introduction

The paramount value of artificial intelligence (AI) and specifically machine learning (ML) and deep learning (DL) systems for healthcare ecosystems is today extensively acknowledged. AI systems and techniques are indeed increasingly deployed for a wide array of tasks in the healthcare and clinical domain, both *strictly medical tasks*, such as the prediction of occurrence risk and development of a specific pathology, image interpretation, drug discovery, and purely *administrative healthcare tasks*,

S. Tiribelli (✉)
University of Macerata, Macerata, Italy
e-mail: simona.tiribelli@unimc.it

M. C. Altman and D. Schwan (eds.), *Ethics and Medical Technology*, The International Library of Bioethics 113, https://doi.org/10.1007/978-3-031-94690-5_3

from interactive notetaking to clinician-patient communication management (Goh et al. 2016; Larrazabal et al. 2020; Nwanosike et al. 2022; Zhou et al. 2023). Because of their unprecedented capabilities to process huge volumes of data and discover predictive patterns invisible to the human eye, AI has the potential to promote preventive and personalized healthcare (Ahmed 2020) and to address today's main challenges arising from contemporary healthcare systems, the increasing demand for health services from an aging population, healthcare access inequities, and the shortage of healthcare staff and socioeconomic resources (Bajwa et al. 2021). However, other studies are less promising and point instead in a different direction, by showing how AI can worsen healthcare systems by reinforcing biases, especially gender and ethnic biases, exacerbating existing healthcare disparities, social inequality, and discrimination (Obermeyer et al. 2019).

Indeed, one of today's main challenges with the use of AI ML and DL systems in healthcare research, practice, and industry is bias: their vulnerability to not only be imprecise and inaccurate but to be so especially against certain minorities and vulnerable groups (or as also called in the AI and ethics literature, disadvantaged groups), producing morally wrongful or unfair discrimination at scale (O'Neil 2016; Benjamin 2019). The word *bias* belongs to cognitive studies as well as to statistics and informatics: in the former field, bias refers to a cognitive distortion, or better, to those heuristics, cognitive shortcuts, and cognitive traps we make as human decision-makers that are rationally bounded, thus undermining our rational decision-making processes (Kahneman and Tversky 1979, 2000; Simon 2000; Kahneman 2011); in the latter field, bias mainly refers to a systematic tendency of some methods of collecting data to present distorted and flawed measurements of the matter analyzed. Both meanings are relevant and often mutually entrenched for the specific kinds of flaws affecting healthcare AI systems. There are cases when biases of the models refer to specific statistical techniques (e.g., aggregation bias such as the Simpson's Paradox). However, the most controversial and problematic ways of perpetuating and exacerbating harmful discrimination are those we can distinguish within the category of cognitive biases (as distorted correlations) that are culturally and socially shaped, what we know as *unfair and discriminating stereotypes and prejudices* such as ethnic and gender biases.

These culturally embedded, often historically rooted, and socially stratified biases can affect both the *design* of healthcare AI systems and the *datasets* used to develop, test, and train them. Indeed, while the list of biases that have been outlined in healthcare and medicine is quite dense (Giovanola and Tiribelli 2023), two prominent biases have been shown to lead to unfair discrimination based on sensitive attributes (such as race, gender, or sex) in healthcare AI. The first pertains to the design of AI models, and it is known as *minority bias*: the non- or insufficient consideration of certain minorities (e.g., ethnic groups) and related socio-contextual, fine-grained characteristics when designing healthcare AI models (including the choice of adequate, that is, also non-stereotyped or prejudiced, data labels and variables). The second bias concerns the choice of the training dataset when this already embeds historical biases, leading AI models to learn unfairly biased patterns and correlations and use them to produce certain outcomes (i.e., historical bias and bias by proxy).

Such issues have spurred the AI and ethics community to develop a substantial number of technical and non-technical methods to eliminate biases to create fairer AI tools. However, such methods have been widely revealed to be inadequate for the design of fairer healthcare AI systems and often even counterproductive. As I argue in this chapter, the problem is a passive understanding of biases as mere errors and technical bugs in AI systems and the related solutions as mainly aiming at their simple removal, instead of valuing them as proactive signals of socio-relational determinants intangibly shaping healthcare access in societies.

This chapter focuses on gender and ethnic biases in healthcare and medicine AI technology and argues for their value in developing AI-based systems and services as drivers of a truly fairer and more just healthcare ecosystem. Also, drawing on ethical theories of affirmative action, the chapter shows how this understanding of biases enables us to generate novel compensatory design actions for the development of truly fair healthcare AI systems, that is, systems capable of addressing longstanding inequalities in healthcare, and therefore promoting better and fairer healthcare ecosystems.

To this aim, the second section introduces the issue of gender and ethnic biases in healthcare AI and the limits of the current approaches to fix them in order to develop fair healthcare AI systems. The third section argues for the reason behind such limits and proposes a novel consideration of biases as proactive signals of what systemic issues should be fixed in order to create truly fair AI systems. Particularly, the chapter shows how the mitigation of biases in healthcare AI systems is not sufficient alone, especially in societies affected by systemic inequalities, but must be complemented with strategies that enable the development of AI systems that work on dismantling the socio-relational sources of unfair health inequalities within societies. In the fourth section, I argue that such an understanding of biases can help to translate theories of affirmative actions into design strategies to make healthcare AI systems promote social justice in healthcare.

3.2 Biases and Mitigation Measures in Healthcare AI

The issue of biases is one of the most debated in the domain of healthcare and medical AI (Morley et al. 2020; Wiens et al. 2020; Chen et al. 2023; Yang 2024). This considerable focus is particularly due to the rising number of real-world cases and scientific scholarship that denounces AI systems used for a wide array of tasks and activities in healthcare and clinical contexts—from clinical support to disease prediction and healthcare management and decision-making—to be unfair due to biases, and specifically ethnic and gender biases, in their design or training datasets. Examples abound.

A benchmark case is an ML-based software applied in thousands of hospitals in the United States (US) for access to specially resourced care programs, found to be racially biased and to reify social disparities. In this case, the software was favoring white patients over sicker Black patients in determining patients-in-need priority scores due to wrong use of past medical expenditures, which are historically lower among Black patients, as a proxy for determining access to extra medical support (Obermeyer et al. 2019). Another case concerns the use of some applications of ML systems for heart failure risk scores that have been shown to inappropriately categorize Black patients as needing less care (Vyas et al. 2020). Further examples concern the domain of medical image analysis, where AI is increasingly applied. Here ML-based algorithmic models have been revealed to be particularly poor at detecting cancers of Black patients due to a minority bias (lack of data representation) of patients with darker skin (Noor 2020). Other studies have also shown biases related to gender and ethnicity in AI systems used for medical imaging in orthopedics to chest radiography (Seyyed-Kalantari et al. 2021; Gichoya et al. 2023; Vrudhula et al. 2024). For example, Ismaeel Siddiqui et al. (2024) point out biases related to sex and race in the AI-driven segmentation of bony anatomy using radiographs, which is a computational strategy routinely used in orthopedic surgery. Also, recently, large-language models (LLMs) such as GPT-3.5-turbo and GPT-4—whose promise to help doctors and healthcare professionals (HCPs) improve patient care are increasingly emphasized in today's health industry (Morley et al. 2023; Tian et al. 2024; Yu et al. 2024)—have also been proven to be racially biased in predicting health costs and generating medical texts based on real patients' health outcomes. This is problematic insofar as the integration of LLMs for generating medical reports becomes more prevalent (Sun 2023; Chen et al. 2024). Particularly, many LLMs largely in use by HCPs have been disclosed to exhibit racialized medical knowledge (Omiye et al. 2023): specific racial bias manifested in disparities of AI-generated treatment recommendations, hospitalization, and prognosis predictions, favoring white patients with immediate treatments, longer hospitalization stays, and better recovery outcomes (Yang et al. 2024).

Such controversial cases have made the problem of bias and specifically of gender and ethnic biases in healthcare AI an issue of great concern, since fairness in healthcare AI is recognized as one of the most important principles with which to comply (High-Level Expert Group on Artificial Intelligence 2019; Jobin et al. 2019; Corrêa et al. 2023). Looking at the main AI ethics and governance frameworks for AI in health (such as the World Health Organization 2021, 2024), justice as fairness emerges as a strong prerequisite for AI in health. Critics of unfairness in healthcare AI mainly prescribe the removal of biases or the development of non-biased AI systems, with particular attention to ethnic and gender bias.

As a consequence, a growing body of scholarship has been developed to address ethnic and gender biases in order to design fair healthcare AI systems. Particularly, because biases are often described as one of the main problems to be eradicated, healthcare AI and ethics scholarship as well as industry have proposed many initiatives and solutions to achieve algorithmic fairness in healthcare, mainly designed to *eliminate* ethnic and gender biases in healthcare AI.[1]

---

[1] See, for example, the initiatives of the panel of experts set up by the Agency for Healthcare Research and Quality (AHRQ) and the National Institute on Minority Health and Health Disparities (NIMHD)

However, as it has been shown, eliminating biases is not only difficult to achieve; it can be even counterproductive to develop accurate and fair AI solutions, especially in healthcare and medicine. Indeed, most proposed methods to achieve fairness by eliminating biases are based on neutral or parity models (Corbett-Davies et al. 2023): models designed to produce non-discriminatory predictions by constraining biases with respect to predicted outcomes for members of protected groups, often through the removal of sensitive attributes (Friedler et al. 2021; Corbett-Davies et al. 2023). However, such methods have been criticized as inadequate or ineffective for healthcare AI. In healthcare and medicine, including identity attributes is often critical, as there are valid reasons to believe these differences can have a causal impact on health outcomes (McCradden et al. 2020). For example, biological variations between genders can influence the effectiveness of certain medications. Omitting factors such as gender and race may reduce the accuracy of predictions and potentially increase disparities in outcomes. Further, as shown in Ziad Obermeyer et al. (2019), the removal of sensitive attributes or the reliance on neutral correlations neither prevents the development of biased AI systems nor implies that AI systems in healthcare are fairly designed.

In the next section, I show that this apparent deadlock depends on an inadequate, reductive, and mainly mathematical understanding of ethnic and gender biases—that is, as something that can be easily eliminated to achieve fairness in healthcare AI. I argue that this understanding is mainly due to a limited ethical conception of fairness in the debate on healthcare AI, which obscures the value of ethnic and gender biases for the design of AI systems capable of truly contributing to more just and fairer healthcare ecosystems.

3.3 Substantial Fairness over Procedural Equity: On the Value of Biases for Fair Healthcare AI

In the previous section, I showed that bias—especially gender and ethnic biases—is presently one of the main problems in the use of AI in healthcare. I have also pointed out that the emergence of this problem in the health industry, facilities, and in-use healthcare applications has prompted a huge corpus of ethics frameworks and policy guidelines that center algorithmic fairness as a core priority and principle for healthcare AI (World Health Organization 2021, 2024), as well as to a great deal of scholarship focusing on techniques for measuring and ensuring fairness that mainly relies on bias removal.

However, the widespread and now codified understanding of ethnic and gender biases as something to be removed per se is misleading and overly simplistic. Such biases are not merely mathematical bugs and technical errors to fix. Rather, gender and ethnic biases—as morally unfair and harmful correlations—reflect the hidden

to establish principles to prevent healthcare AI from perpetuating and exacerbating existing racial inequalities in medicine (Backman 2023).

patterns of systemic oppression and structural inequalities that unfairly affect healthcare access, quality, and benefits. To put it differently, such biases are social determinants of health and healthcare (Paradies et al. 2017; Ramsoondar et al. 2023). They drive and nurture structural phenomena such as racism, which creates invisible but powerful barriers to the achievement of fair health ecosystems by reinforcing disparities in quality of care and health outcomes. Their acritical or passive removal in healthcare AI development is—and has been shown to be—neither useful nor effective. It might even constitute a missed societal opportunity. Indeed, biases hold tremendous value in the context of healthcare AI to the extent they can allow us to proactively detect, assess, critically investigate, and create measures to address historically embedded and socially stratified sources of health inequity, disparity, and oppression at scale. Further, thanks to AI (ML and DL) access and related capacity to process huge amounts of health data—which are heavily affected by long-standing social, cultural, and institutional inequalities—such biases (that emerge as data patterns) enable us to detect what created and continues to profoundly nurture such unfair asymmetries according to diverse and critical (i.e., epistemic, cognitive, interpersonal, institutional, practical) dimensions of health and care at the micro- (individual), meso- and macro- (systemic) levels, both locally and globally. Gender and racial biases are indeed encoded and perpetuated through medical knowledge, clinical methods (including benchmark scales), traditional tools (e.g., pulse oximeter medical devices), and established health practices, as well as via clinician evaluations and encounters, physician-patient communications, and individual beliefs and attitudes (Smedley et al. 2003; Diao et al. 2021; Sudat et al. 2023)—as in the case of marginalized people who have internalized prejudices and oppression in their health and care perspectives and judgments (Veltman and Piper 2014). For example, half of white medical trainees still believe such myths as Black people have thicker skin or less sensitive nerve endings than white people—biased, often unconscious misbeliefs that lead to unfair medical treatment and healthcare quality for the considered group (Hoffman et al. 2016). It follows that investigating these biases along these dimensions and in correlation with other social determinants of health (e.g., language barriers, poor nutrition, socioeconomic deprivation, lifestyle habits, living and working conditions, and environmental factors such as air pollution) is of paramount importance: it enables us to understand what proxy should be used in the design of specific task-related healthcare AI systems, preventing bias by proxy or "discrimination by association" (Wachter 2020), and most importantly, to create systems capable of subverting them, hence promoting more just and fairer AI-empowered healthcare ecosystems (Giovanola and Tiribelli 2023; Tiribelli 2023).

Conversely, purely removing ethnic and gender biases, for example, through the elimination of sensitive attributes, obscures important information generated by AI systems we can and should harness. Furthermore, removing biases would be effective only in creating solutions that replicate the status quo. Bias-cleaned healthcare AI, when used in real-life situations that are imbued with social inequality and by consciously or unconsciously biased laypersons and healthcare operators, will easily relearn them and be refueled by biased decisions, practices, and data.

Much of such bias removal solutions are linked to a specific idea of fairness they explicitly aim to operationalize that emerges from within the debate on healthcare AI. As I have pointed out (Giovanola and Tiribelli 2022, 2023), algorithmic fairness within this debate exclusively overlaps with non-discrimination and therefore it is understood as mainly achievable through the removal of biases. However, this widespread idea of fairness is quite limited from an ethical perspective. Indeed, it refers mainly or exclusively to a *procedural account of fairness* grounded in *formal* equality of opportunity for people's access and fruition of health and care, as ensured by the legal systems (e.g., antidiscrimination laws).

However, fairness as an ethical value demands more: it entails the substantial promotion of opportunities as real chances for every person to express their agency and therefore the development of adequate conditions for people to afford them (*substantial fairness*) with a specific regard to the worst off. The philosophically thin and oversimplified idea of fairness within the debate on healthcare AI has led to problematic techniques that exclusively treat fairness as a *mathematical affair* (Mittelstadt et al. 2023). In such a debate, indeed, fairness is mainly measured in terms of disparity in performance and outcomes between advantaged or disadvantaged groups (see fairness options in Rajkomar et al. 2018). In other words, in this debate algorithmic fairness entails adjusting the models in order to reduce gaps in performance and outcomes between diverse demographic groups, hence ignoring other social and contextual factors. However, such an account of fairness is not only theoretically but also practically problematic. Algorithmic fairness measures that are purely formal suffer from both "fairness and performance degradation, or *levelling down*, where fairness is achieved by making every group worse off, or by bringing better performing groups down to the level of the worst off" (Mittelstadt et al. 2023, 56). This translates into measures counteracting fairness because they unnecessarily harm advantaged groups (with multiple examples in medical AI) without improving outcomes for historically disadvantaged, vulnerable, or marginalized groups, which is what fairness should aim for, and failing to address longstanding social inequalities.

The limits of such a vague and simplified idea of fairness can be overcome by endorsing a more complex and sounder account of justice as fairness, rooted in moral philosophy and ethical reasoning, that is, *substantial fairness*, which asks to guarantee substantial fair equality of opportunity with special regard to the worst off in the development of healthcare AI systems. Fair equality of opportunity needs to be thought of along with the difference principle, which emphasizes the attention to the expectations and conditions of the least advantaged, not just to access but also to enjoy those chances substantially (Giovanola and Tiribelli 2022). This entails the design of compensatory tools that, rather than just adjusting the model (a task that auditing meta-algorithms can perform), can be used to mitigate social disparities and individuals' capacity to enjoy opportunities, specifically for the least advantaged. In other words, to achieve substantial fairness, healthcare AI systems should be designed by considering and addressing the background conditions of justice within a society, and particularly systemic sources of oppression and harms that affect people unfairly and create asymmetric knowledge and agency conditions for historically deprived and harmed groups (Mhlambi and Tiribelli 2023; Tiribelli

2023). Therefore, compensatory tools are needed for operationalizing substantial fairness in healthcare AI. These tools can be created by harnessing the disclosing value of biases emerging from ML and DL processing to unmask large-scale patterns and correlations of unfair inequalities affecting healthcare ecosystems at different levels.

Following this line, Brent Mittelstadt et al. (2023) contend that the current fairness methods that focus on tweaking a system to make two numbers equal between groups might be "mathematically fair" but do not benefit the worst off. Similarly to what is argued by other scholars, they claim that "the challenge for the future of fairness in AI is to create systems that are substantively fair through levelling up, not only procedurally fair through levelling down" (48; see also Giovanola and Tiribelli 2022, 2023).

In the next section, I propose framing this challenge in philosophical terms as *substantial algorithmic fairness* through *affirmative action by AI design*. I clarify why substantial affirmative action by AI design is needed for developing fairer AI systems, capable of contributing to more just healthcare ecosystems, and what these dynamic actions entail for healthcare AI development, deployment, and use lifecycle.

3.4 Affirmative Action for Fairer AI-Based Healthcare Ecosystems

In the previous section, I argued for the inadequacy of a purely mathematical understanding of biases and fairness in favor of a *substantial conception of fairness* as fair equality of opportunity. I have also argued that biases in this sense instead of being passively removed as mathematical bugs should be *decoded* to investigate deep sources and patterns of inequalities they can disclose, which disproportionally affect historically marginalized or vulnerable groups (worst off) in healthcare access, quality, and substantive fruition, in order to design "compensatory" (Giovanola and Tiribelli 2022) or "levelling up" actions (Mittelstadt et al. 2023). In this section, I explain what that means from a philosophical and technical standpoint and what open challenges ought to be addressed.

Mittelstadt et al. (2023) conclude their critical essay on the "unfairness of fair ML" by stating that AI should be substantively, not just mathematically, fair; this entails designing systems that are fair through levelling up actions, that help (historically) disadvantaged groups. In practice, such actions consist of increasing by design decision rates or recalls to the required level for those groups usually harmed by decision rates or recalls that are too low (37)—that is, levelling up the rate, precision, or recall for a certain (disadvantaged) group to a minimum rate constraint (MRC), that is, a minimally acceptable performance threshold. In practice, these can be achievable by post-processing methods that allow different versions of a model by adjusting thresholds for each group—adjustments that help control the proportion of individuals in each group that receive a positive decision (Corbett-Davies et al. 2017; Petersen et al.

2021). By doing so, such levelling up actions better satisfy the real goal of fairness, from achieving strict parity between groups to ensuring a minimum fair performance threshold is met (Mittelstadt et al. 2023, 45).

In previous essays, after criticizing parity or neutral models proposed for achieving fairness in healthcare AI, Benedetta Giovanola and I (2022, 2023) proposed that, to promote substantial fairness (that is, real chances for every person to enjoy equally health and care resources and facilities), sensitive traits (e.g., gender and ethnicity) should not be obscured in healthcare AI, as they are critical from a medical and social justice standpoint (that is, for both accuracy and fairness). Indeed, they can function as decisional nodes to signal and evaluate who in a certain health domain may necessitate compensatory tools (the implementation of extra health measures, support, or facilities, etc.), as belonging to historically disadvantaged groups—usually harmed by AI. We concluded by calling for further work in the AI and ethics field to work on methods focusing on both extending these sensitive attributes (also to health issues, e.g., mental health issues) and making them reliable proxies for the need for compensatory tools or options. Such methods would intervene—on the basis of the healthcare AI tool—through an explicit clause[2] (for example, semi-structured interviews), while implementing meta-algorithms capable to detect and fix pernicious biases reflecting historical inequalities arising from them. Here, I provide an example of this proposal.

Consider a healthcare AI decision-making system designed to support clinicians or HCPs in determining priority access to first aid facilities, designed using as a proxy patients' reported pain levels. In this context, historical data show that women and individuals from ethnic minority groups often have their pain underestimated compared to white men (Hoffman et al. 2016). If the AI system is solely trained on historical data, it will easily inherit and perpetuate these biases, leading to a biased prioritization process, widening existing inequalities by negatively affecting historically deprived categories. Such bias still depends on misbeliefs that are to date very common among clinical trainers and residents. Therefore, even if the system would be trained on controlled (i.e., deprived of biases) data samples, it will easily re-learn biases through the new data produced from the interaction with clinicians and patients (a phenomenon called "automation bias"). To prevent this risk, the AI model could be designed by intentionally leveraging sensitive attributes such as gender and ethnicity, utilizing them as decision nodes to identify and signal the possible risk of underestimation or inadequate treatment of patients from minoritized and historically disadvantaged groups. For instance, if the system assesses a Black woman reporting severe pain, it can signal to the clinician and patient that this is an "at-risk demographic" for the specific task to evaluate: the system would flag this patient as belonging to a demographic group that faces a higher likelihood of pain underestimation, based on reported scientific evidence of historical biases in this

[2] Think about a healthcare AI system used for the elderly. Not everyone in such a category needs extra support or to be categorized as vulnerable. Therefore, especially for healthcare AI systems that do not include human, physician, or HCP in the loop, such as eHealth systems for treatment recommendation or health monitoring, it is necessary to ask the user whether such profiling is correct and whether extra measures or compensation options are needed, is necessary. With an explicit clause, the user is explicitly informed of such interventions and agree to them.

regard over time. The systems can be trained using flags for second-order proxies for the possible need for compensatory tools. The systems can then display compensatory tools, such as additional options whose outputs can be introduced in the assessment, weighted along with others, so as to calibrate the model toward a more accurate and fair decision for the specific patient. Such compensatory tools can be, for instance, semi-structured assessments based on diverse parameters and indicators. This is very relevant because, for example, the experience of pain differentially activates stress-related physiological responses across various ethnic groups, and members of different ethnic groups use different coping strategies in managing pain complaints, which therefore need to be considered (Campbell and Edward 2012).

Throughout this process, meta-algorithms can be implemented to work in real time to detect any other known patterns of bias, thereby finetuning the healthcare AI model's accuracy and fairness over time without obscuring sensitive attributes that are critical to understanding potential disparities. This compensatory tool by design would allow us to benefit from AI (make more efficient urgency management) while also promoting fair health access and treatment for those negatively impacted on a large scale in this domain. Further, it prompts a process of sensitization to such phenomenon that, over time, can produce better and fairer cohorts of physicians and healthcare operators (i.e., dismantle such biased misbeliefs) and more accurate health data for AI systems and the entire healthcare ecosystem.

In this section, I propose that actions of this kind can be understood as "affirmative actions" (AA); here, I focus specifically on what I define as *substantial affirmative actions by AI design*. The concept of AA sounds particularly important based on what I contended in the previous pages; however, it is poorly explored in the debate on the ethics of AI and almost unexplored for healthcare AI. Broadly speaking, AA is a concept used in many fields to refer to a set of proactive interventions (usually policy interventions) that recognize asymmetries in the equality of opportunity and act in a multiplicity of ways to correct or compensate for those deficiencies. The concept has been widely debated within moral philosophy and applied ethics (Fullinwider 2024; see also Fullinwider 1980, 13; Cohen and Sterba 2003, 279; Anderson 2010, 135; Lippert-Rasmussen 2020, 2–21). From a philosophical perspective, I endorse Kasper Lippert-Rasmussen's (2020) definition of AA: a policy, an act, or an intervention (etc.) is an AA if and only if it prescribes and enacts positive steps to increase the representation of women and minorities in a relevant area from which they have been historically excluded and/or aims to reasonably address the disadvantages they suffer in some ways other than boosting their representation (e.g., through quotas). In this sense, AA is understood as reducing the degree to which minority people have worse opportunities than majority people (clearly where this inequality does not simply reflect differential choices). As pointed out by the American Civil Liberties Union (2008), "AA helps to ensure equal access to opportunities and brings our nation closer to the ideal of giving everyone a fair chance."

From this standpoint, AA is broadly claimed within philosophical debates as a requirement for social justice. However, it is a requirement for social justice and hence it is ethically justifiable if and only if it is a *substantive equality of opportunity-promoting affirmative action* (Lippert-Rasmussen 2023, 5). That is, AA aims not only to reduce asymmetries that unfairly affect certain groups but also to address their sources. An example of non-substantive equality of opportunity-promoting AA could be a hiring program in a hospital aimed at increasing ethnic diversity in the medical staff by reserving quotas to hire a minimum number of individuals from ethnic minority groups, without addressing the structural and indirect barriers these groups might face. The hospital may hire medical staff from diverse ethnic backgrounds but without providing any training or support to tackle internal biases and racialized assumptions among existing clinicians, including those from minority groups. As a result, new hires may still find themselves in a discriminatory or hostile environment that lacks support for their professional growth or for addressing systemic biases and even quit their jobs. This AA initiative, therefore, would not promote substantive equality of opportunity because it fails to address the root causes of unfair disparities. It merely removes a direct barrier (lack of representation) without tackling the indirect sources of discrimination or bias that impact healthcare access, quality, and fruition.

Another key distinction is that there are diverse types of AA: AA can be numerical and not numerical. One of the most well-known examples of numerical AA is quotas for underrepresented groups. Quotas are often described as strong AA. There are also non-numerical AAs that do not set quotas, such as outreach AA programs involving special efforts to advertise open positions to underrepresented groups or remedial training programs. They are widely claimed as weak AA and therefore are more readily accepted.[3]

The value of AA is acknowledged in healthcare. This is because past and present injustices have impacted the health of individuals from disadvantaged groups in myriad ways, shaping social determinants of health, the broad set of forces and systems shaping the conditions of daily life (Jones 1985). As reported (Ong and Norris 2023), phenomena such as racism and the inequitable distribution of the social determinants of health are major driving forces in health disparities and major root causes in the racial and ethnic disparities in the access to and quality of health care. For this reason, the elimination of AA in the healthcare and medical fields have been condemned as justifying and exacerbating health disparities for minoritized groups (Rice et al. 2023). Similarly, the COVID-19 pandemic had a disproportionately negative impact on Black and Hispanic people, who were five times more likely to be hospitalized from COVID-19 than white people. Therefore, ethicists have proposed placing Black and Hispanic people high on the list for vaccine priority and giving more weight to individual members of disadvantaged racial groups so they have a higher chance of accessing ventilators (Zohny et al. 2022 see also Sederstrom 2020).

Despite this work on AA in healthcare, the integration of substantive equality of opportunity-promoting AA through healthcare AI design and deployment has not been proposed or investigated. Nonetheless, we can understand some of the latest design actions proposed in healthcare AI to be forms of AA, but of different kind.

[3] I do not focus on the debate between strong or weak AA here, as that would lead us astray, but such a clarification can be of particular utility for further studies called to justify AA in the AI development not only from an ethical but also a legal perspective.

For example, levelling up actions by AI design that aim to augment the number of positive rates, precision, or recall for a certain underrepresented group can be understood as numerical AA. This AA can be important for substantive fairness but it is not a *substantive equality of opportunity-promoting* AA. They can be important insofar as augmenting representation of certain historically disadvantaged groups to a minimum acceptable threshold[4] is key in healthcare, where nonrepresentation (especially in the AI design) translates into inaccuracy, beyond unfairness: having worse health-related outcomes, and as a consequence a lower chance of accessing certain goods associated with good health, including quality of life and life expectancy. However, such measures do not address the roots of the problems of social inequalities perpetuating over time. This is because such AA measures mainly focus on the distributive dimension of justice (as access and distribution of benefits and opportunities) but do not encompass its socio-relational dimension (even though practices of distribution are mainly shaped and revised by individuals and social groups), which is where the biases, power, and knowledge that propagate unfair asymmetries are fueled.

By contrast, the compensatory actions by AI design described above can be understood as non-numerical AA (e.g., cases of outreach AA programs or remedial training). They do not aim only to foster the representation of the categories they target numerically or quantitatively; they work also on the qualitative dimension. That is, they are designed to address the historical sources of disparities from a distributive and socio-relational standpoint. By doing so, such actions can promote substantial fair equality of opportunity, mitigating the sources of unfair oppression that hamper substantial fairness. Therefore, such actions can be classified as substantive equality of opportunity-promoting AA, and hence, their ethical justification for healthcare AI design can be construed as a requirement for social justice, to achieve more socially just healthcare ecosystems.

First technical and theoretical attempts are ongoing in this regard and have a strong justification and sound application for promoting the value of fairness in healthcare. For example, attempts to investigate the social determinants of health through AI and LLMs specifically have been made (Guevara et al. 2024), attempts that can be extended and investigated through the lenses of ethnic and gender biases. For example, Cindy Zhang et al. (2023) propose algorithm models that can identify discriminatory samples in the data that could cause disparities in systems' predictions, then re-used to retrain DL models for more fair predictions. All these efforts constitute prominent technical steps and propaedeutic layers for the development and operationalization of substantive equality of opportunity-promoting AA by design. Nevertheless, they cannot be deployed in an ethical and social vacuum. If they are not informed by philosophical, ethical, and sociological analyses, such algorithm

[4] What actually constitutes an acceptable minimum threshold is a fundamental question that ought to be discussed and contextually analyzed.

models will be ineffective and damaging instead of fixing the societal problems they aim to address.[5]

To conclude, the proposed taxonomy framework for AA for the design of truly fair healthcare AI—that is, capable of contributing to better, more just, and fairer healthcare ecosystems—does not aim to be exhaustive. Much work needs to be done on this issue. However, it has the potential to generate novel, less purely mathematical, and more complex and demanding technical and ethical research, on how to promote fairness in and through AI-based healthcare systems, that is, in a way that truly deals with a broken and historically damaged system and makes AI systems tools for social justice in healthcare.

3.5 Conclusion

In this chapter, I have claimed that AI systems currently deployed for healthcare purposes can contribute to the promotion of more just healthcare ecosystems if they are redesigned and deployed by harnessing the value of ethnic and gender biases to understand the unfair, historically rooted, and socially stratified hindrances to the achievement of substantial fairness in healthcare. In particular, I have argued that biases can disclose invisible patterns of unfair inequalities that hamper fair equality of opportunity in healthcare for the most vulnerable and historically mostly deprived. Therefore, I claimed we ought to harness such biases and hence the data processing and knowledge discovery capacities of AI systems as they flag what is deeply problematic and need to be fixed within our societies. In doing so, we will create fair AI systems in unfair societies and healthcare ecosystems. I concluded by showing how such information about what is morally wrong in our societies can enable us to redesign more effective and adequate healthcare AI systems through dynamic and context-specific substantial affirmative action schemes with the capacity to repair a broken system and promote social justice in healthcare.

[5] It is important to note that such actions should be dynamic and time-sensitive. For example, once the systemic structures of injustice have been eradicated and substantial equality of opportunity has been achieved in healthcare, such affirmative schemes can also end. AA efforts are generally not intended to be permanent or fixed solutions but rather as time-bound interventions designed to address deeply embedded injustices. When these structural barriers to fairness are effectively dismantled and substantial equality of opportunity established, the need for such affirmative measures will naturally diminish.

References

Ahmed, Zeeshan. 2020. "Practicing Precision Medicine with Intelligently Integrative Clinical and Multi-Omics Data Analysis." *Human Genomics* 14 (35). https://doi.org/10.1186/s40246-020-00287-z.

American Civil Liberties Union. 2008. "Striving for Equal Opportunity: Why the ACLU Supports Affirmative Action." March 21. https://www.aclu.org/documents/striving-equal-opportunity-why-aclu-supports-affirmative-action.

Anderson, Elizabeth. 2010. "The Fundamental Disagreement between Luck Egalitarians and Relational Egalitarians." *Canadian Journal of Philosophy* 40 (Supplement 1): 1–23. https://doi.org/10.1080/00455091.2010.10717652.

Backman, Isabella. 2023. "Eliminating Racial Bias in Health Care AI: Expert Panel Offers Guidelines." Yale School of Medicine. December 21. https://medicine.yale.edu/news-article/eliminating-racial-bias-in-health-care-ai-expert-panel-offers-guidelines/.

Bajwa, Junaid, Usman Munir, Aditya Nori, and Bryan Williams. 2021 "Artificial Intelligence in Healthcare: Transforming the Practice of Medicine." *Future Healthcare Journal* 8 (2) (July): e188–e1894. https://doi.org/10.7861/fhj.2021-0095.

Benjamin, Ruha. 2019. *Race after Technology: Abolitionist Tools for the New Jim Code.* Medford, MA: Polity.

Campbell, Claudia M., and Robert R. Edwards. 2012. "Ethnic Differences in Pain and Pain Management." *Pain Management* 2 (3): 219–230. https://doi.org/10.2217/pmt.12.7.

Chen, Richard J., Judy J. Wang, Drew F. K. Williamson, Tiffany Y. Chen, Jana Lipkova, Ming Y. Lu, Sharifa Sahai, and Faisal Mahmood. 2023 "Algorithmic Fairness in Artificial Intelligence for Medicine and Healthcare." *Nature Biomedical Engineering* 7 (6) (June): 719–742. https://doi.org/10.1038/s41551-023-01056-8.

Chen, Yuxuan, Haoyan Yang, Hengkai Pan, Fardeen Siddiqui, Antonio Verdone, Qingyang Zhang, Sumit Chopra, Chen Zhao, and Yiqiu Shen. 2024. "BURExtract-Llama: An LLM for Clinical Concept Extraction in Breast Ultrasound Reports." In *Proceedings of the 1st International Workshop on Multimedia Computing for Health and Medicine (MCHM'24)*, 53–58. New York: Association for Computing Machinery. https://doi.org/10.1145/3688868.3689200.

Cohen, Carl, and James P. Sterba. 2003. *Affirmative Action and Racial Preference.* New York: Oxford University Press.

Corbett-Davies, Sam, Emma Pierson, Avi Feller, Sharad Goel, and Aziz Huq. 2017. "Algorithmic Decision Making and the Cost of Fairness." In *KDD '17: Proceedings of the 23rd ACM SIGKDD International Conference on Knowledge Discovery and Data Mining*, eds. Stan Matwin, Shipeng Yu, and Faisal Farooq, 797–806. New York: Association for Computing Machinery. https://doi.org/10.1145/3097983.3098095.

Corbett-Davies, Sam, Johann D. Gaebler, Hamed Nilforoshan, Ravi Shroff, and Sharad Goel. 2023. "The Measure and Mismeasure of Fairness." *Journal of Machine Learning Research* 24 (312) (January): 1–117.

Corrêa, Nicholas Kluge, Camila Galvão, James William Santos, Carolina Del Pino, Edson Pontes Pinto, Camila Barbosa, et al. 2023. "Worldwide AI Ethics: A Review of 200 Guidelines and Recommendations for AI Governance." *Patterns* 4 (10) (October 13). https://doi.org/10.1016/j.patter.2023.100857.

Diao, James A., Gloria J. Wu, Herman A. Taylor, John K. Tucker, Neil R. Powe, Isaac S. Kohane, and Arjun K. Manrai. 2021. "Clinical Implications of Removing Race from Estimates of Kidney Function." *JAMA: Journal of the American Medical Association* 325 (2) (December 2): 184–186. https://doi.org/10.1001/jama.2020.22124.

Friedler, Sorelle A., Carlos Scheidegger, and Suresh Venkatasubramanian. 2021. "The (Im)possibility of Fairness: Different Value Systems Require Different Mechanisms for Fair Decision Making." *Communications of the ACM* 64 (4) (April): 136–143. https://doi.org/10.1145/3433949.

Fullinwider, Robert K. 1980. *The Reverse Discrimination Controversy*. Totowa, NJ: Rowman and Littlefield.

Fullinwider, Robert K. 2024. "Affirmative Action." In *Stanford Encyclopedia of Philosophy* (Fall 2024 edition), eds. Edward N. Zalta and Uri Nodelman. http://plato.stanford.edu/entries/affirmative-action/.

Gichoya, Judy Wawira, Kaesha Thomas, Leo Anthony Celi, Nabile Safdar, Imon Banerjee, John D. Banja, Laleh Seyyed-Kalantari, Hari Trivedi, and Saptarshi Purkayastha. 2023. "AI Pitfalls and What Not to Do: Mitigating Bias in AI." *British Journal of Radiology* 96 (1150) (October 1). https://doi.org/10.1259/bjr.20230023.

Giovanola, Benedetta, and Simona Tiribelli. 2022. "Weapons of Moral Construction? On the Value of Fairness in Algorithmic Decision-Making." *Ethics and Information Technology* 24 (3). https://doi.org/10.1007/s10676-022-09622-5.

Giovanola, Benedetta, and Simona Tiribelli. 2023. "Beyond Bias and Discrimination: Redefining the AI Ethics Principle of Fairness in Healthcare Machine-Learning Algorithms." *AI & Society* 38 (2) (April): 549–563. https://doi.org/10.1007/s00146-022-01455-6.

Goh, Gabriel, Andrew Cotter, Maya Gupta, and Michael Friedlander. 2016 "Satisfying Real-World Goals with Dataset Constraints." *arXiv*: 1606.07558. https://doi.org/10.48550/arXiv.1606.07558.

Guevara, Marco, Shan Chen, Spencer Thomas, Tafadzwa L. Chaunzwa, Idalid Franco, Benjamin H. Kann, et al. 2024. "Large Language Models to Identify Social Determinants of Health in Electronic Health Records." *NPJ Digital Medicine* 7 (6). https://doi.org/10.1038/s41746-023-00970-0.

High-Level Expert Group on Artificial Intelligence. 2019. "Ethics Guidelines for Trustworthy AI." European Commission. https://digital-strategy.ec.europa.eu/en/library/ethics-guidelines-trustworthy-ai.

Hoffman, Kelly M., Sophie Trawalter, Jordan R. Axt, and M. Norman Oliver. 2016. "Racial Bias in Pain Assessment and Treatment Recommendations, and False Beliefs about Biological Differences Between Blacks and Whites." *PNAS* 113 (16) (April 19): 4296–4301. https://doi.org/10.1073/pnas.1516047113.

Jobin, Anna, Marcello Ienca, and Effy Vayena. 2019. "The Global Landscape of AI Ethics Guidelines." *Nature Machine Intelligence* 1 (9) (September): 389–399. https://doi.org/10.1038/s42256-019-0088-2.

Jones, Gary E. 1985. "Preferential Treatment and the Allocation of Scarce Medical Resources." *Philosophical Quarterly* 35 (141) (October): 382–393. https://doi.org/10.2307/2219473.

Kahneman, Daniel. 2011. *Thinking, Fast and Slow*. New York: Farrar, Straus and Giroux.

Kahneman, Daniel, and Amos Tversky. 1979. "Prospect Theory: An Analysis of Decision under Risk." *Econometrica* 47 (2) (March): 263–291. https://doi.org/10.2307/1914185.

Kahneman, Daniel, and Amos Tversky, eds. 2000. *Choices, Values, and Frames*. Cambridge: Cambridge University Press.

Larrazabal, Agostina J., Nicolás Nieto, Victoria Peterson, and Enzo Ferrante. 2020. "Gender Imbalance in Medical Imaging Datasets Produces Biased Classifiers for Computer-Aided Diagnosis." *PNAS* 117 (23) (May 26): 12592–12594. https://doi.org/10.1073/pnas.1919012117.

Lippert-Rasmussen, Kasper. 2020. *Making Sense of Affirmative Action*. New York: Oxford University Press.

Lippert-Rasmussen, Kasper. 2023. "Equality of Opportunity and Affirmative Action." In *Handbook of Equality of Opportunity*, eds. Mitja Sardoč, 1–22. Cham: Springer. https://doi.org/10.1007/978-3-319-52269-2_87-1.

McCradden, Melissa D., Shalmali Joshi, Mjaye Mazwi, and James A. Anderson. 2020. "Ethical Limitations of Algorithmic Fairness Solutions in Health Care Machine Learning." *Lancet Digital Health* 2 (5) (May): e221–e223. https://doi.org/10.1016/S2589-7500(20)30065-0.

Mhlambi, Sábëlo, and Simona Tiribelli. 2023. "Decolonizing AI Ethics: Relational Autonomy as a Means to Counter AI Harms." *Topoi* 42 (3) (July): 867–880. https://doi.org/10.1007/s11245-022-09874-2.

Mittelstadt, Brent, Sandra Wachter, and Chris Russell. 2023. "The Unfairness of Fair Machine Learning: Levelling Down and Strict Egalitarianism by Default." *Michigan Technology Law Review* 30 (1): 3. https://repository.law.umich.edu/mtlr/vol30/iss1/3.

Morley, Jessica, Caio C.V. Machado, Christopher Burr, Josh Cowls, Indra Joshi, Mariarosaria Taddeo, and Luciano Floridi. 2020. "The Ethics of AI in Health Care: A Mapping Review." *Social Science & Medicine* 260 (September). https://doi.org/10.1016/j.socscimed.2020.113172.

Morley, Jessica, Nicholas J. DeVito, and Joe Zhang. 2023. "Generative AI for Medical Research." *BMJ* 382 (July 12): 1551. https://doi.org/10.1136/bmj.p1551.

Noor, Poppy. 2020. "Can We Trust AI Not to Further Embed Racial Bias and Prejudice?" *BMJ* 368. https://doi.org/10.1136/bmj.m363.

Nwanosike, Ezekwesiri Michael, Barbara R. Conway, Hamid A. Merchant, and Syed Shahzad Hasan. 2022. "Potential Applications and Performance of Machine Learning Techniques and Algorithms in Clinical Practice: A Systematic Review." *International Journal of Medical Informatics* 150 (March). https://doi.org/10.1016/j.ijmedinf.2021.104679.

Obermeyer, Ziad, Brian Powers, Christine Vogeli, and Sendhil Mullainathan. 2019. "Dissecting Racial Bias in an Algorithm Used to Manage the Health of Populations." *Science* 366 (6464) (October 25): 447–453. https://doi.org/10.1126/science.aax2342.

Omiye, Jesutofunmi A., Jenna Lester, Simon Spichak, Veronica Rotemberg, and Roxana Daneshjou. 2023. "Beyond the Hype: Large Language Models Propagate Race-Based Medicine." *medRxiv*. https://doi.org/10.1101/2023.07.03.23292192.

O'Neil, Cathy. 2016. *Weapons of Math Destruction: How Big Data Increases Inequality and Threatens Democracy*. New York: Crown.

Ong, Michael K, and Keith C. Norris. 2023. "Advancing Equity Research in the Quality of and Access to Health Care in a Post-Affirmative Action Era." In *Achieving Healthcare Equity in the United States*, eds. Alexander N. Ortega. Supplement, *Health Services Research* 58 (S3) (December): 281–283. https://doi.org/10.1111/1475-6773.14249.

Paradies, Yin, João Luiz Bastos, and Naomi Priest. 2017. "Prejudice, Stigma, Bias, Discrimination, and Health." In *The Cambridge Handbook of the Psychology of Prejudice*, eds. Chris G. Sibley and Fiona Kate Barlow, 559–581. Cambridge: Cambridge University Press. https://doi.org/10.1017/9781316161579.025.

Petersen, Felix, Debarghya Mukherjee, Yuekai Sun, and Mikhail Yurochkin. 2021. "Post-Processing for Individual Fairness." *arXiv*: 2110.13796. https://doi.org/10.48550/arXiv.2110.13796.

Rajkomar, Alvin, Michaela Hardt, Michael D. Howell, Greg Corrado, and Marshall H. Chin. 2018. "Ensuring Fairness in Machine Learning to Advance Health Equity." *Annals of Internal Medicine* 169 (12) (December 18): 866–872. https://doi.org/10.7326/M18-1990.

Ramsoondar, Nusha, Alex Anawati, and Erin Cameron. 2023. "Racism as a Determinant of Health and Health Care: Rapid Evidence Narrative from the SAFE for Health Institutions Project." *Canadian Family Physician/Médecin de Famille Canadien* 69 (9) (September 1): 594–598. https://doi.org/10.46747/cfp.6909594.

Rice, Valerie Montgomery, Martha L. Elks, and Mark Howse. 2023. "The Supreme Court Decision on Affirmative Action—Fewer Black Physicians and More Health Disparities for Minoritized Groups." *JAMA: Journal of the American Medical Association* 330 (11) (August 25): 1035–1036. https://doi.org/10.1001/jama.2023.15515.

Sederstrom, Nneka. 2020. "The 'Give Back': Is There Room for It?" *Bioethics Today*. July 16. http://www.bioethics.net/2020/07/the-give-back-is-there-room-for-it/.

Seyyed-Kalantari, Laleh, Haoran Zhang, Matthew B. A. McDermott, Irene Y. Chen, and Marzyeh Ghassemi. 2021. "Underdiagnosis Bias of Artificial Intelligence Algorithms Applied to Chest Radiographs in Under-served Patient Populations." *Nature Medicine* 27 (12) (December): 2176–2182. https://doi.org/10.1038/s41591-021-01595-0.

Siddiqui, Ismaeel A., Nickolas Littlefield, Luke A. Carlson, Matthew Gong, Avani Chhabra, Zoe Menezes, et al. 2024. "Fair AI-Powered Orthopedic Image Segmentation: Addressing Bias and Promoting Equitable Healthcare." *Scientific Reports* 14: article no. 16105. https://doi.org/10.1038/s41598-024-66873-6.

Simon, Herbert A. 2000. "Bounded Rationality in Social Sciences: Today and Tomorrow." *Mind & Society* 1 (1) (March): 25–39. https://doi.org/10.1007/BF02512227.

Smedley, Brian D., Adrienne Y. Stith, and Alen R. Nelson, eds. 2003. *Unequal Treatment: Confronting Racial and Ethnic Disparities in Health Care*. Washington, DC: National Academies. https://doi.org/10.17226/12875.

Sudat, Sylvia E. K., Paul Wesson, Kim F. Rhoads, Stephanie Brown, Noha Aboelata, Alice R. Pressman, Aravind Mani, and Kristen M. J. Azar. 2023. "Racial Disparities in Pulse Oximeter Device Inaccuracy and Estimated Clinical Impact on COVID-19 Treatment Course." *American Journal of Epidemiology* 192 (5) (May): 703–713. https://doi.org/10.1093/aje/kwac164.

Sun, Zhongxiang. 2023. "A Short Survey of Viewing Large Language Models in Legal Aspect." *arXiv*: 2303.09136. https://doi.org/10.48550/arXiv.2303.09136.

Tian, Shubo, Qiao Jin, Lana Yeganova, Po-Ting Lai, Qingqing Zhu, Xiuying Chen, et al. 2024. "Opportunities and Challenges for ChatGPT and Large Language Models in Biomedicine and Health." *Briefings in Bioinformatics* 25 (1) (January): bbad493. https://doi.org/10.1093/bib/bbad493.

Tiribelli, Simona. 2023. "Inequalities and Artificial Intelligence." *Filosofia Morale/Moral Philosophy* 1 (3): 185–196. https://mimesisjournals.com/ojs/index.php/MF/article/view/2722.

Veltman, Andrea, and Mark Piper. 2014. *Autonomy, Oppression, and Gender*. Oxford: Oxford University Press.

Vrudhula, Amey, Alan C. Kwan, David Ouyang, and Susan Cheng. 2024. "Machine Learning and Bias in Medical Imaging: Opportunities and Challenges." *Circulation: Cardiovascular Imaging* 17 (2) (February). https://doi.org/10.1161/CIRCIMAGING.123.015495.

Vyas, Darshali A., Leo G. Eisenstein, and David S. 2020. Jones. "Hidden in Plain Sight—Reconsidering the Use of Race Correction in Clinical Algorithms." *New England Journal of Medicine* 383 (9) (August 27): 874–882. https://doi.org/10.1056/NEJMms2004740.

Wachter, Sandra. 2020. "Affinity Profiling and Discrimination by Association in Online Behavioural Advertising." *Berkeley Technology Law Journal* 35 (2). https://doi.org/10.2139/ssrn.3388639.

Wiens, Jenna, W. Nicholson Price II, and Michael W. Sjoding. 2020. "Diagnosing Bias in Data-Driven Algorithms for Healthcare." *Nature Medicine* 26 (1) (January): 25–26. https://doi.org/10.1038/s41591-019-0726-6.

World Health Organization. 2021. *Ethics and Governance of Artificial Intelligence for Health: WHO Guidance*. https://www.who.int/publications/i/item/9789240029200.

World Health Organization. 2024. *Ethics and Governance of Artificial Intelligence for Health: Guidance on Large Multi-modal Models*. https://www.who.int/publications/i/item/9789240084759.

Yang, Yuzhe, Yujia Liu, Xin Liu, Avanti Gulhane, Domenico Mastrodicasa, Wei Wu, Edward J. Wang, Dushyant W. Sahani, and Shwetak Patel. 2024. "Demographic Bias of Expert-Level Vision-Language Foundation Models in Medical Imaging." *arXiv*: 2402.14815. https://doi.org/10.48550/arXiv.2402.14815.

Yu, Qinkai, Mingyu Jin, Dong Shu, Chong Zhang, Lizhou Fan, Wenyue Hua, et al. 2024. "Health-LLM: Personalized Retrieval-Augmented Disease Prediction System." *arXiv*: 2402.00746. https://doi.org/10.48550/arXiv.2402.00746.

Zhang, Cindy Y., Sarah H. Cen, and Devavrat Shah. 2023. "Matrix Estimation for Individual Fairness." In *ICML'23: Proceedings of the 40th International Conference on Machine Learning*, eds. Andreas Krause, Emma Brunskill, Kyunghyun Cho, Barbara Engelhardt, Sivan Sabato, and Jonathan Scarlett, 40871–40887. Honolulu, HI: Journal of Machine Learning Research.

Zhou, Hongjian, Fenglin Liu, Boyang Gu, Xinyu Zou, Jinfa Huang, Jinge Wu, et al. 2023. "A Survey of Large Language Models in Medicine: Principles, Applications, and Challenges." *arXiv*: 2311.05112. https://doi.org/10.48550/arXiv.2311.05112.

Zohny, Hazem, Ben Davies, and Dominic Wilkinson. 2022. "Affirmative Action in Healthcare Resource Allocation: Vaccines, Ventilators and Race." *Bioethics* 36 (9) (November): 970–977. https://doi.org/10.1111/bioe.13067.

Simona Tiribelli is tenure-track Assistant Professor in Ethics at the University of Macerata, Italy, and Director for Artificial Intelligence (AI) Ethics at the Institute for Technology and Global Health, the PathCheck Foundation policy research and innovation center founded at the Massachusetts Institute of Technology (MIT), USA. Previously, she held visiting positions in the NYU Center for Bioethics at New York University and the MIT Media Lab at MIT. Her research interests are in moral philosophy and applied ethics, with a focus on the ethics of AI. On these topics, she has authored more than thirty articles and two books.

Chapter 4
Advanced Technologies in Medicine: Safeguarding Physician Skill, Knowledge, and Character in the AI-Enhanced Clinic

Amitabha Palmer and David Schwan

Abstract As AI moves rapidly into medicine, we explore how these technologies may over time erode core physician competencies through various stages of the clinical encounter: from preparation and diagnosis to treatment planning and patient monitoring. We identify three critical areas at risk: clinical skills (*techne*), where AI automation may lead to dangerous deskilling; medical knowledge (*episteme*), where overreliance on AI systems can erode diagnostic reasoning abilities; and moral character (*ethos*), where AI-mediated patient interactions may compromise empathetic care. Our analysis demonstrates how AI tools, while promising improved efficiency and accuracy, can paradoxically undermine physician expertise through automation bias, alert fatigue, and the displacement of essential human-to-human interactions. To address these challenges, we introduce a novel framework for the ethical deployment of advanced technologies in healthcare: participatory deliberative conservatism (PDC). This model emphasizes broad stakeholder participation, deliberative decision-making processes, and the preservation of core medical values.

Keywords Artificial intelligence in medicine · Clinical decision support systems · Provider-patient relationship · Medical ethics · Technological deskilling

4.1 Introduction

The rapid advancement of artificial intelligence (AI) and robotic technologies in healthcare presents both unprecedented opportunities and profound ethical challenges (Palmer and Schwan 2024). As these advanced technologies increasingly permeate clinical settings, they promise to revolutionize medical practice, potentially

A. Palmer
MD Anderson Cancer Center, Houston, TX, USA
e-mail: apalmer1@mdanderson.org

D. Schwan (✉)
Central Washington University, Ellensburg, WA, USA
e-mail: david.schwan@cwu.edu

M. C. Altman and D. Schwan (eds.), *Ethics and Medical Technology*, The International Library of Bioethics 113, https://doi.org/10.1007/978-3-031-94690-5_4

improving patient accessibility, enhancing health outcomes, and reducing healthcare costs (Matheny et al. 2022). In addition, they may serve to alleviate the burdens on an overstressed healthcare system faced with increasing healthcare worker shortages (American Association of Colleges of Nursing 2024; see also Association of American Medical Colleges 2024) and burnout (Ortega et al. 2023). At the same time, the adoption of advanced technologies into medical practice also raises critical questions about the future role of physicians, the nature of clinical expertise, and the fundamental values that ground the practice of medicine.

This chapter examines the relationship between advanced technologies, such as AI and robotics (defined below), and the central attributes of an ideal physician: core clinical skills (*techne*), expert medical knowledge (*episteme*), and moral character (*ethos*). We explore how these technologies may augment or erode these essential qualities through various stages of the clinical encounter: from preparation and diagnosis to treatment planning and patient monitoring. We argue that the integration of advanced technologies in medicine offers significant benefits but also poses substantial risks, such as the atrophy of critical clinical skills, overreliance on opaque AI systems, and dehumanization of patient care.

To address these challenges, we introduce a novel framework for the ethical deployment of advanced technologies in healthcare: participatory deliberative conservatism (PDC). This model emphasizes broad stakeholder participation, deliberative decision-making processes, and the preservation of core medical values. To illustrate how the framework functions, we apply it to a hypothetical AI tool that generates diagnoses and treatment plans. We demonstrate how this framework can help healthcare institutions deploy emerging technologies without undermining the development of physicians' core clinical skills, expert knowledge, and moral character.

4.2 The Rise of Advanced Technologies in Clinical Care

In the past decade, the ethics of AI and robotic technologies have received increased attention (see Turkle 2011; Vallor 2016; Coeckelbergh 2020). This is to be expected given that these technologies have the potential to profoundly reshape fundamental aspects of human life. As noted in the United Nations' *Resource Guide on Artificial Intelligence (AI) Strategies*, "AI-based technologies blur the boundary between human subjects and technological objects [and] not only have societal implications … but they also affect the central categories of ethics: our concepts of agency and responsibility, and our value frameworks" (2021, 6–7; see also Ho 2023).

In medicine, numerous researchers have explored how advanced technologies can be ethically designed (van Wynsberghe 2013) and applied (Topol 2019) in a variety of care contexts, such as nursing (Barnard and Sandelowski 2001; Etzioni and Etzioni 2017; Archibald and Barnard 2018; Briganti and Le Moine 2020; Stokes and Palmer 2020) and elder care (Sparrow and Sparrow 2006; Sharkey and Sharkey 2012; Coeckelbergh 2016). Researchers from several disciplines have explored how advanced technologies raise normative issues surrounding autonomy, dignity, welfare, privacy, safety, deception, capability, social interaction, and the care relationship (Vandemeulebroucke et al. 2018; see also Secinaro et al. 2021).

We understand AI to be "any kind of artificial computational system that shows intelligent behavior, i.e., complex behavior that is conducive to reaching goals" (Müller 2020). AI has its roots in the early twentieth century, though the concept of simulated intelligence was not formalized until the Dartmouth Workshop organized by John McCarthy in 1956 (McCarthy et al. 1955). For our purposes here, we distinguish among machine learning, which is a "subset of AI that involves systems that can learn by themselves"; deep learning, which is "a subset of machine learning that uses models built on deep neural networks to detect patterns with minimal human involvement"; and natural language processing, which is a "branch of AI focused on teaching machines to understand, interpret, and generate human language" (Alowais et al. 2023). In healthcare, AI has expanding applications in imaging, drug discovery, predictive analytics, personalized medicine, clinical decision support, virtual assistance, surgery, and both patient and remote monitoring (Alowais et al. 2023).

By contrast, we understand robotic technologies as "agentive [devices] in a broad sense, purposed to act in the physical world in order to accomplish one or more tasks" (IEEE 2015). In the domain of medicine, we follow Noel Sharkey and Amanda Sharkey (2010) in referring to general robotic technologies as "assistive robots," and in some contexts "carebots" (Stokes and Palmer 2020). Presently, robotic technologies are assisting medical providers with surgery, patient rehabilitation, nursing assistance, and dispensing pharmaceuticals. In addition, carebots can provide companionship for patients and promote their independence and autonomy (Palmer and Schwan 2022).

4.3 Three Attributes of an Ideal Physician: *Techne*, *Episteme*, *Ethos*

Medical technology stands not only to support physicians and extend their abilities but also to fundamentally alter the way that medicine has long been practiced. These changes may not be innocuous. When basic activities are displaced by machines, there is a risk that physicians' skills in these areas will atrophy. Whether we ought to be concerned depends upon a conception of the ideal physician's skills, knowledge, and character, and how these attributes may be altered by the introduction of advanced technologies.

In the model that we favor, skills, knowledge, and character traits are acquired through specific practices that, with repetition, foster practical wisdom and habituation (Aristotle 2019). These attributes involve knowing when, how, and to whom to apply actions in particular contexts. Cultivating these attributes depends on factors such as having good role models, supportive cultural norms, personal motivation, and opportunities for practice. Advanced technologies stand to disrupt the acquisition and maintenance of skills, knowledge, and character traits because they can diminish the presence of these role models, cultural norms, personal motivation, and opportunities for practice.

Moreover, advanced technologies stand to displace goods that are internal to basic activities in medicine. Advanced technologies are primarily outcome-based. That is, they aim to diagnose, prognosticate, and develop treatment plans more quickly and accurately than their human counterparts. Critically, the *processes* by which these technologies arrive at their outcomes are opaque to humans. While these tools may, for example, diagnose more accurately and quickly than a human, they also displace the activities that a physician would have engaged in were they to develop the diagnosis themselves. Such activities might include physical touch, empathetic listening, and dialectic communication. Introducing a diagnostic tool that automatically draws information from an electronic health record (EHR) displaces or diminishes all these "human" activities. The main point is that although technologies may deliver instrumentally better outcomes, their presence may displace important caring aspects of medicine that are internal to its core activities (e.g., diagnosing, prognosticating, and developing treatment plans) and, importantly, the opportunity for physicians[1] (and medical students) to practice, develop, and maintain these skills.

Following the Medical School Objectives Project (MSOP) Learning Objectives for Medical Student Education, we stipulate three core areas of competence that physicians need to embody to meet society's expectations and practice good medicine (Association of American Medical Colleges 1998). These include:

1. *Techne*: *Physicians must be skillful.* They need excellent clinical skills to obtain medical histories, perform physical exams, interpret diagnostic tests, reason deductively to solve clinical problems, and communicate effectively with patients and families.
2. *Episteme*: *Physicians must be knowledgeable.* They must have a strong scientific understanding of the human body, diseases, and therapeutic options. They need to engage in lifelong learning to stay current with scientific advances.
3. *Ethos*: *Physicians must be intellectually and morally virtuous.* They must be compassionate, empathetic, and trustworthy, and they must act with integrity in caring for patients. They need to understand medical ethics and always advocate for patients' interests over their own. They should collaborate with other health professionals and understand the limits of their own knowledge. They need to understand disease prevention, evidence-based medicine, healthcare systems, and barriers faced by underserved populations.

In what follows, we explore the ways in which the introduction of advanced technologies in the core activities of a clinical encounter may either augment or adversely affect physicians' abilities to cultivate *techne*, *episteme*, and *ethos*.

[1] In the paper, we focus on tasks typically performed by physicians. However, our arguments extend to any healthcare worker who engages in the activities that we discuss.

4.4 Physicians, Diagnostic Support, and AI

In this section, we discuss some of the ways that new and emerging AI technologies impact the structure of the physician-patient clinical interaction, traditionally conceptualized as involving "opening, problem presentation, history-taking, physical examination, diagnosis, treatment and closing" (Khazen et al. 2022, 3). Practically speaking, this process often involves reviewing previous patient notes, updating patient health history through conversation, and performing a physical examination, before diagnosis and discussion of treatment plans. Our goal at each stage is to identify and illustrate how existing (and emerging) AI technologies stand to both promote and detract from the aforementioned attributes of the ideal physician. In many concrete cases, the application of concepts such as medical *techne* or *episteme* will overlap, but for the sake of clarity we will address them as distinct attributes.

4.4.1 Preparing for the Clinical Encounter

Ideally, before an appointment, a physician has time to review a patient's notes and history. However, given the practical and economic constraints of modern medicine, this kind of review is not always possible. To meet growing needs in this area, AI developers have created "smart" EHR systems that use machine learning to provide accessible data, streamline workflows, and supplement clinical decisions (Shickel et al. 2018). Such smart EHRs can assist medical providers in pre-visit planning, identify updated or relevant health information for a patient, locate potential diagnoses (pertinent to recent visits), and even identify care gaps or risks based on the existing records (Waldren and Billings 2024).

Recent research in this area shows promising results. For example, the American Academy of Family Physicians followed a large group of physicians (n = 1,836) who used the Navina smart EHR system to create more efficient workflows. Researchers found that use of the Navina EHR tool reduced "chart review burden" by 29.5% and provider burnout by 23%, and increased the practice satisfaction of physicians by 21.7%. Given that paperwork and EHR maintenance is fairly closely associated with burnout among medical providers (Budd 2023), "smarter" EHR tools will likely emerge as a welcome advance in clinical preparation and organization.

4.4.2 Analysis of Clinical Preparation Stage

It is a central skill (*techne*) in medicine to review detailed reports and patient records. In the near future, it is likely that AI will perform these functions in a preliminary manner. As physicians increasingly rely on AI to summarize medical records, we should expect that their skill of synthesis may atrophy in clinical settings. Growing reliance on such tools also disincentivizes physicians from investigating the "raw" notes and reports themselves. These new behaviors generate risks. First, failure to independently read the notes and reports risks the exclusion of relevant information not captured by AI, which in turn may lead to incorrect diagnosis, inaccurate prognosis, or inappropriate treatment plans. Second, the AI summary itself may include inaccurate or irrelevant information. Overreliance on machine-generated summaries (i.e., automation bias [Goddard et al. 2012]) generates risks of providing diagnoses, prognoses, and treatment plans that draw on irrelevant information.

These risks are not insurmountable; nevertheless, they highlight the need for physicians to engage with patients during clinical encounters to confirm the relevance of the information in the AI-generated summary. Moreover, it is important to acknowledge that these risks are in the context of tradeoffs with time. Because these technologies save physicians time, they may allow physicians to spend more time with each patient or to see more patients per day (Topol 2019).

As noted above, it is vital that physicians possess and maintain a deep knowledge (*episteme*) of the human body, diseases, and therapeutic options. Smart EHR systems may provide initial diagnostic options, which in some cases will expand physicians' understanding of the potential conditions before an encounter. However, such tools also stand to narrow the physician's attention by nudging them toward a particular diagnosis in advance of the patient encounter.

Overall, machine-generated patient summaries will save time. However, in terms of impact on *ethos*, the use of AI tools may also condense or flatten the provider's concept of the patient as a full human before the clinical encounter. Ideally, a physician should "seek to understand the meaning of the patients' stories in the context of the patients' beliefs and family and cultural values" (American Association of Medical Colleges 1998, 4).

4.4.3 The Clinical Encounter: Clinical Decision Support and Diagnostic Testing

Within the clinical encounter itself, AI tools can serve multiple ends. Consider that one prominent frustration with "manual entry" EHR systems is that their design and the time required to enter data (which typically involves accessing submenus, removing pop-ups, and responding to alerts) detracts from face-to-face interactions with patients (Friedberg et al. 2014). In addition, medical providers argue that they still spend a disproportionate amount of time on paperwork and administrative tasks each week, often related to EHR systems.[2] To help reduce these burdens, tools such as MIT's Medknowts use machine learning to automatically complete medical terms, include relevant information (such as lab results), and autopopulate data fields to

[2] According to a recent report in *Becker's Hospital Review*, physicians currently spend 15.5 hours per week on paperwork, with EHR documentation taking 9 hours (Cass 2023; see also Arndt et al. 2017).

save time. Further, in combination with the smart EHR systems described above, AI assistants such as Freed and DeepScribe can use natural language processing to transcribe conversations and update the EHR in real time (see Siwicki 2023). While smarter notetaking systems and ambient AI scribes are still in the early stages of implementation, they show significant potential for alleviating the administrative burden on clinicians, particularly by minimizing the time required to create and maintain patient notes (Tierney et al. 2024).

4.4.3.1 Clinical Decision Support

In addition to diagnostic testing, AI tools can serve to improve clinical decision-making. A computerized clinical decision support system (CDSS) is a health information technology system designed to assist healthcare providers in making clinical decisions for patient care. These tools use patient-specific information, combined with an established medical knowledge base, to generate patient-specific assessments or recommendations that are presented to clinicians for consideration. While CDSSs have existed since the 1970s, physicians did not have meaningful access to computerized versions until the 1980s (Sutton et al. 2020). The CDSSs presently in use tend to be classified based on how they generate outputs. For example, a CDSS may be "knowledge-based," using conditional logic or Bayesian inference over a fixed dataset, to generate helpful outputs (Martinez-Franco et al. 2018). Alternatively, the system may be "non-knowledge-based," powered by machine learning to generate outputs (Sutton et al. 2020). In more recent literature, such systems are also referred to as machine learning clinical decision support systems (ML-CDSSs) (Heyen and Salloch 2021).

Non-knowledge-based ML-CDSSs currently exist at the level of proof of concept (Moazemi et al. 2023), as prototypes (Timiliotis et al. 2022), or to address narrow problems (Wang et al. 2023). For example, one research team used AI tools trained on a large EHR dataset ($n = 17{,}556$) to accurately predict patient responses to different classes of antidepressants (Alowais et al. 2023; Sheu et al. 2023). Having this form of accessible predictive information available to physicians clearly has the potential to improve clinical decision-making, efficiency, and accuracy. This is particularly important in contexts such as emergency medicine where life-saving decisions must be made quickly with little or no patient information or background, or where triage of complex cases is required without much time to deliberate (Chenais et al. 2023).

4.4.3.2 Diagnostic Testing

The use of AI and machine learning in medicine is still in its relative infancy, but some of the more impressive developments have occurred in diagnostic testing (see Alowais et al. 2023). Given the rich EHR datasets available, AI systems have been developed to detect or monitor a wide variety of conditions such as cancer (Esteva et al. 2017; Urban 2018; McKinney et al. 2020), retinopathy (Gulshan et al. 2016), heart disease

(Alfaras et al. 2019), Alzheimer's disease (Ding et al. 2019), pneumonia (Becker et al. 2022), stroke (Lee et al. 2020), and depression (Nickson et al. 2023). Among other values (such as efficiency), such technologies show great promise for early detection of disease and for reducing human error. For example, researchers analyzed mammograms using AI tools and were able to reduce both false positives and false negatives (5.7 and 9.4%, respectively) (McKinney et al. 2020). In a related study, AI was more sensitive than radiologists in diagnosing breast cancer (Kim et al. 2020). While these diagnostic tools continue to improve, they are already having impacts on standards of care in some fields of medicine. For example, an autonomous AI system designed to detect diabetic retinopathy received de novo authorization from the US Food and Drug Administration (FDA) in 2020 and now serves as the benchmark for relevant standards of care in diabetes treatment (Abramoff 2021).

As we have reviewed, the integration of machine learning and AI into the clinical encounter, diagnostics, and testing holds great promise for improving the experiences of both physicians and patients. Smart EHR systems, combined with AI scribes or notetaking tools, have the potential to substantially streamline the clinical workflow, reduce paperwork and bureaucratic burdens, and thereby reduce the burnout often associated with those activities. In addition, being able to outsource some of the unimportant data-entry and EHR navigation to machines would allow physicians to engage more mindfully with patients during the clinical encounter even if they spend the same amount of time with them.

In the realm of diagnosis, AI tools now regularly serve as powerful adjuncts to the human interpretation of imaging, laboratory, and pathology reports. In addition to reducing medical errors and increasing efficiency, the predictive power of these tools will likely continue to help physicians identify early indications of disease. Not only is this desirable from the perspective of the patient, but it will also likely serve to contain costs and optimize scarce resources in many clinical contexts. For example, according to a 2024 estimate from the National Bureau of Economic Research, "AI adoption within the next five years using today's technologies could result in savings of 5 to 10% of health care spending, or $200 billion to $360 billion annually in 2019 dollars, without sacrificing quality and access" (Sahni et al. 2024, 50).

4.4.3.3 Analysis of the Clinical Encounter

We expect that as these technologies continue to evolve and improve, they will serve an increasingly central role in clinical practice. However, use of AI in clinical care also poses significant ethical and social concerns.

For example, as clinicians outsource tasks such as data entry, EHR use, note-taking, and transcription, it is likely that they will become less adept at the skills (*techne*) required to perform these tasks on a regular basis. While this may seem like a relatively minor change, this loss of technical proficiency will be problematic in cases in which the technology fails or is unavailable temporarily. In addition, an increased reliance on AI tools for transcription may negatively impact clinicians' active listening skills. Since AI tools may serve to automatically transcribe conversations (or update records in EHR systems), clinicians will no longer need to pay as much attention to the nuances and details of conversations with patients. In some cases, knowing that notes can be effortlessly synthesized and retrieved could disincentivize clinicians from committing the information to working memory. In theory, outsourcing otherwise mechanical tasks to AI could free a physician to focus more directly on active listening. However, unless clinicians act intentionally, use of AI tools may also serve to diminish the kind of engagement that is essential for accurate diagnosis and empathetic care.

Perhaps a greater risk is that overreliance on AI automation in the clinical encounter will negatively affect core epistemic features (*episteme*) of physician training such as diagnostic reasoning or the maintenance and retention of medical knowledge. Consider a practice such as diagnostic reasoning. The traditional epistemic scaffolding for a diagnosis begins to be constructed as a physician reviews patient notes, conducts an examination, and engages in conversation with the patient. By relying on their advanced medical training and experience, the physician synthesizes this rich stream of information into a working diagnosis which may be refined with further information or testing.

As AI tools improve in their abilities to provide differential diagnoses (based on reported symptoms or available tests), it may be tempting for physicians to outsource more of this cognitive processing to machines. Such a state of affairs could produce a vicious cycle of "deskilling" over time. Here is how one clinician frames the issue in the context of reading radiology scans:

> My research has shown that the higher the case load, the better you get at this. …What [early career providers] actually need is high case numbers. So if you're taking away high case numbers from them to reduce the workload [by having a machine read the scan], you actually have the potential to deskill in that visual perception task. (Aquino et al. 2023, 5)

This result would be quite troubling over time, especially in the context of calls for human oversight of machine evaluations. But for the sake of argument, grant that AI tools will not displace the training process required to develop relevant domain-specific expertise. The remaining problem is that well-trained providers may still be unduly influenced by the outputs of their diagnostic tools (Cabitza et al. 2017). For example, one study found that while computer-aided detection (CAD) benefited less experienced mammography readers, there was a noticeable decrease in diagnostic sensitivity when more experienced readers were presented with CAD-tagged images (Povyakalo et al. 2013). More recently, researchers found that diagnostic accuracy increased (4.4%) when clinicians reviewed a patient clinical vignette with an accurate AI model but decreased (11.3%) when clinicians were shown systematically biased AI model predictions (Jabbour et al. 2023). In short, patterns of deference to AI models help clinicians moderately when the AI is accurate but can be harmful when it is not.

These issues are not insurmountable, though one final challenge remains. Even if clinical AI tools could always be built on high-quality (and unbiased) datasets, the complex nature of AI systems is often inaccessible to medical providers (i.e., the "black box" problem)—especially when they are integrated with large language models (Yang et al. 2022b). Large language models provide justifications post hoc as a function of the statistical relationship between words. In some cases, it will be "challenging or impossible to convey the specific logic behind an alert or recommendation" (Henry et al. 2022, 1). In cases of human-to-human disagreement, providing the relevant reasons for a judgment may allow for resolution or identification of relevant errors. However, the kind of transparency that comes from reason-giving and reason-sensitivity is not presently possible with available AI tools, and as AI tools become more complex, it is even less likely.

In addition, it may be unclear how to proceed when the professional judgment of a physician and the outputs of AI are in conflict or apparent disagreement (Kempt et al. 2023). Currently, the physician takes moral and legal responsibility for any clinical judgments even if ML-CDSS tools are employed, though recent work is now exploring the extent to which physicians should provide reasons for rejecting the diagnosis of an AI tool (when the AI systems are well-designed) (Kempt et al. 2023, 1412). How these potential situations (i.e., physician-AI disagreement) will impact physicians' willingness to adopt new tools[3] and how such apparent tensions will impact patient trust are open questions and ones that require further research and exploration. Finally, the idea that AI or machine learning may eventually fully outpace the diagnostic abilities of human physicians also has substantial implications for wider standards of care and medical malpractice law (Froomkin et al. 2019).

Lastly, we should consider how these technological changes stand to impact the intellectual and moral virtues (*ethos*) of future physicians. We have noted above that the expansion of AI use in clinical care could serve to deskill physicians in some domains of practice. We have also detailed some evidence that the presence of powerful AI tools (or quasi-agents) can encourage overreliance on the outputs of AI and serve to undermine the independent judgment of clinicians. This state of affairs will likely produce a series of downstream effects. First, if and when physicians are unable to explain a clear rationale for AI judgments, it will likely undermine patient trust in their care. A second, and deeper, issue is that in cases of physician-AI disagreement, physicians may implicitly shift moral responsibility to AI judgments without having access to the relevant scope of reasons that would justify that deference. While the current norms around technology require physicians to take responsibility for any clinical decisions, the power of AI systems trained on large amounts of data may make AI-generated verdicts nearly irresistible.

In addition, while having tools such as ambient scribes or smart EHR systems would theoretically free a physician to engage in deeper listening or empathetic engagement with patients, this is not inevitable (Schwan 2018). In some cases, the belief that a machine is monitoring for important details or data may lead a physician to attend *less* to the lived experiences of the patient. This form of distraction will be compounded by any AI tools that output real-time analyses. For example, physicians

[3] One illustrative comment from a physician is provided in Segal et al.: "I am really concerned about the malpractice implications. Having to defend even one lawsuit stemming from the use of the CDSS would negate any time saved" (2017, 15).

in these contexts will likely be subjected to new forms of "alert fatigue." This occurs when "too many alerts consume time and mental energy," causing important alerts to be "ignored along with clinically unimportant ones" (Peterson and Bates 2001). Within the last decade, physicians have identified alert fatigue as an increasingly pressing concern. One survey of 2,590 physicians found that approximately 87% deemed the quantity of alerts "excessive," and 70% noted that they received more alerts than "they could effectively manage" (Singh et al. 2013).[4]

While advances in AI stand to improve the clinical encounter, they may also profoundly disrupt a physician's basic moral attention. Our worry is that technologies favoring the representation of patients as objective data points and of their concerns as engineering problems may strain the moral attention required to represent patients in their full subjectivity. As machines become more embedded in clinical settings, this approach is likely to increasingly dominate medical training and practice. The physician-patient relationship is fundamental for ensuring effective communication, building trust, and providing personalized, humanistic care that addresses individual patient needs.

The virtuous physician of the future will need training and habituation (*ethos*) to develop their moral attention and avoid the pitfalls noted above. That is, they will need to actively attend to patients' subjectivity in order to maintain the crucial human connection required for the practice of empathetic, patient-centered medicine. For this to be fully effective, medical institutions must develop policies and practices that encourage physicians to inquire into and consider a patient's subjective concerns, such as how their illness affects meaningful activities, personal goals, emotional well-being, and relationships.

4.4.3.4 Treatment Plans, Monitoring, and Targeted Intervention

Our final topic of discussion is the use of AI tools to develop treatment plans, predict or monitor for complications, or provide targeted interventions. For example, machine learning systems can compare a patient's profile to those of similar cases (disease severity and progression) and generate a variety of customized treatment plans (Dubey et al. 2023). In addition, one emerging area of research is how to integrate a patient's existing genomic data into the standard EHR workflow (Linder et al. 2021). Much of the present research in this area is focused on AI-assisted treatment planning for cancer, though these technologies also have applications to other conditions (van de Sande et al. 2021; Jiang et al. 2022; Yang et al. 2022a).

New technologies have also contributed to advancements in treatment monitoring with the widespread use of smartwatches and other health tracking devices by patients. The data collected by many consumer-grade devices can predict health complications such as atrial fibrillation (Perez et al. 2019), and more targeted medical applications can provide continuous monitoring of diabetes, hemodynamics, electroencephalogram activity, and sleep (Dubey and Tiwari 2023; Shaik et al. 2023;

[4] Some progress has been made, but the problem still remains. See Payne (2019).

Shajari et al. 2023). One advantage of these advanced monitoring techniques is that physicians are now better placed to consider early interventions or provide helpful nudges to improve adherence to treatment plans or medication regimens (Killian et al. 2019, Babel et al. 2021; see also Chap. 13 in this volume).

4.4.3.5 Analysis of Treatment Plans, Monitoring, and Targeted Intervention

These tools offer significant promise in terms of truly personalized medicine and improved safety and outcomes. As with other elements of medical practice, the widespread introduction of these monitoring and intervention tools will involve tradeoffs in the domains of physician *techne*, *episteme*, and *ethos*.

Introducing these monitoring technologies raises several risks with respect to the development and maintenance of physicians' *techne*. First, these tools may reduce physicians' ability to interpret complex data. With AI handling much of the data analysis and pattern recognition, clinicians may become less adept at interpreting complex test results, imaging studies, and other clinical data on their own. As AI increasingly suggests likely diagnoses and complications, physicians may exercise their diagnostic reasoning skills less frequently, potentially weakening this core clinical ability over time. Finally, reliance on AI and smart devices for continuous patient monitoring could cause the atrophy of clinicians' skills in detecting subtle changes in patients' conditions through direct observation and examination.

Smart tools that generate treatment plans and interventions and monitor patients also introduce concerns surrounding physicians' *episteme*. Developing personalized treatment planning requires that physicians have a deep knowledge of the diverse range of treatment options and the reasons for proposing one over another. Moreover, a personalized approach to treatment planning demands that physicians creatively combine aspects of different treatment protocols. Insofar as introducing AI tools diminishes this domain of knowledge, it could adversely affect physicians' proficiency in developing comprehensive, personalized treatment plans that integrate subjective patient goals and values.

Moreover, if AI systems routinely handle treatment planning, clinicians may develop gaps in their knowledge of those areas and have diminished incentives to stay current on new practices and processes. Research on automation bias suggests that physicians—especially those early in their careers—may become overly dependent on AI-filtered information, potentially missing important new research or treatment options that fall outside the AI's parameters (Khera et al. 2023). Based on this research, we can infer that clinicians may fail to inculcate or maintain the nuanced, contextual knowledge that experienced clinicians acquire over time about how different factors interact in complex cases. This knowledge is particularly important for developing the ability to competently address atypical cases. With reduced understanding of treatment options and their mechanisms, clinicians may fail to acquire or maintain a sophisticated understanding of underlying disease mechanisms.

An essential trait of the virtuous physician (*ethos*) is a sense of responsibility to patients and for their health outcomes. As AI systems take on more decision-making roles, clinicians may feel less personally responsible for patient outcomes, potentially impacting their sense of professional ethics and duty. This sense of responsibility is closely tied to an empathetic and caring disposition. As AI tools are increasingly used for treatment plan generation and wearable devices collect patient data, the replacement of interpersonal interactions by these technologies reduces or eliminates many of the activities in which empathy and caring are instantiated in clinical practice.

In the case of treatment plan development, for example, rather than beginning by eliciting a patient's goals and values around which to develop a treatment plan, an algorithm may generate a "menu" of treatment plan options based entirely on biomedical factors. Although patient goals and values can still figure into the eventual care plan, automated treatment plan generation alters the process by which such plans are developed and deemphasizes the use of patient values in that process. It inverts the patient-centered approach to medicine that begins with a patient's goals and values into a process that appends those goals and values to an antecedently, algorithmically generated treatment plan. This shifts the center of the conversation from the patient to the treatment. Ultimately, the patient and physician may arrive at the same care plan regardless of the process, but in the machine-generated version, the activities by which the physician can come to know the patient as an individual—precursors to developing empathy and caring—are attenuated.

Monitoring technologies, too, can displace the activities that lead to empathy and personal connection. Rather than engaging the patient in dialogue to elicit their daily activities and attitudes, it is easier simply to use data that is passively collected by a health monitoring device. Moreover, there is a potential loss of richness in what a physician learns if they rely too heavily on device-collected data, especially if those data are predigested before being presented. There is, after all, an allure of objectivity with quantitative data. All of this conspires to flatten the image of the patient's situation from which the physician will develop treatment plans, interventions, diagnosis, and prognosis.

Even if patients and monitoring devices could generate identical data, deferring to monitoring devices displaces important physician-patient interactions that are necessary for the cultivation of empathy and personal connection. Again, it is not that monitoring technologies necessarily eliminate certain kinds of physician-patient conversations, but rather that they make these conversations less likely. They require more effort while the monitoring technology reduces their importance, and therefore reduce the likelihood that the empathy and care-generating activities contained within those conversations occur as frequently or are given as much emphasis.

A related concern involves the potential loss of qualitative aspects of the physician-patient relationship. AI systems tend to focus on discrete, quantifiable data and may implicitly frame patients as a cluster of conditions or a technical challenge to be resolved (Ho 2023, 168). In contrast, well-trained professional physicians have learned to integrate the objective aspects of medicine with the qualitative aspects of patients as embodied persons with values, goals, and concerns. An overreliance on AI tools may detract from the essentially holistic nature of patient care. In addition, without sustained practice in this form of holistic attention, we may expect to see these humanistic aspects of medical care atrophy.

4.5 Participatory Deliberative Conservatism: A Model for Ethical Deployment of Advanced Technologies in Medicine

As advanced technologies continue to reshape medical practice, it is crucial to develop frameworks for their ethical deployment that balance their substantial benefits with medicine's core values. In this final section, we outline our model, called participatory deliberative conservatism (PDC), for the ethical deployment of advanced technologies in healthcare, and we apply it to clinical contexts.

4.5.1 The Participatory Deliberative Conservatism (PDC) Model

The PDC model for the deployment of advanced technologies incorporates three elements: (1) stakeholder *participation* and (2) stakeholder *deliberation*, both of which are (3) constrained by the values inherent in the practice of medicine (*conservative* element) (Palmer and Schwan 2024). The participatory nature of the process ensures that the diverse range of stakeholder interests (e.g., those of providers, patients, and hospital administrators) are involved in decision-making processes. This broad inclusion helps capture a wide range of perspectives and concerns, ensuring that the values and needs of all affected parties are considered. The deliberative element provides stakeholder education and, within this context, encourages them to identify relevant values and concerns. This process allows stakeholders to identify and resolve value conflicts. Finally, this model and form of deliberation preserves core medical values and respects local legal frameworks, cultural values, and economic constraints. Hence, the conservative element of the model ensures that patient and caregiver desires do not contravene local and national healthcare law and ethics. Ideally, the PDC model supports integrating patient perspectives into the deployment of policy while also taking into account the special expertise and responsibility of medical and administrative professionals.

Briefly stated, the PDC model involves a four-step process:

1. *Preliminary identification of values and concerns*

The first step involves the preliminary identification of values and concerns from primary stakeholders. A pilot committee should be composed of a small number of patients, caregivers, medical providers, hospital administrators, and an ethicist (if available).[5] The pilot committee is responsible for the development and continued oversight of deployment plans throughout the lifecycle of the technology. In the first stage, the goal should be to identify both practical and normative concerns that are relevant to the deployment of the new technology. For example, a practical concern might be whether someone with a gloved hand can interact with the technology's screen or interface. Nurses may be concerned that the displacement of human interaction deprives the patient of human care, so a normative concern might be whether a technology replaces a diagnostic test that usually requires face-to-face time with a nurse. To ensure broad representation, the committee should then gather information from larger samples of each of the stakeholder groups through various methods such as surveys, interviews, and focus groups, depending on the context. This step ensures that initial values and concerns are representative.

2. *Deliberation about values, concerns, and ranking*

Next, the stakeholders should be asked to deliberate about their concrete concerns, attempt to identify the broader values that ground or motivate them, and generate a provisional ordering of the relevant values. For instance, a nurse's practical concern about reduced facetime with patients might be understood as reflecting the broader value of caring. By focusing on underlying values, this process will also reveal more avenues for the resolution of potential value conflicts, since there are multiple ways to instantiate the same value. During this process, the expertise of ethicists is critical, as they are trained in reconciling and mediating value conflicts.

3. *Formulation of initial deployment policy*

If the pilot committee decides to adopt and deploy the relevant technology, they should formulate an initial deployment plan that best promotes and preserves the values identified in the previous step. In addition, they should generate provisional success criteria and assessment tools and determine the intervals at which the plan will be reassessed. While this process is participatory, it is not strictly populist. While patient values serve a central role in this deliberative process, the final authority and responsibility regarding deployment rests with medical practitioners and administrators because they bear the legal and moral consequences of the deployment policy. This *conservative* element of the process ensures that established medical values and relevant legal and economic concerns are not overlooked.

[5] Generally, we do not anticipate that more than one ethicist will be required for this deliberative process. Following the American Society for Bioethics and Humanities (ASBH) guidelines, ethicists in the medical context primarily serve as facilitators. They draw out stakeholder concerns, highlight normative tradeoffs and conflicts, and propose processes for their resolution. When policy enters uncharted ethical territory, clinical ethicists function as facilitators translating the stakeholder's ethical concerns into a common mutually understandable language. However, their role is not to impose "from above" ethical solutions but to point out the ethical guardrails of established medical ethics when stakeholder proposals fall outside of them. Having more than one ethicist-facilitator does not clearly improve this facilitation process.

4. *Deployment and iterative evaluation*

The final step involves the deployment of the new technology and the subsequent iterative evaluation of its impact in relation to the previously identified goals and values. The deployment should be monitored for unintended consequences, and the pilot committee should meet regularly to assess the efficacy of the technology and whether adjustments are required over time.

4.5.2 Virtues of the PDC Model

Before applying this model to the present discussion, consider a few virtues of this approach. First, practically speaking, it helps to resolve the ambiguity that is often associated with applying abstract ethical principles to concrete situations by ensuring that the relevant values are understood in ways that reflect local cultural, economic, and social contexts. In addition, it provides a non-ad hoc process for ordering values and resolving the expected conflicts between them in practical settings.

Second, this approach provides a clear justification for the inclusion of some values and concerns over others. Those subject to the effects of the new technology decide which values and concerns are most relevant and in which order of priority. Unlike some institutional approaches to technology, PDC explicitly involves patient voices. At the same time, the diversity of stakeholders and the deliberative process ensures that concerns of any given group are not overrepresented. For example, it is a longstanding concern that if deployment decisions are primarily made by hospital administrators, then economic concerns may be given disproportionate attention. Yet, if patient voices are given overriding influence in many medical contexts, then core medical values (or economic concerns) may not receive appropriate consideration.

Finally, the PDC approach is not rigid but rather is sensitive to the local cultural context in which deployment decisions function. For example, a decision whether to deploy carebots in rural Thailand will be informed by regional cultural, religious, or political values and may differ from a similar decision in rural Texas.

The PDC model addresses a variety of epistemic challenges inherent to healthcare contexts. Even within a single hospital or clinic, there are often numerous divisions, each with distinct priorities, staffing, and technological needs. By including a diverse set of stakeholders, this process ensures that decision-makers have access to fine-grained information about how new technologies will likely augment and displace existing values and concerns. Since individual stakeholders typically have narrow concerns, the multi-stakeholder deliberative process ensures that decision-makers are not insulated from the impacts of their priorities on other stakeholder groups. In addition, the iterative nature of PDC's evaluation process ensures that new information and challenges are continuously integrated into the deliberative process.

Having briefly outlined the central contours of the model, let us consider how it might structure the process of deployment of several advanced technologies that we have previously discussed in terms of physician *techne*, *episteme*, and *ethos*: A large cancer center in the southern US is interested in adopting a new AI-powered clinical decision support system (AI-CDSS) to help diagnose and generate treatment plans for breast cancer. The pilot committee identifies numerous concerns related to efficacy and patient safety, economic issues, and the role of physician deskilling. To ensure representativeness, members of each stakeholder group complete surveys eliciting their goals and concerns for the AI-CDSS. After deliberation, patient stakeholders are satisfied that the deployment of the technology will improve patient outcomes, and the hospital administration is confident that the technology will reduce costs within a ten-year window. While medical providers are optimistic about the potential to improve patient outcomes, they remain concerned that the AI-CDSS will complicate the process of diagnosis and treatment. In particular, they remain concerned that patients will lose trust in them if their professional judgments conflict with the AI-CDSS and about potential deskilling over time.

As a result of the PDC process, the pilot committee generates several recommendations. First, given physicians' concerns about deskilling (*techne* and *episteme*), the committee recommends that the AI-CDSS-generated recommendations are only to be consulted after a physician has formed and entered their own independent assessment. In cases where the attending physician and the AI-generated diagnosis disagree, the physicians develop an institutional process in which additional colleagues are consulted to resolve the conflict.

Second, the physicians of the future require a new kind of knowledge (*episteme*): that is, the knowledge of how to best integrate AI-CDSS into their clinical practice. This requires learning when an AI-CDSS works well, when it does not, and how to work with such systems. Such learning is only possible when communities of clinicians share their successes and failures. Hence, the physicians propose a monthly meeting akin to morbidity and mortality (M&M) meetings. In these meetings, the physicians openly discuss cases in which errors occurred because of how they used the AI-CDSS and cases in which they discovered novel and successful ways of integrating AI-CDSS into their workflow. These open and frank meetings provide the opportunity for physicians to learn from each other how to best work with these new tools.

Finally, physicians will need to resist the temptation to merely issue machine-generated treatment plans that only incorporate the biomedical profile of the patient. The committee recommends that physicians foreground the psychosocial and subjective aspects of patient concerns by structuring the clinical encounter around empathetic, patient-centered communication. In this way, the activity of eliciting patient goals and values supports the preservation and development of a disposition to see patients as individuals (*ethos*). Moreover, it ensures better patient outcomes since treatment plans will reflect individual patient goals, values, and lifestyles. While this final treatment plan is a function of patient values and concerns, the physician maintains final moral and legal authority for the AI-assisted diagnosis, treatment plans, and follow-up.

This illustration involves a simplified scenario in which intractable disagreements do not arise. In cases where there are recalcitrant normative or practical disagreements, our model is neutral on approaches to conflict resolution. Each institution, depending on its history, culture, and legal environment, should in advance incorporate conflict resolution processes.

4.6 Conclusion

The integration of advanced technologies into healthcare represents a radical change in medical practice, offering immense potential to enhance diagnostic accuracy, treatment efficacy, and overall patient care. However, as we have argued, this technological revolution also presents significant challenges to the traditional roles and competencies of physicians.

We have examined how advanced technologies impact the core attributes of an ideal physician—*techne*, *episteme*, and *ethos*—across various stages of the clinical encounter. While these technologies can significantly improve efficiency and accuracy in diagnosis and treatment planning, they also risk diminishing critical clinical skills and may encourage overreliance on these systems. Moreover, these technologies may interfere with and atrophy the development of moral dispositions, which in turn risks weakening the moral relationship between the patient and physician.

To address these concerns, we introduce a novel framework for the ethical deployment of advanced technologies in healthcare: participatory deliberative conservatism. We propose this model to ensure broad stakeholder participation and deliberative decision-making processes, while preserving core values and goods inherent in the practice of medicine. This approach provides a practical, context-sensitive procedure for helping local institutions deploy advanced technologies in a manner that captures the benefits of these tools while mitigating the harms we have detailed. As advanced technologies continue to improve and are deployed more widely in healthcare, it is critical that deployment policies be sensitive to the ways in which these technologies can enhance or compromise the central attributes of the ideal physician.

References

Abramoff, Michael D. 2021. "Autonomous Artificial Intelligence Safety and Trust." In *Artificial Intelligence in Ophthalmology*, ed. Andrzej Grzybowski, 55–67. Cham: Springer. https://doi.org/10.1007/978-3-030-78601-4_4.

Alfaras, Miquel, Miguel C. Soriano, and Silvia Ortín. 2019. "A Fast Machine Learning Model for ECG-Based Heartbeat Classification and Arrythmia Detection." *Frontiers in Physics* 7 (July): article no. 103. https://doi.org/10.3389/fphy.2019.00103.

Alowais, Shuroug A., Sahar S. Alghamdi, Nada Alsuhebany, Tariq Alqahtani, Abdulrahman I. Alshaya, Sumaya N. Almohareb, et al. 2023. "Revolutionizing Healthcare: The Role of Artificial Intelligence in Clinical Practice." *BMC Medical Education* 23: article no. 689. https://doi.org/10.1186/s12909-023-04698-z.

American Association of Colleges of Nursing. 2024. "Nursing Shortage." Last modified May 2024. https://www.aacnnursing.org/news-data/fact-sheets/nursing-shortage.

Aquino, Yves Saint James, Wendy A. Rogers, Annette Braunack-Mayer, Helen Frazer, Khin Than Win, Nehmat Houssami, Christopher Degeling, Christopher Semsarian, and Stacy M. Carter. 2023. "Utopia versus Dystopia: Professional Perspectives on the Impact of Healthcare Artificial Intelligence on Clinical Roles and Skills." *International Journal of Medical Informatics* 169 (January): 104903. https://doi.org/10.1016/j.ijmedinf.2022.104903.

Archibald, Mandy M., and Alan Barnard. 2018. "Futurism in Nursing: Technology, Robotics and the Fundamentals of Care." *Journal of Clinical Nursing* 27 (11–12) (June): 2473–2480. https://doi.org/10.1111/jocn.14081.

Aristotle. 2019. *Nichomachean Ethics.* Translated by Terence Irwin. Indianapolis: Hackett.

Arndt, Brian G., John W. Beasley, Michelle D. Watkinson, Jonathan L. Temte, Wen-Jan Tuan, Christine A. Sinsky, and Valerie J. Gilchrist. 2017. "Tethered to the EHR: Primary Care Physician Workload Assessment Using EHR Event Log Data and Time-Motion Observations." *Annals of Family Medicine* 15 (5) (September/October): 419–426. https://doi.org/10.1370/afm.2121.

Association of American Medical Colleges. 1998. *Learning Objectives for Medical Student Education: Guidelines for Medical Schools.* January. Washington, DC: Association of American Medical Colleges.

Association of American Medical Colleges. 2024. "New AAMC Report Shows Continuing Projected Physician Shortage." March 21. https://www.aamc.org/news/press-releases/new-aamc-report-shows-continuing-projected-physician-shortage.

Babel, Aditi, Richi Taneja, Franco Mondello Malvestiti, Alessandro Monaco, and Shaantanu Donde. 2021. "Artificial Intelligence Solutions to Increase Medication Adherence in Patients with Non-communicable Diseases." *Frontiers in Digital Health* 3 (June): article no. 669869. https://doi.org/10.3389/fdgth.2021.669869.

Barnard, Alan, and Margarete Sandelowski. 2001. "Technology and Humane Nursing Care: (Ir)reconcilable or Invented Difference?" *Journal of Advanced Nursing* 34 (3) (May): 367–375. https://doi.org/10.1046/j.1365-2648.2001.01768.x.

Becker, Judith, Josua Decker, Christoph Römmele, Maria Kahn, Helmut Messman, Markus Wehler, Florian Schwarz, Thomas Kroencke, and Christain Scheurig-Muenkler. 2022. "Artificial Intelligence-Based Detection of Pneumonia in Chest Radiographs." *Diagnostics* 12 (6) (June): 1465. https://doi.org/10.3390/diagnostics12061465.

Briganti, Giovanni, and Olivier Le Moine. 2020. "Artificial Intelligence in Medicine: Today and Tomorrow." *Frontiers in Medicine* 7 (February): article no. 27. https://doi.org/10.3389/fmed.2020.00027.

Budd, Jeffrey. 2023. "Burnout Related to Electronic Health Record Use in Primary Care." *Journal of Primary Care & Community Health* 14 (January-December). https://doi.org/10.1177/21501319231166921.

Cabitza, Federico, Raffaele Rasoini, and Gian Franco Gensini. 2017. "Unintended Consequences of Machine Learning in Medicine." *JAMA: Journal of the American Medical Association* 318 (6) (August 8): 517–518. https://doi.org/10.1001/jama.2017.7797.

Cass, Andrew. 2023. "The Hours 23 Physician Specialties Spend on Paperwork, Administration." April 19. https://www.beckershospitalreview.com/hospital-physician-relationships/the-hours-23-physician-specialties-spend-on-paperwork-administration.html.

Chenais, Gabrielle, Emmanuel Lagarde, and Cédric Gil-Jardiné. 2023. "Artificial Intelligence in Emergency Medicine: Viewpoint of Current Applications and Foreseeable Opportunities and Challenges." *Journal of Medical Internet Research* 25: e40031. https://doi.org/10.2196/40031.

Coeckelbergh, Mark. 2016. "Care Robots and the Future of ICT-Mediated Elderly Care: A Response to Doom Scenarios." *AI & Society* 31 (4) (November): 455–462. https://doi.org/10.1007/s00146-015-0626-3.

Coeckelbergh, Mark. 2020. *AI Ethics.* Cambridge, MA: MIT Press.

Ding, Yiming, Jae Ho Sohn, Michael G. Kawczynski, Hari Trivedi, Roy Harnish, Nathaniel W. Jenkins, et al. 2019. "A Deep Learning Model to Predict a Diagnosis of Alzheimer Disease by Using 18F-FDG PET of the Brain." *Radiology* 290 (2) (February): 456–464. https://doi.org/10.1148/radiol.2018180958.

Dubey, Ayushmaan, and Anuj Tiwari. 2023. "Artificial Intelligence and Remote Patient Monitoring in US Healthcare Market: A Literature Review." *Journal of Market Access and Health Policy* 11 (1). https://doi.org/10.1080/20016689.2023.2205618.

Dubey, Snigdha, Gaurav Tiwari, Sneha Singh, Saveli Goldberg, and Eugene Pinsky. 2023. "Using Machine Learning for Healthcare Treatment Planning." *Frontiers in Artificial Intelligence* 6: 1124182. https://doi.org/10.3389/frai.2023.1124182.

Esteva, Andre, Brett Kuprel, Roberto A. Novoa, Justin Ko, Susan M. Swetter, Helen M. Blau, and Sebastian Thrun. 2017. "Dermatologist-Level Classification of Skin Cancer with Deep Neural Networks." *Nature* 542 (7639) (February 2): 115–118. https://doi.org/10.1038/nature21056.

Etzioni, Amitai, and Oren Etzioni. 2017. "The Ethics of Robotic Caregivers." *Interaction Studies,* 18 (2) (January): 174–190. https://doi.org/10.1075/is.18.2.02etz.

Friedberg, Mark, Peggy G. Chen, Kristin R. Van Busum, Frances Aunon, Chau Pham, John P. Caloyeras, et al. 2014. *Factors Affecting Physician Professional Satisfaction and Their Implications for Patient Care, Health Systems, and Health Policy.* Rand Corporation and American Medical Association. https://www.rand.org/pubs/research_reports/RR439.html.

Froomkin, A. Michael, Ian Kerr, and Joelle Pineau. 2019. "When AIs Outperform Doctors: Confronting the Challenges of a Tort-Induced Over-reliance on Machine Learning." *Arizona Law Review* 61 (1): 33–99. https://arizonalawreview.org/pdf/61-1/61arizlrev33.pdf.

Goddard, Kate, Abdul Roudsari, and Jeremy C. Wyatt. 2012. "Automation Bias: A Systematic Review of Frequency, Effect Mediators, and Mitigators." *Journal of the American Medical Informatics Association* 19 (1) (January): 121–127. https://doi.org/10.1136/amiajnl-2011-000089.

Gulshan, Varun, Lily Peng, Marc Coram, Martin C. Stumpe, Derek Wu, Arunachalam Narayanaswamy, et al. 2016. "Development and Validation of a Deep Learning Algorithm for Detection of Diabetic Retinopathy in Retinal Fundus Photographs." *JAMA: Journal of the American Medical Association* 316 (22) (December 13): 2402–2410. https://doi.org/10.1001/jama.2016.17216.

Henry, Katherine E., Rachel Kornfield, Anirudh Sridharan, Robert C. Linton, Catherine Groh, Tony Wang, Albert Wu, Bilge Mutlu, and Suchi Saria. 2022. "Human-Machine Teaming is Key to AI Adoption: Clinicians' Experiences with a Deployed Machine Learning System." *NPJ Digital Medicine* 5: article no. 97. https://doi.org/10.1038/s41746-022-00597-7.

Heyen, Nils B., and Sabine Salloch. 2021. "The Ethics of Machine Learning-Based Clinical Decision Support: An Analysis through the Lens of Professionalisation Theory." *BMC Medical Ethics* 22: article no. 112. https://doi.org/10.1186/s12910-021-00679-3.

Ho, Anita. 2023. *Live Like Nobody Is Watching: Relational Autonomy in the Age of Artificial Intelligence Health Monitoring.* New York: Oxford University Press.

Institute of Electrical and Electronics Engineers (IEEE). 2015. "IEEE Standard Ontologies for Robotics and Automation." In *IEEE Standards 1872–2015*, 1–60. https://doi.org/10.1109/IEEESTD.2015.7084073.

Jabbour, Sarah, David Fouhey, Stephanie Shepard, Thomas S. Valley, Ella A. Kazerooni, Nikola Banovic, Jenna Wiens, and Michael W. Sjoding. 2023. "Measuring the Impact of AI in the Diagnosis of Hospitalized Patients: A Randomized Clinical Vignette Survey Study." *JAMA: Journal of the American Medical Association* 330 (23) (December 19): 2275–2284. https://doi.org/10.1001/jama.2023.22295.

Jiang, Shengpeng, Yi Xue, Ming Li, Chengwen Yang, Daguang Zhang, Qingxin Wang, at al. 2022. "Artificial Intelligence-Based Automated Treatment Planning of Postmastectomy Volumetric Modulated Arc Radiotherapy." *Frontiers in Oncology* 12: 871871. https://doi.org/10.3389/fonc.2022.871871.

Kempt, Hendrik, Jan-Christoph Heilinger, and Saskia K. Nagel. 2023. "'I'm Afraid I Can't Let You Do That, Doctor': Meaningful Disagreements with AI in Medical Contexts." *AI & Society* 38 (4) (August): 1407–1414. https://doi.org/10.1007/s00146-022-01418-x.

Khazen, Maram, Erin E. Sullivan, Jason Ramos, Maria Mirica, Mark Linzer, Gordon D. Schiff, and Andrew P. J. Olson. 2022. "Anatomy of Diagnosis in a Clinical Encounter: How Clinicians

Discuss Uncertainty with Patients." *BMC Primary Care* 23: article no. 153. https://doi.org/10.1186/s12875-022-01767-y.

Khera, Rohan, Melissa A. Simon, and Joseph S. Ross. 2023. "Automation Bias and Assistive AI: Risk of Harm from AI-Driven Clinical Decision Support." *JAMA: Journal of the American Medical Association* 330 (23) (December 19): 2255–2257. https://doi.org/10.1001/jama.2023.22557.

Killian, Jackson A., Bryan Wilder, Amit Sharma, Vinod Choudhary, Bistra Dilkina, and Milind Tambe. 2019. "Learning to Prescribe Interventions for Tuberculosis Patients Using Digital Adherence Data." In *Proceedings of the 25th ACM SIGKDD International Conference on Knowledge Discovery and Data Mining*, eds. Ankur Teredesai, Vipin Kumar, Ying Li, Rómer Rosales, Evimaria Terzi, and George Karypis, 2430–2438. New York: Association for Computing Machinery. https://doi.org/10.1145/3292500.3330777.

Kim, Hyo-Eun, Hak Hee Kim, Boo-Kyung Han, Ki Hwan Kim, Kyunghwa Han, Hyeonseob Nam, Eun Hye Lee, and Eun-Kyung Kim. 2020. "Changes in Cancer Detection and False-Positive Recall in Mammography Using Artificial Intelligence: A Retrospective, Multireader Study." *Lancet Digital Health* 2 (3) (March): E138–E148. https://doi.org/10.1016/s2589-7500(20)30003-0.

Lee, Hyunna, Eun-Jae Lee, Sungwon Ham, Han-Bin Lee, Ji Sung Lee, Sun U. Kwon, Jong S. Kim, Namkug Kim, and Dong-Wha Kang. 2020. "Machine Learning Approach to Identify Stroke within 4.5 Hours." *Stroke* 51 (3) (March): 860–866. https://doi.org/10.1161/STROKEAHA.119.027611.

Linder, Jodell, Lisa Bastarache, Jacob J. Hughey, and Josh F. Peterson. 2021. "The Role of Electronic Health Records in Advancing Genomic Medicine." *Annual Review of Genomics and Human Genetics* 22: 219–238. https://doi.org/10.1146/annurev-genom-121120-125204.

Martinez-Franco, Adrian Israel, Melchor Sanchez-Mendiola, Juan Jose Mazon-Ramirez, Isaias Hernandez-Torres, Carlos Rivero-Lopez, Troy Spicer, and Adrian Martinez-Gonzalez. 2018. "Diagnostic Accuracy in Family Medicine Residents Using a Clinical Decision Support System (DXplain): A Randomized Controlled Trial." *Diagnosis* 5 (2): 71–76. https://doi.org/10.1515/dx-2017-0045.

Matheny, Michael, Sonoo Thadaney Israni, Mahnoor Ahmed, and Danielle Whicher, eds. 2022. *Artificial Intelligence in Health Care: The Hope, the Hype, the Promise, the Peril.* Washington, DC: National Academy of Medicine.

McCarthy, J., M. L. Minsky, N. Rochester, and C. E. Shannon. 1955. *A Proposal for the Dartmouth Summer Research Project on Artificial Intelligence.* August 31. https://www-formal.stanford.edu/jmc/history/dartmouth/dartmouth.html.

McKinney, Scott Mayer, Marcin Sieniek, Varun Godbole, Jonathan Godwin, Natasha Antropova, Hutan Ashrafian, et al. 2020. "International Evaluation of an AI System for Breast Cancer Screening." *Nature* 577 (7788) (January 2): 89–94. https://doi.org/10.1038/s41586-019-1799-6.

Moazemi, Sobhan, Sahar Vahdati, Jason Li, Sebastian Kalkhoff, Luis J. V. Castano, Bastian Dewitz, et al. 2023. "Artificial Intelligence for Clinical Decision Support for Monitoring Patients in Cardiovascular ICUs: A Systematic Review." *Frontiers in Medicine* 10: 1109411. https://doi.org/10.3389/fmed.2023.1109411.

Müller, Vincent C. 2020. "Ethics of Artificial Intelligence and Robotics." *Stanford Encyclopedia of Philosophy* (Fall 2023 Edition), eds. Edward N. Zalta and Uri Nodelman. https://plato.stanford.edu/archives/fall2023/entries/ethics-ai/.

Nickson, David, Caroline Meyer, Lukasz Walasek, and Carla Toro. 2023. "Prediction and Diagnosis of Depression Using Machine Learning with Electronic Health Records Data: A Systematic Review." *BMC Medical Informatics and Decision Making* 23: article no. 271. https://doi.org/10.1186/s12911-023-02341-x.

Ortega, Marcus V., Michael K. Hidrue, Sara R. Lehrhoff, Dan B. Ellis, Rachel C. Sisodia, William T. Curry, Marcela G. del Carmen, and Jason H. Wasfy. 2023. "Patterns in Physician Burnout in a Stable-Linked Cohort." *JAMA Network Open* 6 (10) (October 6): e2336745. https://doi.org/10.1001/jamanetworkopen.2023.36745.

Palmer, Amitabha, and David Schwan. 2022. "Beneficent Dehumanization: Employing Artificial Intelligence and Carebots to Mitigate Shame-Induced Barriers to Medical Care." *Bioethics* 36 (2) (February): 187–193. https://doi.org/10.1111/bioe.12986.

Palmer, Amitabha, and David Schwan. 2024. "More Process, Less Principles: The Ethics of Deploying AI and Robotics in Medicine." *Cambridge Quarterly of Healthcare Ethics* 33 (1) (January): 121–134. https://doi.org/10.1017/S0963180123000087.

Payne, Thomas H. 2019. "EHR-related Alert Fatigue: Minimal Progress to Date, but Much More Can Be Done." *BMJ Quality and Safety* 28 (1) (January): 1–2. https://doi.org/10.1136/bmjqs-2017-007737.

Perez, Marco V., Kenneth W. Mahaffey, Haley Hedlin, John S. Rumsfeld, Ariadna Garcia, Todd Ferris, et al. 2019. "Large-Scale Assessment of a Smartwatch to Identify Atrial Fibrillation." *New England Journal of Medicine* 381 (20) (November 14): 1909–1917. https://doi.org/10.1056/NEJMoa1901183.

Peterson, Josh, and David W. Bates. 2001. "Preventable Medication Errors: Identifying and Eliminating Serious Drug Interactions." *Journal of the American Pharmacists Association* 41 (2) (March-April): 159–160. https://doi.org/10.1016/S1086-5802(16)31243-8.

Povyakalo, Andrey A., Eugenio Alberdi, Lorenzo Strigini, and Peter Ayton. 2013. "How to Discriminate between Computer-Aided and Computer-Hindered Decisions: A Case Study in Mammography." *Medical Decision Making* 33 (1) (January): 98–107. https://doi.org/10.1177/0272989X12465490.

Sahni, Nikhil R., George Stein, Rodney Zemmel, and David Cutler. 2024. "The Potential Impact of Artificial Intelligence on Health Care Spending." In *The Economics of Artificial Intelligence: Health Care Challenges*, eds. Ajay Agrawal, Joshua Gans, Avi Goldfarb, and Catherine E. Tucker, 49–86. Chicago: University of Chicago Press.

Schwan, David. 2018. "Should Physicians Be Empathetic? Rethinking Clinical Empathy." *Theoretical Medicine and Bioethics* 39 (5) (October): 347–360. https://doi.org/10.1007/s11017-018-9463-y.

Secinaro, Silvana, Davide Calandra, Aurelio Secinaro, Vivek Muthurangu, and Paolo Biancone. 2021. "The Role of Artificial Intelligence in Healthcare: A Structured Literature Review." *BMC Medical Informatics and Decision Making* 21: article no. 125. https://doi.org/10.1186/s12911-021-01488-9.

Segal, Michael M., Alanna K. Rahm, Nathan C. Hulse, Grant Wood, Janet L. Williams, Lynn Feldman, et al. 2017. "Experience with Integrating Diagnostic Decision Support Software with Electronic Health Records: Benefits versus Risks of Information Sharing." *Journal for Electronic Health Data and Methods* 5 (1): article no. 23. https://doi.org/10.5334/egems.244.

Shaik, Thanveer, Xiaohui Tao, Niall Higgins, Lin Li, Raj Gururajan, Xujuan Zhou, and U. Rajendra Acharya. 2023. "Remote Patient Monitoring Using Artificial Intelligence: Current State, Applications, and Challenges." *WIREs Data Mining and Knowledge Discovery* 13 (2) (March-April): e1485. https://doi.org/10.1002/widm.1485.

Shajari, Shaghayegh, Kirankumar Kuruvinashetti, Amin Komeili, and Uttandaraman Sundararaj. 2023. "The Emergence of AI-Based Wearable Sensors for Digital Health Technology: A Review." *Sensors* 23 (23) (December 1): 9498. https://doi.org/10.3390/s23239498.

Sharkey, Amanda, and Noel Sharkey. 2012. "Granny and the Robots: Ethical Issues in Robot Care for the Elderly." *Ethics and Information Technology* 14: 27–40. https://doi.org/10.1007/s10676-010-9234-6.

Sharkey, Noel, and Amanda Sharkey. 2010. "The Crying Shame of Robot Nannies: An Ethical Appraisal." *Interaction Studies* 11 (2) (January): 161–190. https://doi.org/10.1075/is.11.2.01sha.

Sheu, Yi-han, Colin Magdamo, Matthew Miller, Sudeshna Das, Deborah Blacker, and Jordan W. Smoller. 2023. "AI-Assisted Prediction of Differential Response to Antidepressant Classes Using Electronic Health Records." *NPJ Digital Medicine* 6: article no. 73. https://doi.org/10.1038/s41746-023-00817-8.

Shickel, Benjamin, Patrick James Tighe, Azra Bihorac, and Parisa Rashidi. 2018. "Deep EHR: A Survey of Recent Advances in Deep Learning Techniques for Electronic Health Record (EHR) Analysis." *IEEE Journal of Biomedical and Health Informatics* 22 (5) (September): 1589–1604. https://doi.org/10.1109/JBHI.2017.2767063.

Singh, Hardeep, Christiane Spitzmueller, Nancy J. Petersen, Mona K. Sawhney, and Dean F. Sittig. 2013. "Information Overload and Missed Test Results in Electronic Health Record-Based Settings." *JAMA Internal Medicine* 173 (8) (April 22): 702–704. https://doi.org/10.1001/2013.jamainternmed.61.

Siwicki, Bill. 2023. "How Epic Is Using AI to Change the Way EHRs Work." *Healthcare IT News*. November 28. https://www.healthcareitnews.com/news/how-epic-using-ai-change-way-ehrs-work.

Sparrow, Robert, and Linda Sparrow. 2006. "In the Hands of Machines? The Future of Aged Care." *Minds and Machines* 16: 141–161. https://doi.org/10.1007/s11023-006-9030-6.

Stokes, Felicia, and Amitabha Palmer. 2020. "Artificial Intelligence and Robotics in Nursing: Ethics of Caring as a Guide to Dividing Tasks Between AI and Humans." *Nursing Philosophy* 21 (4) (October): e12306. https://doi.org/10.1111/nup.12306.

Sutton, Reed T., David Pincock, Daniel C. Baumgart, Daniel C. Sadowski, Richard N. Fedorak, and Karen I. Kroeker. 2020. "An Overview of Clinical Decision Support Systems: Benefits, Risks, and Strategies for Success." *NPJ Digital Medicine* 3: article no. 17. https://doi.org/10.1038/s41746-020-0221-y.

Tierney, Aaron A., Gregg Gayre, Brian Hoberman, Britt Mattern, Manuel Ballesca, Patricia Kipnis, Vincent Liu, and Kristine Lee. 2024. "Ambient Artificial Intelligence Scribes to Alleviate the Burden of Clinical Documentation." *NEJM Catalyst Innovations in Care Delivery* 5 (3) (March). https://doi.org/10.1056/CAT.23.0404.

Timiliotis, Joanna, Bibiana Blümke, Peter Daniel Serfözö, Stephen Gilbert, Marta Ondrésik, Ewelina Türk, Martin Christian Hirsch, and Jens Eckstein. 2022. "A Novel Diagnostic Decision Support System for Medical Professionals: Prospective Feasibility Study." *JMIR Formative Research* 6 (3) (March): e29943. https://doi.org/10.2196/29943.

Topol, Eric. 2019. *Deep Medicine: How Artificial Intelligence Can Make Healthcare Human Again*. New York: Basic Books.

Turkle, Sherry. 2011. *Alone Together: Why We Expect More from Technology and Less from Each Other*. New York: Basic Books.

United Nations Department of Economic and Social Affairs. 2021 *Resource Guide on Artificial Intelligence (AI) Strategies*. 2021. https://sdgs.un.org/sites/default/files/2021-06/Resource%20Guide%20on%20AI%20Strategies_June%202021.pdf.

Urban, Gregor, Priyam Tripathi, Talal Alkayali, Mohit Mittal, Farid Jalali, William Karnes, and Pierre Baldi. 2018. "Deep Learning Localizes and Identifies Polyps in Real Time with 96% Accuracy in Screening Colonoscopy." *Gastroenterology* 155 (4) (October): 1069–1078.e8. https://doi.org/10.1053/j.gastro.2018.06.037.

Vallor, Shannon. 2016. *Technology and the Virtues: A Philosophical Guide to a Future Worth Wanting*. New York: Oxford University Press.

Vandemeulebroucke Tijs, Bernadette Dierckx de Casterlé, and Chris Gastmans. 2018. "The Use of Care Robots in Aged Care: A Systematic Review of Argument-Based Ethics Literature." *Archives of Gerontology and Geriatrics* 74 (January): 15–25. https://doi.org/10.1016/j.archger.2017.08.014.

van de Sande, Dennis, Marjan Sharabiani, Hanneke Bluemink, Esther Kneepkens, Nienke Bakx, Els Hagelaar, Maurice van der Sangen, Jacqueline Theuws, and Coen Hurkmans. 2021. "Artificial Intelligence Based Treatment Planning of Radiotherapy for Locally Advanced Breast Cancer." *Physics and Imaging in Radiation Oncology* 20 (October): 111–116. https://doi.org/10.1016/j.phro.2021.11.007.

van Wynsberghe, Aimee. 2013. "A Method for Integrating Ethics into the Design of Robots." *Industrial Robot*. 40 (5): 433–440. https://doi.org/10.1108/IR-12-2012-451.

Waldren, Steven E., and Edmund Billings. 2024. *AI Assistant for Clinical Review and Value-Based Care*. American Academy of Family Physicians. January. https://www.aafp.org/dam/AAFP/documents/practice_management/innovation_lab/report-navina-ai-clinical-review-phase2.pdf.

Wang, Lu, Xinyi Chen, Lu Zhang, Long Li, Yongbiao Huang, Yinan Sun, and Xianglin Yuan. 2023. "Artificial Intelligence in Clinical Decision Support Systems for Oncology." *International Journal of Medical Sciences* 20 (1): 79–86. https://doi.org/10.7150/ijms.77205.

Yang, D., C. Murr, S. Yoo, L. O'Neill, S. Catalano, R.C. Blitzblau, S. McDuff, F. F. Yin, Q. J. J. Wu, and Y. Sheng. 2022a. "Prospective Clinical Integration of AI Based Treatment Planning Tool for Whole Breast Radiation Therapy (WBRT): A Single Institution's Three-Year Experience." *International Journal of Radiation Oncology, Biology, Physics* 114 (3S) (November 1): S33.

Yang, Guang, Qinghao Ye, and Jun Xia. 2022b. "Unbox the Black-Box for the Medical Explainable AI via Multi-modal and Multi-centre Data Fusion: A Mini-review Two Showcases and Beyond." *Information Fusion* 77 (January): 29–52. https://doi.org/10.1016/j.inffus.2021.07.016.

Amitabha (Ami) Palmer is an Assistant Professor and clinical ethicist at MD Anderson Cancer Center's Center for Clinical Ethics in Cancer Care, USA. He also holds an Affiliate Faculty position at the Institute for Data Science in Oncology, where he provides ethical guidance and education for the development and design pipeline of new AI tools. His primary areas of research within the ethics of AI in healthcare include participatory design, human-machine interaction, and deployment policy. A longtime researcher of medical misinformation, he has developed a conversation guide to help providers engage fruitfully with patients who endorse medical misinformation about cancer care.

David Schwan is a Senior Lecturer in the Department of Philosophy and Comparative Religion at Central Washington University, USA. In addition, he serves as the Director of the EthicsLab initiative at CWU. His research focuses on the intersection between applied ethics and moral psychology. He has published on empathy in medicine, the ethics of electronic health records, and medical scribes. His current research focuses on the ethics of advanced technology (AI/carebots) in medical care.

Chapter 5
Telehealth as a Window into the Future: Ethical Lessons for AI in Healthcare

Amitabha Palmer and Christopher F. Masciari

Abstract This chapter examines how telehealth's rapid and widespread deployment into medical practice offers valuable insights for understanding the ethical dimensions of implementing new technologies in healthcare, particularly artificial intelligence. We argue that telehealth is not merely a tool for improving healthcare accessibility and clinical effectiveness; it serves as a critical case study for understanding how technology reshapes medicine and affects non-medical domains in unexpected ways. Through analysis of telehealth's impact on medical adherence, provider-patient relationships, and the medicalization of personal spaces, we identify three key lessons for the ethical deployment of healthcare technologies: First, while benefits are often readily quantifiable, risks to normative aspects of medicine—such as patient autonomy and identity—are subtler and harder to measure. Second, technologies affect different populations and specialties in varying and unexpected ways, demanding context-sensitive implementation strategies rather than universal solutions. Third, new technologies shape not just what we can do but who we become as healthcare providers and patients. As healthcare becomes increasingly technology-dependent, we must balance innovation with the preservation of human values and relationships that lie at the foundation of good care. These insights are particularly relevant for the ongoing integration of AI systems into healthcare practice.

Keywords Telehealth · Medical ethics · Healthcare technology · Provider-patient relationship · Healthcare access

---

A. Palmer (✉) · C. F. Masciari
MD Anderson Cancer Center, Houston, TX, USA
e-mail: apalmer1@mdanderson.org

C. F. Masciari
e-mail: cfmasciari@mdanderson.org

M. C. Altman and D. Schwan (eds.), *Ethics and Medical Technology*, The International Library of Bioethics 113, https://doi.org/10.1007/978-3-031-94690-5_5

5.1 Introduction

Telemedicine has rapidly grown over the past several years. Some centers experienced close to a 9,000% increase in video visit use during the COVID-19 pandemic compared to the same period the year before (Ramaswamy et al. 2020). Telemedicine and telehealth technologies (we use these terms interchangeably moving forward) are thus important topics for ethical inquiry and fertile ground from which to extract general lessons about the ethical dimensions of rapid and widespread deployment of new technologies into medicine—such as is occurring right now with medical AI.

The introduction of new technologies into medicine can sometimes have predictable effects that are ethically insignificant beyond their intended purpose. For example, the introduction of a new surgical adhesive will improve clinical outcomes and have little impact on norms surrounding provider-patient interactions or patient autonomy. Conversely, other technologies can have unpredictable effects that extend to matters of ethical concern beyond clinical effectiveness. In this chapter, we examine telehealth, which falls into the latter category. For this reason, we argue that telehealth is not just a tool for improving healthcare accessibility and clinical effectiveness; it is a critical case study for understanding how the rapid and widespread integration of a technology reshapes medicine in surprising and unpredictable ways—especially norms surrounding clinical relationships and patient autonomy. By examining telehealth's sometimes surprising and unintended effects, we extrapolate lessons and strategies to navigate the ethical challenges of implementing new technologies and suggest how these lessons might be applied to the next wave of rapid and widespread medical technology—namely, medical AI.

At a high level of abstraction, some of the lessons we draw can be seen as mundane: we should not forget to consider risks; recognize that there is no one universal rule for all people, technologies, and specialties; and think about how technology changes norms and practices. However, we hope to persuade the reader that the specific ways in which these general lessons are instantiated in telehealth's deployment are surprising, interesting, and unlikely to have been anticipated from the armchair. Moreover, these lessons are of significance to ethicists writing about the deployment of new technologies—such as AI in healthcare—because of important similarities between the two technologies: both have a similar rapid and widespread deployment pattern, both mediate provider-patient interactions, and both will, in surprising and ethically significant ways, affect aspects of medicine beyond their intended goals of improving accessibility and clinical efficacy.

Three key themes emerge from our analysis. First, the benefits of new technologies are often easier to identify and quantify than their risks, especially when those risks involve subtle changes to the normative foundations of medicine, provider-patient relationships, and patient identity. Second, our analysis challenges the tendency to treat healthcare technologies as universal solutions with predictable impacts. A recurring theme in telehealth research is how technological effectiveness depends heavily on psychological differences, social embeddedness, and disease profile—a finding that undermines simplistic narratives about technological progress in medicine.

Instead of asking whether a technology "works," we must examine how its benefits and risks manifest differently across various communities, specialties, and individual circumstances, demanding deployment strategies as diverse as the populations they serve.

Finally, and perhaps most importantly, new technologies shape not just what we can do but who we become as healthcare providers and patients. As healthcare becomes increasingly mediated by and dependent on technology, we must carefully consider how these changes affect the roles, responsibilities, and relationships at the heart of medicine. The progressive expansion of technology into healthcare—while often driven by laudable goals of efficiency and accessibility—risks transforming medical institutions from centers of human care into mere dispensaries of depersonalized, technologized medicine. As we move forward with AI and other advanced technologies in healthcare, we must balance innovation with preservation of medicine's fundamental human elements.

Our chapter proceeds in the following way. In Sect. 5.2, we provide a brief history of telehealth technology. In Sect. 5.3, we argue that even if telehealth is clinically effective and improves nonadherence, it can restructure the nature of care delivery in ways that affect other ethically significant domains. In Sect. 5.4, we argue that telehealth can reshape medical norms, care, relationships, and identities in interesting and unexpected ways. Finally, in Sect. 5.5, we reflect on generalizable lessons from telehealth and how they can help to guide ethicists working on medical AI.

5.2 A Brief History of Telehealth Technologies

Telehealth is defined by D. W. Nickelson as "the use of telecommunications and information technology to provide access to health assessment, intervention, consultation, supervision, education, and information across distance" (1998, 527). These technologies can include things such as the telegraph, landline phone, fax machine, cellular telephone, email, video conferencing technologies such as Zoom, and online chat services.

Telehealth technologies saw an explosion in use during the COVID-19 pandemic; however, their origins date back much further. In fact, telehealth can be traced to the American Civil War, with the deployment of the telegraph to help coordinate the transmission of medical supplies (Tang and Reddy 2022). Other seminal events took place during the late nineteenth and early twentieth centuries, which mark the beginning of telehealth's perceived usefulness and promise for increasing the quality of and access to personalized care. For example, in 1879, shortly after the Civil War ended, the *Lancet* presented a case report of a physician who used the telephone to provide medical care to an infant (Tang and Reddy 2022). Telehealth's prominence in modern medicine is obvious, but without these early successes its value and promise might not have been widely acknowledged.

The COVID-19 pandemic created an unprecedented opportunity to deploy telehealth technologies in the West, as quarantines and social distancing made traditional, in-person medical care difficult to access. The opportunity to deploy telehealth technologies also depended in part on the sheer ubiquity of internet access, at least in the US. Since the beginning of the 2010s, smartphones, tablets, and laptop computers have entered many households. According to recent census data, 91.2% of US households had access to the internet in 2022 (Taylor 2023). Policy changes at the federal and state levels during COVID-19 were significant for the rapid expansion of telehealth. For instance, Medicare expanded coverage for the approved list of telehealth services through the end of 2024 (US Department of Health and Human Services 2023). But more importantly, permanent Medicare changes also occurred. These include the following: (1) Federally Qualified Health Centers (FQHCs) and Rural Health Clinics (RHCs) can serve as distant site providers for mental and behavioral health services, (2) patients can now receive telehealth services for mental and behavioral healthcare in their homes, (3) geographic restrictions for originating site for mental and behavioral services have been removed, (4) mental and behavioral services can be audio only, and (5) rural emergency hospitals (REHs) are now eligible originating sites for telehealth services (US Department of Health and Human Services 2023).

The benefits of telehealth are well known and well understood. The result, then, is that telehealth technologies are likely here to stay. However, despite their obvious promise of improving the accessibility of healthcare, we should remain cautious. As with all good medicine, benefits should be weighed against burdens. If a technology presents disadvantages, we should be keenly aware of them and look to mitigate them. Below, we discuss some of the major ethical dimensions of telehealth. In doing so, we draw out broader lessons about the ethics of new technologies in healthcare and apply them to AI-based technologies.

5.3 Telehealth, Nonadherence, and Unintended Ethical Impacts

Medicine is heavily outcome-oriented. Hence, when a medical technology is evaluated, significant weight is rightly placed on clinical effectiveness but with less concern for how it might affect other domains. In this section, we argue that even if telehealth is as clinically effective as face-to-face care, the widespread deployment of telehealth raises significant ethical questions about surveillance, patient motivation, and the broader place of medicine in a person's life. All these effects are ethically significant and some not easily anticipated. To illustrate these points, we discuss how telehealth can influence the problem of nonadherence and patient motivation.

The problem of nonadherence is ubiquitous across medicine: sometimes patients do not adhere to their treatment plans, even if the patient played an essential role in its construction (Masciari 2025). For illnesses that are primarily managed though medication, nonadherence is associated with poor health outcomes, suboptimal management, and significant financial burdens on patients and healthcare systems due to emergency room visits and hospitalizations. Some studies of the US suggest that each year 125,000 deaths and $100–200 billion in healthcare costs are attributable to medical nonadherence. Telehealth technologies have been suggested as one potential remedy for this problem. Indeed, the World Health Organization has made statements about the use of such technologies for improving adherence (WHO Global Observatory for eHealth 2011).

The literature divides the problem of nonadherence into two types: *intentional* and *nonintentional* nonadherence. The former occurs when a patient decides not to engage in an activity that is constitutive of their treatment plan, while the latter occurs when a patient forgets. These classifications are distinct from *primary* and *secondary* nonadherence. The latter distinction marks the difference between the patient never beginning their treatment and the patient not faithfully following the treatment plan after they have started it. Telemedicine addresses each category of nonadherence differently. For example, some technologies may reduce unintentional nonadherence but not intentional nonadherence. Some may improve primary adherence but not secondary. And some may help with adherence in the context of mental health but not for physiological conditions.

Several studies have found positive effects of using telehealth to improve adherence. For example, one meta-analysis showed a significant reduction of Hemoglobin A1c (HbA1c)—a blood test that measures the average blood sugar (glucose) levels—in patients with diabetes who participated in telehealth, compared to a non-telehealth group (Anderson et al. 2022). Other reviews and meta-analyses showed a positive correlation between telehealth and improved health outcomes. For instance, one concluded that 59% of studies involving telehealth showed an improvement in drug adherence for patients with affective disorders (Leiz et al. 2022), and another showed positive effects of various telehealth interventions on weight loss (Ufholz and Bhargava 2021). Additionally, a meta-analysis investigating HIV patients' adherence rates to antiretroviral therapy found that those who received telehealth interventions improved adherence by an average of 18% compared to those who did not (Esmaeili et al. 2023). So, it seems that for at least a subset of medical problems, telehealth can be an effective intervention for increasing adherence.

One major theme found among the studies reviewed was the use of the telephone to monitor participants' activities and to send reminders. Telephones are common and inexpensive, so they can be used to check in with patients, send reminders to take medications, and so on. Other notification-based technologies such as SMS have similar effects (Jayasree et al. 2024). However, some obvious limitations are that they will not directly affect intentional nonadherence. If patients do not trust their doctors, it is unclear that receiving repeated phone calls would positively affect adherence. This is especially true if a patient is experiencing paranoia, for instance.

Even if we suppose that telehealth unambiguously improves adherence, telehealth itself restructures the nature of care delivery in ways that affect other ethically significant domains, including privacy, security, accessibility, autonomy, and identity. Unaddressed privacy and security concerns can impede accessibility. In fact, for at least some people, a lack of internet access does not explain why they do not use telehealth. Indeed, Robin Adams et al. (2021) found a strong correlation between general concerns about privacy and security and a resistance to telehealth in older adults. Hence, the introduction of telehealth bears on values outside of clinical effectiveness and improving access.

The regular check-ins facilitated by telehealth imply that one's daily activities will be regularly monitored and registered in a way they were not previously. This medical encroachment into a patient's life raises ethical concerns about patient information and activities that may unintentionally transmitted to providers (Hall and McGraw 2014). Moreover, the constant monitoring of one's daily life can have significant positive or negative effects on one's sense of autonomy and identity. Telehealth can enhance autonomy when it helps to motivate patients to adhere to their treatment goals. However, when telehealth monitoring and alerts shift a patient's attention away from other important non-medical goals, it can undermine autonomy. Identity is also affected because the regular check-ins and alerts can increasingly direct attention to one's medical condition relative to and in ways that interfere with other sources of identity. Regular monitoring and alerts can lead one to fixate on physiological aspects of themselves that were previously unknown or unnoticed. We discuss both in more detail in Sect. 5.4. What we want to emphasize at this juncture is that the effects of telehealth extend beyond its intended targets to other normatively important domains.

The broader lessons here concern the ethics of surveillance and motivation and the extent to which medical technologies enter aspects of a person's life that were previously independent. This example also illustrates the interdependence of values: the ways in which some medical technologies affect other values (e.g., security and privacy) can adversely affect the target value (improving adherence). In the context of medical AI, even if patient privacy concerns can be adequately addressed, new AI tools offer unprecedented access to monitor and manipulate patient behaviors in the name of addressing nonadherence. For example, mHealth apps monitor everything from sleep and menstrual cycle to blood sugar levels and mood. Since many such devices are not covered by HIPAA, such devices may not only transmit sensitive information to providers but to app and device developers—especially if the app or device's development was financed through data sharing with third parties (Hall and McGraw 2014). Without thoughtful deployment and adequate regulatory oversight, privacy and security concerns surrounding these new technologies stand to worsen distrust between patient and provider, or at the very least, will make some patient populations apprehensive about their use.

5.4 Provider-Patient Relationship

Although most telehealth research examines whether telehealth and face-to-face encounters generate clinically similar outcomes and align with patient and provider preferences (Snoswell et al. 2021), another dimension is underexplored: how technologically mediated interactions affect the therapeutic relationship. Especially in the ethics of nursing literature, there is concern that telemedicine supplants human and empathetic touch (Ftouni et al. 2022). Physical touch is an important means of conveying psychological support and has therapeutic effects that cannot be replaced by other means (Ftouni et al. 2022). The ethical dimensions of provider-patient interactions often elude quantifiability and include effects on the role of patients and healthcare providers, the significance of new patterns of communications, and the significance of in-person care (Frittgen and Haltaufderheide 2022).

In this section, we claim that telemedicine, in surprising and important ways, affects the norms underpinning the therapeutic relationship in the context of psychotherapy and palliative care. We focus on these two medical specialties because, unlike routine medicine, the quality of the relationships is central to their clinical success (Del Re et al. 2021; Tang and Reddy 2022). Provider-patient interactions in these specialties are characterized by the fact that they are particularly private, personal, and highly emotional. Crucially, patient adherence and outcomes often depend on whether there is a strong and stable therapeutic relationship, since distrust is an important predictor of nonadherence (Krupnick et al. 2006). We close this section by arguing that telehealth in palliative care affects a patient's relationship with themselves and their home environment.

5.4.1 *Psychotherapy and Psychiatry*

A naïve view of telehealth might suppose that technology which mediates the provider-patient interaction will have negligible effects on the nature of that interaction. However, research from telepsychiatry reveals that providers must work harder to read nonverbal cues and support emotional connections through video calls, leading to increased mental fatigue. This finding matters for all telehealth services since empathy and strong patient relationships are essential to medical care across all specialties, but especially psychotherapy (Myronuk 2022).

The patient's perspective is sometimes different, however. Under certain conditions, telehealth can either be unproblematic or even promote the development of trust in provider-patient relationships. A recent systematic review found that trusting relationships were easier to establish for patients if they had met their therapist prior to telehealth visits (Moeller et al. 2022). This suggests that telehealth technologies are not perceived by patients to be outright detrimental to their goals. Second, some patients may even prefer to develop therapeutic relationships in person instead of on video—even though both are equally clinically effective (Ftouni et al. 2022; Moeller et al. 2022). Third, patients were more open to telehealth if they had established, trustful relationships with their therapists (Hensel et al. 2020). This trust extended to therapists that patients had not met so long as the patient was supported in person by a mental health nurse or general practitioner. One study found that although patients were able to develop strong therapeutic relationships with therapists they had never met in person, patients preferred to have in-person sessions until rapport was established (Simpson et al. 2015). Our main point here is that the introduction of telehealth into provider-patient interactions affects the nature of the therapeutic relationship in normatively important ways that could not have been predicted from the armchair.

5.4.2 *Palliative and Supportive Care*

As we noted with psychotherapy, palliative care clinicians also experienced technologically mediated interactions as detrimental to their practice. For them, distance increased their hesitancy to raise sensitive emotional issues with patients because they worried that they would not be able to comfort them (van Gurp et al. 2015).

Although early literature on telehealth speculated that it may lead to detached, dehumanized relationships, Michael Tang and Akhila Reddy (2022) found that palliative care patients can form trusting relationships with palliative care teams even when interactions are mediated by technology. Variables that supported the development of provider-patient trust included (1) the repetitive nature of teleconsults (which suggest to patients that the provider will "still be there") and (2) co-developing a medical and interpersonal history with the same team of providers (van Gurp et al. 2015). In addition, Jelle van Gurp et al. (2015) found that, for palliative care patients, telehealth created "valuable free space" within which they could "pour out their hearts, define their own roles, and co-design their own care in more equal patient-professional relationships" (2015, 10). That is, the distance and at-home privacy afforded by the technology supported patients' ability to emote then quickly return to their "normal" lives.

In palliative care and psychotherapy, predictions about patients' attitudes toward new technologies that mediate their clinical relationships are influenced by whether patients have existing relationships with their providers and the nature of those relationships. Importantly, acceptance of technology seems to emerge from existing trusting relationships with providers. However, the acuteness of psychiatric need also influences openness to provider-patient mediating technologies (Trondsen et al. 2018).

5.4.3 *Medicalization of the Home and Self*

Until recently, medicine was largely practiced "out there," with one's home or work environments being distinct domains and free from constant reminders about one's health status. But telehealth technology can expand the domain of medicine into these previously unmedicalized environments. This might be a worry or a benefit. The effects of this expansion provide further examples of how the rapid and widespread introduction of telehealth affects areas of normative importance beyond its intended targets.

For instance, some patients prefer to avoid telehealth for palliative care since it draws their attention to their inevitable decline (Pols 2012; van Gurp et al. 2015).

The home was traditionally a sanctuary from one's medical reality, but with the advent of telehealth, the distinction between the doctor's office and home has eroded. This perspective is not universal, however. Indeed, some palliative care and hospice patients *prefer* telemedicine because having to take a trip to a hospital often causes distress (van Gurp et al. 2015). Their distress may be explained by a variety of factors, including the physical discomfort of having to travel and the stigma of being considered a "sick person" upon entering the hospital or clinic. One patient was quoted as saying that their home is "the place where [they were] not dying men" (van Gurp et al. 2015). This latter point may seem counterintuitive, but we interpret it as suggesting that at-home patients have more liberty to define their own existence. After all, home is where many people feel most comfortable and in control.

Some general lessons emerge from this literature. Early critiques of telehealth arose before the widespread deployment of tablets, so they offer valuable insight into how a novel technology is sometimes perceived; it may remind patients of their current condition or distract from their sense of well-being if the technology is not already embedded into one's life. This suggests that when conceiving of new technologies and their respective deployment strategies, people should think about who is receiving the technology, how they are receiving the technology, and what sort of message the technology may deliver. It is not intuitively obvious, for example, that many palliative care patients will prefer telehealth to in-person care, and the reasons for these preferences are even less obvious. Moreover, predictions about future technologies should consider how ubiquitous a particular interface or medium may be, since whether a piece of technology is already employed in people's lives will make a difference to its reception. Although these considerations are not specific to medicine, their implications are more ethically significant in such contexts.

Since medicine should aspire to be person-centered, institutions should be hesitant to introduce telehealth for psychotherapy or palliative care unless a patient either has an already established trusting relationship or they indicate a preference for it. Typically, this will require that a patient first has a consultation to establish their preferences. Of course, this condition is most apt for medical conditions that require regular care over longer time periods. It will be less important for acute short-term medical problems.

These lessons extend to conversations surrounding the ethical deployment of healthcare artificial intelligence (HCAI). We think that more caution and empirical studies are needed when we consider the deployment of HCAI—especially those that continually monitor patients and their behaviors in their homes. One of the main differences between the use of a smartphone or tablet for telehealth visits and surveillance HCAI is that the former devices do not monitor one's life continuously or as extensively. There are some continuous non-AI monitoring devices such as glucose monitors, but they are not as "existentially invasive" since they do not monitor a wide range of activities and behaviors in one's home environment or elsewhere (Ho 2023). As we noted above, some patients prefer telehealth because it affords them greater control over their environment and personal identity, but continuous surveillance HCAI devices can undermine that advantage. The sort of continuous and invasive monitoring from some surveillance HCAI is apt to increase self-consciousness and critically alter one's practical identity (see Ho 2023, ch. 2).

5.5 Guiding Lessons

In this chapter, we have argued that telemedicine affects normatively important domains of medicine in unexpected and significant ways. For these reasons and similarities with some HCAI, telehealth functions as a fruitful case study from which to draw lessons about rapid and widespread ethical deployment of technologies that alter provider-patient interactions. In addition to the lessons above, we believe that assessing the ethics of telemedicine reveals three broad themes that can guide ethicists working on the ethics of AI in healthcare:

1. The benefits of new technologies are often easier to identify and quantify than their risks, especially when those risks involve subtle changes to the normative foundations of medicine, provider-patient relationships, and patient identity.
2. Ethicists should resist treating healthcare technologies as universal solutions with predictable impacts.
3. New technologies shape not just what we can do but who we become as healthcare providers and patients.

5.5.1 Rapid Deployment and the Relative Invisibility of Normative Risks

Telehealth demonstrates that medical technologies can be widely deployed in healthcare more quickly than robust ethical analyses can be performed. We suspect this trend is explained in part by the ease with which potential benefits are identified (compared to risks) and the weight of institutional values (compared to other stakeholder values) in decisions to adopt a particular technology. That is, like pharmaceutical products, medical technologies are often only evaluated in terms of narrowly defined medical risks and benefits prior to being deployed.

The benefits of telehealth are easy to identify and articulate: patients with mobility, transportation, and scheduling challenges have easier access to healthcare; and telehealth introduces efficiency and cost savings for healthcare institutions. But the risks are not so easy to identify since they often (but not always) involve considerations related to the normative dimensions of provider-patient interactions, which often elude quantifiability (Frittgen and Haltaufderheide 2022). Moreover, healthcare institutions typically place significant weight on efficiency and other economic criteria. Since these institutions are the decision-makers regarding whether a technology is deployed, their (more easily quantifiable) values will be disproportionately represented in deployment decisions.

Ethicists working on HCAI should take these general observations to heart. Tech entrepreneurs eagerly tout the benefits of new HCAI tools, and institutions are keen to increase safety, reduce costs, and increase efficiency. The claimed benefits are rarely hard to spot. Some risks are also conspicuous. For example, privacy and security concerns receive the most attention, and for good reason. However, there are other areas of concern, especially with surveillance and monitoring technologies. Consider medication-monitoring devices that "report" to a physician's dashboard or an electronic health record. These devices may help patients improve adherence, but the monitoring technology cannot evaluate the many reasons why a patient may have altered their regimen. This can shift the traditional ethical stance of the therapeutic relationship in which patients are assumed to be truthful and reasonable. With every pill monitored, every deviation from the prescription is recorded, and every deviation demands justification. Moreover, it is not hard to imagine the development of coercive pressure to accept the monitoring once its use is widespread. Patients who decline could become targets of suspicion: "Why don't they want help ensuring proper adherence? What are they hiding?" Such technologies also threaten to overturn the traditional presumption in favor of patient privacy about their lives outside of medical facilities (Ho 2023).

A corollary of HCAI's massive expansion into healthcare is how it stands to displace and change provider-patient interactions. On one hand, we can imagine that HCAI may diminish the need for frequent interactions and discussion of certain topics. There is no need to ask the patient how they are doing when all the "objective" data has been collected and assembled in an eye-pleasing way in the chart. Again, the administrative values of efficiency, quantifiability, and economy reign supreme. Who could be against efficiency and cost savings? But surely something is lost when, instead of speaking with patients and administering various tests, the provider just glances at their screen of data collected by the wearable or swallowable smart device. More attention needs to be placed on how HCAI displaces and affects provider-patient interactions and how this may alter the nature of the therapeutic relationship, the role of the physician, and the patient's role.

While technology can displace and replace certain activities, it can also lead to their increase. Technology makes certain tasks easier. And when tasks become easier (i.e., less costly), the expectation for them increases. This lesson is readily apparent in the exponential demand for documenting everything. As electronic health records made documentation easier—with checkboxes and drop-down menus—the demand for documentation exploded. The chat function in electronic health records has similarly increased patients' (and administrators') expectation of frequent and timely communication with their providers.

5.5.2 *Against Universalism*

Another persistent theme in the ethics of telehealth literature revolves around the relationship between the technology itself and the socio-cultural environments and patient populations where it is deployed. Hence, the ethical issues that arise in one location or population may not be the same as those that arise in another for the same technology. Moreover, benefits (or harm) for one group of people might not apply to other groups. This fact speaks to how ethical issues ought to be addressed when considering implementation. As other authors have argued, implementation policy must have broad stakeholder involvement to ensure that local values, goals, and concerns are addressed in a way that fits the community in question (Palmer and Schwan 2024). It follows that different communities will make different value tradeoffs given distinct background commitments or goals. This process also invites us to think about why one population may be resistant to a new technology when others welcome it.

Not only can a patient's socioeconomic status make a difference to the appropriateness of reliance on telehealth technology; a patient's health status or mental state can make a difference as well. If technologically mediated interactions are interchangeable one-for-one with face-to-face interactions—that is, if they differ only in clinically unimportant ways—then replacing one with the other is ethically permissible, assuming of course that the technology itself is morally unproblematic. However, whether they are clinically interchangeable depends on several context-dependent features. As we saw in our discussion of medical adherence, even if an intervention benefits one group, it does not follow that it will help another despite their shared medical needs.

Exploring these nuances requires deep, domain-specific knowledge. For example, it is unlikely that ethicists could have hypothesized, let alone been confident in the effects of telehealth on psychiatric or palliative care patients. Hence, an important lesson for ethicists of technology in medicine is to collaborate with medical specialists to ensure nuanced and accurate predictions rather than gross generalizations. Gross generalizations risk (1) creating barriers for novel technologies in narrow applications which might deliver important benefits to patients and healthcare systems, or (2) allowing the deployment of technologies that adversely affect provider-patient relationships, patient autonomy, and patients' identity. Interdisciplinary collaboration is even more pressing in a context where early ethical analyses have frequently treated HCAI as a homogenous category and often made broad assumptions about what may work for all individuals or patient populations.

5.5.3 *Unanticipated Effects of Technology on the Normative Foundations of Medicine*

The last theme that we will touch on is the relationship between new technologies and the roles and responsibilities of providers and patients. Telehealth can affect provider-patient norms, relationships, and expectations, as well as patient identities and the extent to which the domain of medicine occupies other aspects of one's life.

Ethicists evaluating HCAI can apply these insights to their own work. Consider for example continuous glucose monitors, which allow patients with diabetes to easily monitor and regulate their blood sugar in real time. This and similar monitoring technologies empower patients to take control of aspects of their health that they would not otherwise be expected to be responsible for, at least not as extensively. This newly accessible knowledge can provide some patients with a sense of relief that they can now control their own health situation. On the other hand, some patients may find the constant flood of information overwhelming, as they may obsess over every fluctuation of their blood insulin level.

Note that this technology is not neutral about which norms may govern the roles and responsibilities of individuals over their health. If this technology becomes cheap and easily accessible, norms surrounding responsibility for managing diabetes (for example) may shift even more responsibility onto individuals rather than being a shared endeavor with healthcare providers. By implication, this shift in responsibility toward individuals may shift norms surrounding blameworthiness for one's health status (even further) onto individuals. Whether this is a good or bad outcome is an open question.

It is reasonable to predict that HCAI will eventually outperform physicians on diagnosis, prognosis, and treatment plan development. When the fundamental activities of medicine are best performed by machines, we will be forced to reimagine the role of physicians. Do they become more like technicians who are experts in using these new technologies? Will they become more like genetic counsellors, who excel in helping patients understand and interpret complex medical facts? Or will physicians become more like nurses, who focus on the "caring" aspect of medicine—now that the machines have surpassed humans in its epistemic and skill-based aspects. The medical professions must wrestle with these questions, especially in medical education. Whatever the answer, one thing is clear: the role of the future physician will differ in important ways from what it is now.

The growing implementation of AI in healthcare risks reducing medical institutions to dispensaries of technology rather than centers of human care. While these tools may increase efficiency, they could also shift responsibilities in ways that reduce medicine to a mere transaction between consumer and service provider. As we develop and deploy intelligent medical systems, we should heed Shannon Vallor's (2014) insight: rather than focusing solely on what machines can do for us, we must consider how they shape who we become.

5.6 Conclusion

Telehealth's rapid and widespread integration into medical practice offers valuable lessons for understanding how new technologies reshape healthcare beyond their intended purposes. Our analysis reveals that technological innovation in medicine requires careful consideration along three critical dimensions. First, while the benefits of new technologies—such as improved accessibility and efficiency—are often readily apparent and quantifiable, their risks to the normative foundations of medicine are subtler and harder to measure. The ways in which new technologies can expand medicine into previously non-medical environments and affect provider-patient relationships, patient autonomy, personal identity, often emerge only through careful empirical study and may not be easily predictable in advance.

Second, the impact of healthcare technologies varies significantly across different contexts, populations, and specialties. The effectiveness and appropriateness of telehealth, for instance, depends heavily on factors such as existing provider-patient relationships, the nature of the medical condition, and the patient's social and psychological circumstances. This heterogeneity undermines simplistic narratives about technological progress in medicine and calls for nuanced, context-sensitive deployment strategies.

Third and perhaps most fundamentally, new technologies reshape not just what healthcare providers and patients can do but who they are and how they relate to one another. As healthcare becomes increasingly mediated by and dependent on technology, we must carefully consider how these changes affect the core human elements of medicine. The introduction of AI systems into healthcare amplifies these concerns. While such technologies promise unprecedented capabilities for diagnosis, monitoring, and treatment, they also risk reducing medicine to a series of technological transactions rather than a fundamentally human enterprise centered on care and healing.

As we move forward with implementing AI and other advanced technologies in healthcare, the lessons from telehealth remind us to balance innovation with preservation of medicine's essential human character and to be alert to unintended effects on non-medical normative concerns. Success in this endeavor will require ongoing collaboration between ethicists, healthcare providers, and technology developers to ensure that new technologies enhance rather than diminish the therapeutic relationship. The future of healthcare lies not in merely choosing between human care, on the one hand, and technological advancement, on the other hand, nor between efficiency and privacy, but in finding ways to integrate new technologies while preserving and strengthening the human values and relationships that lie at the foundation of good care.

References

Adams, Robin B., Victoria R. Nelson, and Bree E. Holtz. 2021. "Barriers for Telemedicine Use among Nonusers at the Beginning of the Pandemic." *Telemedicine Reports* 2 (1): 211–216. https://doi.org/10.1089/tmr.2021.0022.

Anderson, Andrew, Samantha S. O'Connell, Christina Thomas, and Rishab Chimmanamada. 2022. "Telehealth Interventions to Improve Diabetes Management among Black and Hispanic Patients: A Systematic Review and Meta-analysis." *Journal of Racial and Ethnic Health Disparities* 9 (6) (December): 2375–2386. https://doi.org/10.1007/s40615-021-01174-6.

Del Re, A. C., Christoph Flückiger, Adam O. Horvath, and Bruce E. Wampold. 2021. "Examining Therapist Effects in the Alliance-Outcome Relationship: A Multilevel Meta-analysis." *Journal of Consulting and Clinical Psychology* 89 (5) (May): 371–378. https://doi.org/10.1037/ccp0000637.

Esmaeili, Elham Davtalab, Hosein Azizi, Saeed Dastgiri, and Leila R. Kalankesh. 2023. "Does Telehealth Affect the Adherence to ART among Patients with HIV? A Systematic Review and Meta-analysis." *BMC Infectious Diseases* 23: article no. 169. https://doi.org/10.1186/s12879-023-08119-w.

Ftouni, Racha, Baraa AlJardali, Maya Hamdanieh, Louna Ftouni, and Nariman Salem. 2022. "Challenges of Telemedicine during the COVID-19 Pandemic: A Systematic Review." *BMC Medical Informatics and Decision Making* 22: article no. 207. https://doi.org/10.1186/s12911-022-01952-0.

Frittgen, Eva-Maria, and Joschka Haltaufderheide. 2022. "'Can You Hear Me?': Communication, Relationship, and Ethics in Video-Based Telepsychiatric Consultations." *Journal of Medical Ethics* 48 (1) (January): 22–30. https://doi.org/10.1136/medethics-2021-107434.

Hall, Mark A., and Deirdre McGraw. 2014. "For-Profit Enterprise in Health Care: Can It Contribute to Health Reform?" *Health Affairs* 33 (5) (May): 1489–1495. https://doi.org/10.1377/hlthaff.2013.0997.

Hensel, Jennifer M., Rebecca Yang, Simone N. Vigod, and Laura Desveaux. 2020. "Videoconferencing at Home for Psychotherapy in the Postpartum Period: Identifying Drivers of Successful Engagement and Important Therapeutic Conditions for Meaningful Use." *Counselling & Psychotherapy Research* 21 (3) (September): 535–544. https://doi.org/10.1002/capr.12372.

Ho, Anita. 2023. *Live Like Nobody Is Watching: Relational Autonomy in the Age of Artificial Intelligence Health Monitoring.* New York: Oxford University Press.

Jayasree, Arya, Padmavathi Shanmuganathan, Parthasarathy Ramamurthy, and M. C. Alwar. 2024. "Types of Medication Non-adherence and Approaches to Enhance Medication Adherence in Mental Health Disorders: A Narrative Review." *Indian Journal of Psychological Medicine* 46 (6) (November): 503–510. https://doi.org/10.1177/02537176241233745.

Krupnick, Janice L., Stuart M. Sotsky, Irene Elkin, Sam Simmens, Janet Moyer, John Watkins, and Paul A. Pilkonis. 2006. "The Role of the Therapeutic Alliance in Psychotherapy and Pharmacotherapy Outcome: Findings in the National Institute of Mental Health Treatment of Depression Collaborative Research Program." *Focus* 4 (2) (April): 269–277. https://doi.org/10.1176/foc.4.2.269.

Leiz, Maren, Nils Pfeuffer, Laura Rehner, Ulrike Stentzel, and Neeltje van den Berg. 2022. "Telemedicine as a Tool to Improve Medicine Adherence in Patients with Affective Disorders: A Systematic Literature Review." *Patient Preference and Adherence* 16: 3441–3463. https://doi.org/10.2147/PPA.S388106.

Masciari, Christopher F. 2025. "Motivational Barriers to Care and the Ethics of Encouragement." *American Journal of Bioethics Neuroscience* (March): 1–13. https://doi.org/10.1080/21507740.2025.2474228.

Moeller, Anne Marie, Lone F. Christensen, Jens Peter Hansen, and Pernille T. Andersen. 2022. "Patients' Acceptance of Video Consultations in the Mental Health Services: A Systematic Review and Synthesis of Qualitative Research." *Digital Health* 8. https://doi.org/10.1177/20552076221075148.

Myronuk, Lonn. 2022. "Effect of Telemedicine via Videoconference on Provider Fatigue and Empathy: Implications for the Quadruple Aim." *Healthcare Management Forum* 35 (3) (May): 174–178. https://doi.org/10.1177/08404704211059944.

Nickelson, D. W. 1998. "Telehealth and the Evolving Health Care System: Strategic Opportunities for Professional Psychology." *Professional Psychology: Research and Practice* 29 (6) (December): 527–535. https://doi.org/10.1037/0735-7028.29.6.527.

Palmer, Amitabha, and David Schwan. 2024. "More Process, Less Principles: The Ethics of Deploying AI and Robotics in Medicine." *Cambridge Quarterly of Healthcare Ethics* 33 (1) (January): 121–134. https://doi.org/10.1017/S0963180123000087.

Pols, Jeannette. 2012. *Care at a Distance: On the Closeness of Technology*. Amsterdam: Amsterdam University Press.

Ramaswamy, Ashwin, Miko Yu, Siri Drangsholt, Eric Ng, Patrick Culligan, Peter Schlegel, and Jim Hu. 2020. "Patient Satisfaction with Telemedicine during the COVID-19 Pandemic: Retrospective Cohort Study." *Journal of Medical Internet Research* 22 (9) (September): e20786. https://doi.org/10.2196/20786.

Simpson, Susan, Lorenzo Guerrini, and Shirley Rochford. 2015. "Telepsychology in a University Psychology Clinic Setting: A Pilot Project." *Australian Psychologist* 50 (4): 285–291. https://doi.org/10.1111/ap.12131.

Snoswell, Centaine L., Georgina Chelberg, Keshia R. De Guzman, Helen M. Haydon, Emma E. Thomas, Liam J. Caffery, and Anthony C. Smith. 2021. "The Clinical Effectiveness of Telehealth: A Systematic Review of Meta-analyses from 2010 to 2019." *Journal of Telemedicine and Telecare* 29 (9) (October): 669–684. https://doi.org/10.1177/1357633X211022907.

Stoll, Julia, Jonas Adrian Müller, and Manuel Trachsel. 2020. "Ethical Issues in Online Psychotherapy: A Narrative Review." *Frontiers in Psychiatry* 10: 933. https://doi.org/10.3389/fpsyt.2019.00993.

Tang, Michael, and Akhila Reddy. 2022. "Telemedicine and Its Past, Present, and Future Roles in Providing Palliative Care to Advanced Cancer Patients." *Cancers* 14 (8) (April 2): 1884. https://doi.org/10.3390/cancers14081884.

Taylor, Petroc. 2023. "U.S. Households with Internet Subscription 1997–2022." *Statista.* Last modified December 13, 2023. https://www.statista.com/statistics/189349/us-households-home-internet-connection-subscription/.

Tran, Steven, Lorraine Smith, and Stephen Carter. 2024. "Understanding Patient Perspectives on the Use of Gamification and Incentives in mHealth Applications to Improve Medication Adherence: Qualitative Study (Preprint)." *JMIR Mhealth and Uhealth* 12: e50851. https://doi.org/10.2196/50851.

Trondsen, Marianne V., Aksel Tjora, Alex Broom, and Graham Scambler. 2018. "The Symbolic Affordances of a Video-Mediated Gaze in Emergency Psychiatry." *Social Science & Medicine* 197 (January): 87–94. https://doi.org/10.1016/j.socscimed.2017.11.056.

Tyson, Alec, Giancarlo Pasquini, Alison Spencer, and Cary Funk. 2023. "60% of Americans Would Be Uncomfortable with Provider Relying on AI in Their Own Health Care." Pew Research Center. February 22. https://www.pewresearch.org/science/2023/02/22/60-of-americans-would-be-uncomfortable-with-provider-relying-on-ai-in-their-own-health-care/.

Ufholz, Kelsey, and Daksh Bhargava. 2021. "A Review of Telemedicine Interventions for Weight Loss." *Current Cardiovascular Risk Reports* 15: article no. 17. https://doi.org/10.1007/s12170-021-00680-w.

US Department of Health and Human Services. 2023. "Telehealth Policy Changes after the COVID-19 Public Health Emergency." Last modified December 19, 2023. https://telehealth.hhs.gov/providers/telehealth-policy/policy-changes-after-the-covid-19-public-health-emergency.

Vallor, Shannon. 2014. "Moral Deskilling and Upskilling in a New Machine Age: Reflections on the Ambiguous Future of Character." *Philosophy & Technology* 28: 107–124. https://doi.org/10.1007/s13347-014-0156-9.

van Gurp, Jelle, Martine van Selm, Kris Vissers, Evert van Leeuwen, and Jeroen Hasselaar. 2015. "How Outpatient Palliative Care Teleconsultation Facilitates Empathic Patient-Professional Relationships: A Qualitative Study." *PLOS One* 10 (4): e0124387. https://doi.org/10.1371/journal.pone.0124387.

WHO Global Observatory for eHealth. 2011. *mHealth: New Horizons for Health through Mobile Technologies: Second Global Survey on eHealth.* World Health Organization. https://iris.who.int/handle/10665/44607.

Amitabha (Ami) Palmer is an Assistant Professor and clinical ethicist at MD Anderson Cancer Center's Center for Clinical Ethics in Cancer Care, USA. He also holds an Affiliate Faculty position at the Institute for Data Science in Oncology, where he provides ethical guidance and education for the development and design pipeline of new AI tools. His primary areas of research within the ethics of AI in healthcare include participatory design, human-machine interaction, and deployment policy. A longtime researcher of medical misinformation, he has developed a conversation guide to help providers engage fruitfully with patients who endorse medical misinformation about cancer care.

Christopher F. Masciari is a postdoctoral fellow in clinical ethics at The University of Texas, MD Anderson Cancer Center in Houston, USA. He works mainly in the philosophy of mind; philosophy of the psychological, cognitive, and brain sciences; and biomedical ethics. Specifically, he works on questions to do with decision-making, autonomy, and consciousness. His approach is largely empirical, and much of his focus is on recent work in cognitive neuroscience and experimental psychology. Before coming to MD Anderson Cancer Center, he earned a PhD in Philosophy from the University of Maryland, College Park.

Chapter 6
On the Possible Impact of Robotic Childcare on Children's Brain Development and the Relevance of Social Structures

Kathinka Evers and Michele Farisco

Abstract Childcare robots are robotic devices designed to assist parents and caregivers in taking care of children. These robots can be equipped with various features such as telepresence and other remote monitoring capabilities, functions for entertainment and interactive play, educational content, and basic caregiving functions such as feeding or changing diapers. An application area of special interest focuses on supporting parenting in dual-income home environments, where both parents work and have limited time to be with their children and perform parenting tasks. In this paper, we discuss risks and benefits of childcare robots with the goal of identifying key factors relevant to the assessment of robotic childcare from psychological, neuroscientific, ethical, cultural, and sociopolitical perspectives. We propose a three-dimensional approach to the assessment of robotic childcare in terms of three distinct perspectives: type, context, and extent. Specifically, we focus primarily on the child's perspective and argue for the relevance of considering (1) the nature of the physical body of the child's caretaker, including the presence versus absence of a mind, that notably permits (or not) mutual psychological relationships; and (2) the effects that the introduction of robotic childcare may have on the broader cultural, economic, and sociopolitical context.

Keywords Childcare · Robotics · Brain development · Neuronal epigenesis · Neuroethics · Social structures

K. Evers · M. Farisco (✉)
Uppsala University, Uppsala, Sweden
e-mail: michele.farisco@uu.se

K. Evers
e-mail: kathinka.evers@uu.se

M. C. Altman and D. Schwan (eds.), *Ethics and Medical Technology*, The International Library of Bioethics 113, https://doi.org/10.1007/978-3-031-94690-5_6

6.1 Introduction: How and Why Robots Are Used in Childcare

For the sake of the present analysis, we define social robots as types of robots capable of performing tasks that generate responses in people who use them (Breazeal 2003; de Graaf et al. 2016; David et al. 2022). Importantly, social robots exhibit communicative skills, either linguistic or nonlinguistic, which facilitate their social interaction with users (Naneva et al. 2020). The acceptability of social robots depends on different factors, including the physical safety of using the robots (De Santis et al. 2008) and their psychological comfort for the user (Zanchettin et al. 2013). To increase their acceptability, social robots may be designed with a humanoid appearance (Eyssel et al. 2011). Overall, data tend to show a tendency toward accepting the use of social robots in a number of contexts (Sarda Gou et al. 2021; David et al. 2022; Dosso et al. 2022a, 2022b).

Childcare robots are robotic devices specifically designed to assist parents and caregivers in taking care of children. These robots can be equipped with various features such as telepresence and other remote monitoring capabilities, functions for entertainment and play, educational content, and basic caregiving functions such as feeding or changing diapers. Jieon Lee et al. (2022) provide an extensive overview of proposed child-robot connections, describing ways in which robotic devices can be used in childcare. For example, in relation to babies and toddlers (Abe et al. 2018), robots can potentially promote effective learning in classroom environments (Belpaeme et al. 2013; Fridin and Belokopytov 2013; Li 2015), enhance the persuasive quality of conveyed messages (for better or for worse) (Bainbridge et al. 2011; Jo et al. 2014), reduce stress, provide emotional relief for children, and even act as their friends and help them build social bonds (Belpaeme et al. 2013), going beyond mere educational purposes and functioning as effective tools for helping children to develop their personalities. Robots can also support parent-child communication (Oonaka 2013), provide entertainment (Kahn et al. 2012; Mwangi et al. 2017; Venture et al. 2017), help with the maintenance of children's behavioral records (Shiomi and Hagita 2017), and be used for mental health interventions (Cabibihan et al. 2013; Clabaugh et al. 2018; Kabacinska et al. 2021). The authors argue that, in view of these possible benefits, social robots can play important roles in child development, combining both the acquisition of specific notions (i.e., educational/intellectual development) and the capacity for mature social and relational skills (i.e., wide sociocultural development).

Different reasons may justify the use of robots in childcare, including technical (e.g., the robots' reliability and functional efficiency), social (e.g., limited time for childcare in some families), and moral (e.g., the robots may avoid or minimize risks of misconduct such as harassment or verbal violence) reasons. On the other hand, objections to their use can be similarly construed: the robots may be technically unreliable and functionally inefficient, create an incentive for parents to spend even less time with and caring for the children, or make parents less sensitive to the importance of physically interacting with their children. The use of robots may also reduce the tenderness of personal contact, physical or verbal. An application area of special interest focuses on supporting parenting in dual-income home environments, where both parents work and have limited time to be with their children and perform parenting tasks. This is especially relevant in societies that do not offer easy and affordable access to high-quality childcare. These parents may be concerned that their limitations in this regard might hinder the children's intellectual and emotional development (Henrich 2014; Hsin and Felfe 2014), and consequently may be more prone to use social robots designed to bridge this gap in nurturing (Kwak et al. 2008; Arroyo et al. 2017), in addition to, or instead of, other alternative forms of childcare.

The question arises how this partial replacement of human care by machine actions might affect the infant or child. As mentioned above, childcare robots can be equipped with systems for telepresence, offering parents the possibility to compensate for their physical distance, but the fact remains that robots physically replace human caretakers. Since the human physicality (the presence of a human body) of parental relationships may arguably be considered as crucial for their effectiveness (e.g., to fulfill a number of children's needs [see below]), its virtualization through childcare robots raises issues analogous to its complete replacement. That is to say, to the extent that children need body contact with their caretakers, the virtualization and the complete absence of the relationship with them have similar, if not the same, negative ethical valence.

Assuming, for the sake of the discussion, that the machines are technically safe (that they will not put the baby in the oven instead of the chicken, or put the diapers over the infant's face, for example), is this technical and social development positive from the child's point of view? For instance, does the use of childcare robots lead to the enrichment of psychological and social skills, or may it instead prevent or hinder them? Can we anticipate any significant societal benefits or drawbacks?

We shall address this kind of question from psychological, neuroscientific, ethical, cultural, and sociopolitical perspectives. Acknowledging that the use of robots to complement or replace human caregivers may have great value for caretakers (whether parents or significant others), not least in liberating women who presently carry most of the burden for childcare globally, our analyses will focus primarily on the needs of children. However, in the course of the discussion, broader sociopolitical implications of introducing human-machine replacements in childcare will also briefly be mentioned.

6.2 The Infant Brain

In order properly to evaluate the possible benefits and risks of introducing robots into childcare, there are several specific needs of infants and children that are important to consider in terms of infant brain development. The extent to which these needs are or can be met by robots is crucial to the relevance and value of using robots in childcare. There are several academic disciplines studying this, notably psychology and neuroscience. We shall describe some relevant neuroscientific data and theories that are well established and not subject to notable controversy.

Human brain maturation, including the formation of synapses, is both prenatal and postnatal; it is far from complete at birth. In the course of growing up, the infant develops a capacity to focus its attention. It learns to distinguish between and recognize objects in its environment, such as faces, and becomes aware of itself as standing in various relations to these objects. Conscious processing develops into auto-distinction (when "this-here" is distinguished from "that-there"). Further developed, the individual becomes aware of itself as a subject of experience and ascribes mental states to itself: auto-distinction evolves into self-awareness (when "this-here" becomes "I"), normally at around one and a half years of age (Lagercrantz 2005), and possibly even earlier (Falck-Ytter et al. 2006). From the age of six to twelve months, the child typically sees a "sociable playmate" in the mirror's reflection. Self-admiring and embarrassment usually begin at twelve months, and at fourteen to twenty months most children demonstrate avoidance behaviors. Finally, at eighteen months, half of the children recognize the reflection in the mirror as their own, and by twenty to twenty-four months, 65% of the children had developed a conception and a memory of their own reflection, revealed for instance by them trying to evince marks on their own nose, taking advantage, in all these instances, of their episodic memory abilities (see Tulving 1983).

Evolutionary and developmental data indicate the following levels of consciousness (Lou et al. 2017):

- *Minimal consciousness*, "characterized by the capacity to display spontaneous motor activity and to create representations, for instance, from visual and auditory experience, to store them in long-term memory and use them, for instance, for approach and avoidance behaviour and for what is referred to as exploratory behaviour" (Changeux 2006, 2240). According to Marco Bartocci et al. (2006) and Lagercrantz and Changeux (2009), the twenty-five-to-thirty-week preterm fetus shows signs of minimal consciousness.
- *Recursive consciousness*, characterized "by functional use of objects and by proto-declarative pointing; … elaborate social interactions, imitation, social referencing and joint attention; … the capacity to hold several mental representations in memory simultaneously, and … to evaluate relations of self; … elementary forms of recursivity in the handling of representations, yet without mutual understanding" (Changeux 2006, 2240). The newborn infant exhibits sensory awareness, the ability to express emotions and processes mental representations (i.e., of a pacifier), and the ability to differentiate between self- and non-self-touch.
- *Explicit self-consciousness*, "characterized by self-recognition in mirror tests and by the use of single arbitrary rules with self-other distinction" (Changeux 2006, 2240). This level of consciousness develops at the end of the second year, together with working and episodic memory and some basic aspects of language (Posner and Rothbart 2007; Lou et al. 2017).

- *Reflective consciousness*, which entails "theory of mind and full conscious experience, with first person ontology and reportability" (Changeux 2006, 2240). This level of consciousness fully develops three to five years after birth.

The postnatal development of the human brain lasts considerably longer than in any other animal and, of particular relevance to our present discussion, social contacts and activities are crucial for this development to take place in an efficient and healthy manner. The most intense development occurs during the first two years, but it continues after puberty, and the highest executive functions that are determined by the frontal lobe are not fully mature until the age of around twenty-five, or even later (Lagercrantz 2005, 145–148). The environment is important for this process to be efficient. If neural networks are not active, they vanish: *Use it or lose it!* as the mantra goes (Lagercrantz 2005, 59). "In the absence of adequate stimulation, the cerebral network suffers irreversible injury" (Changeux 2004, 194). In fact, synapses are literally pruned on the basis of how much they are used.

Torsten Wiesel and David Hubel (1963) have, for example, demonstrated the irreversibility of lesions caused by experimental manipulation of the visual environment. By suturing the eyelid of a newborn monkey during its first six weeks of life, thus narrowing the columns corresponding to the closed eye (resulting in decreased vision or blindness), they established the existence of a sensitive period during which a reduction of sensory stimulation causes irreversible damage to cortical connectivity. Carla Shatz and her colleagues have subsequently shown through experiments with weasels that stimulation is necessary before the eye is even opened in order for synapses to develop adequate connectivity (Katz and Shatz 1996). It has been argued (e.g., by Eric Kandel) that early stimulation of children influences the formation of synapses; conversely, that lack of stimulation, poor nourishment, insecurity or absence of tender physical contact can give rise to serious brain damage (detectable, e.g., by fMRI [Lagercrantz 2005])—damage that can be irreversible.

There are a number of needs that must be satisfied in order for the infant brain to develop in a healthy and harmonious manner, including:

- Tactile stimulation (touch, cuddles, holding, feeling caregivers' skin and heartbeat, notably when being breast- or bottle-fed) (Hertenstein 2011). This is important because the infant is still unable to articulate and communicate its needs linguistically, as well as cognitively to process information from others. In other words, the emotionally salient body contact with caretakers is crucial for them to experience being part of an interactive relationship of care.
- Smell. Among the emotionally salient interactions with caretakers, smell is particularly relevant, since it elicits strong emotional experiences, including the development of valenced memory (Cameron 2018; Ingebretsen Kucirkova and Stray Gausel 2023).
- Eye contact. Another relevant channel for emotionally salient interactions between infants and caretakers is eye contact, which plays an important role for the development of a number of infants' capacities, including empathy and self-other distinction (Çetinçelik et al. 2021; Khaluyan et al. 2021; Wever et al. 2022).

- Facial expressions. Human infants mimic a lot and learn to consistently connect emotions and behavior through observing parents, which is important for their development (Nelson and Modloch 2018; Garcia and Tully 2020). In fact, infants learn through imitation (Wang et al. 2015; Altinok et al. 2023).
- Emotional responses. These include the capacity to learn the most appropriate emotions for the different experiences, as well as the distinction between a private (i.e., emotional) and public (i.e., behavioral) sphere. Again, the infants learn the alphabet of emotions and how to connect them to reality through imitation (Donohue et al. 2020).

The question here arises: to what extent can these needs be met by a machine?

6.3 A Three-Dimensional Approach to the Assessment of Robotic Childcare

For a childcare robot to be effective and its use positive for the child's development, we suggest that it should be able to, at least partly, meet the needs listed above and, in any case, not form an obstacle to their satisfaction. Some of them relate to the constitution (or physical nature) of both infants and caretakers, while others relate to their operational/functional capabilities. While robots can in principle replace humans for the latter, their use for fulfilling the first kind of needs is more challenging, at least to date.

The idea here is that, whereas robots may satisfy some infants' needs that depend only on executing some relevant functions (e.g., singing a lullaby) or for which the emulation of human features (e.g., facial expressions) is sufficient, they may be insufficient/unable to satisfy needs that are more deeply "physical" in both their origin and satisfaction (e.g., emotional bonding mediated by physical touch with a warm-blooded body). We should note that we are here referring to contemporary robots that do not have, for example, heartbeats or a warm-blooded body. If future technical developments alter this, the corresponding human–machine comparisons will have to be adapted.

This line of thought introduces three distinct perspectives that need to be considered: type, context, and extent. The evaluation of using robots in childcare will depend on the type of care it is intended for—and in what context—as well as the extent to which it is supposed to be used. We propose this three-dimensional evaluation as a useful approach to the assessment of childcare robots. Are we, for example, speaking about complementing or replacing human caregivers? And in which context? Relevant factors to consider are: the age of the child, the type of robot-child interaction, the type of family or parent (age, education, socioeconomic status, etc.), the broader social and human environment beyond the family, and the cultural and sociopolitical structures in which the child develops.

Against the background of the epigenetic development of the infant brain (by which we mean the cultural-social influence over the developing brain's architecture) and of the socioeconomic factors impacting the acceptability and effectiveness of using childcare robots, many questions arise about potential risks and benefits of using childcare robots. Before introducing some illustrative issues, we want to highlight the need to avoid an anthropocentric bias against the use of robots—that is, the idea that robotic childcare is intrinsically defective and worse than the direct human involvement in childcare. We propose a more balanced view, for instance, by not depicting human parenting as essentially idyllic while at the same time trying to identify what (if any) only humans can give to children, and examining whether the related limitation of robots is intrinsic to them or rather dependent on the level of presently available technology. We also avoid describing the "family" as a parent–child nuclear family, since in the contemporary world, numerous children grow up in other social formations—for example, with one parent (usually the mother) and an extended family of significant others (other relatives, friends, neighbors, etc.).

In what follows we shall argue specifically for the relevance of (1) the nature of the physical body of the child's caretaker, including the presence versus absence of a mind that notably permits (or not) mutual psychological relationships; and (2) the effects that the introduction of robotic childcare may have on the broader cultural, economic, and sociopolitical context.

6.3.1 *The Importance of Bodies, Minds, and the Capacity for Mutuality*

We identified above a number of infants' needs that are connected to the epigenetic development of their brains. These include the need for tactile stimulation, smell, eye contact, facial expressions, and emotional responses, among others. As mentioned above, the satisfaction of some of these needs (i.e., tactile stimulation, smell, eye contact) requires the kind of physical (i.e., bodily) constitution that is presently typical of humans. With this we are not endorsing any form of biological chauvinism or essentialism, but merely point to certain features that human bodies presently have and that robots presently lack. Also, robots have a body, but that body is (so far) devoid of some features (e.g., warm blood, emotionality, value-based empathy capacity) that appear to be crucial for fulfilling some of the needs of infants in their development. As we said above, this may change in the future.

Importantly, the human body allows a form of mutuality. In fact, mutuality requires that behaviors are not simply the execution of functions but real manifestation of deliberate choices accompanied by subjectively salient experiences. For instance, happy facial expressions or joyful emotions may be displayed by robots while they are actually unable to really experience joy. This may be considered an ethically negative limitation of robots, which goes against their use in childcare, especially in situations where emotional responses are required. It may be objected that this depends on whether "perceived" mutuality is what really counts: in fact, robots may to some extent (and in the future may perfectly) imitate emotions, and this imitation may arguably be sufficient for the appropriate experience of mutuality by the child. Yet the question remains open whether this form of gaming emotionality can replace genuine human emotionality; and, if not, if it is of lesser value from the child's point of view, and if this then is ethically acceptable. As a general criterion, we have previously suggested that the use of AI (including robotics) is ethically problematic in contexts where features and capabilities that are (at least to date) specific to humans are required (Farisco et al. 2020).

That said, we note that human caregivers may engage in various forms of "emotional labor," expressing certain positive attitudes even though they do not feel them, due to fatigue, etc. Moreover, any capacity and characteristic of parents (and human caretakers more broadly) can have negative versions: emotional responses can be negative, and aggressive behavior, including violent educational practices, can cause great damage to children. In these cases, the use of neutral childcare robots would arguably be preferable to (such) human caretakers. While this conclusion may be valid in some cases, we should also note that children can learn the sensitivity to diverse relational/emotional experiences through their parents and/or other human caretakers. While these experiences may be positive or negative, parenthood and other forms of human caretaking help children to avoid becoming "emotionally blind" (i.e., unable to experience, detect, and express emotions, either positive or negative). Moreover, a child who is mostly used to robot company and is not accustomed to the varied, and sometimes intense and rapid, human emotional expressions and reactions, may become less able or even unable to deal with them when they occur (for example, the child may find the human emotionality scary and withdraw). This may then hamper that child's social development and future social capacities to engage maturely in human contexts. Importantly, reliance on social robotics for children (versus developed adults) has a potential for harm in social development that is more substantial at an earlier age and (perhaps) more likely to produce longer-term problems than a similar (social) technology used by adults. Even if social robots develop to the point where they seem to be able to replicate an adult caregiver, their introduction will also be somewhat experimental at key moments of a child's development, and we might imagine that placing tighter restrictions on this use than among adults (e.g., companion robots for adults or elderly individuals) is ethically recommendable.

It is relevant to note here the recent recommendation (2024) issued by COMETS (the ethics committee of the Centre National de la Recherche Scientifique [CNRS]) calling for further research and vigilance regarding the effects that the use of so-called "social" robots have or may have on humans and human relations (Pelachaud et al. 2024).

This point also highlights the relevance of considering the dimension of extent. We have little doubt that both families and children could benefit from using some robotic devices. For example, a cute robot could be a sophisticated and fun toy, sing soothing lullabies, help ensure safety around the house, help children with special needs (e.g., autism), and so on. Such uses would hardly constitute any hindrance for the child's development in any obvious way but can on the contrary support it. Concerns arise when the robotic complement begins to approach an increasingly large and perhaps almost complete *replacement* of human caregivers in contexts where human aspects of care are more crucial, some of which we outline above.

Another ethically salient dimension of using childcare robots is the use of misleading terms that result from an anthropomorphic view of the robots. This is the case, for instance, when the term "interaction" is applied to the child-robot relation or the term "collaboration" applied to the human caretaker-robot relation. In both cases, the question arises whether a real relationship of reciprocity between two agents is in place, or rather the interaction originates from only one of the two involved terms (e.g., from children only, while the robots only more or less automatically react to their inputs). These are not only linguistic details but ethically salient linguistic choices that impact the way we perceive, accept, or refuse (in a word: evaluate) technology.

6.3.2 *Cultural, Political, and Socioeconomic Perspectives on Robotic Childcare*

The social context is highly relevant when assessing robotic childcare. Although our aim in this paper is not primarily focused on the possible societal impacts of this technological development, we still find it useful briefly to draw attention to the relevance of sociopolitical factors for analyzing the use of childcare robots and to some important issues that may arise from such use.

Different societies have very different structures regarding childcare, in part due to deep cultural divergences in how infants/children, parenting, education, gender equity, and families are conceived (Georgas 2003; Bornstein 2012; Lansford 2022; Ria Novianti-Nur 2023). In some societies, a system of high-quality, human-staffed nurseries is well developed. In Sweden, for example, they are widely accessible, with 86% of children age one to five enrolled in 2022 (see Skolverket 2024). In France, the attendance of children in nurseries (free of charge) is obligatory from the age of three (see Ministère de l'Éducation nationale 2024). These nurseries offer children social activities and help with their upbringing and social development whether or not they come from dual-income families. The underlying ideology includes (among other things) the idea that children benefit from contact with other children in organized settings from an early age (see, e.g., Wilford 2009), and the idea that women and men share equal responsibility for childcare and should have equal opportunities to pursue their respective education, career, and so on. In these societies, robotic childcare would probably not be considered necessary, although they could still be considered useful. Moreover, if children have already spent their day away from the parents or primary caregivers, replacing them with robots to care for the children in the evening/night as well may be considered too extensive from the point of view of the child's well-being and sound development, assuming that spending time with human caregivers is better for a child than not spending time with them; and, in particular, assuming that a specific child's family is a good environment for its well-being and development.

In societies with an advanced system of nurseries and politics of parental equity (e.g., assuring paid parental leave for each gender), the introduction of robotic childcare could possibly even be seen as a threat to the system. If, say, robotic childcare would be less expensive for the state than nurseries, one can easily envisage a political push to replace nurseries (no matter how well they function) with home-robots, to save money for the state.

In other countries, such as Italy, where the dominant ideology is more conservative, there are far less developed nursery-systems, and the responsibility for childcare is placed directly on the parents, above all the mother, who receives very little state-funded assistance for the task (notwithstanding some recent attempts by the government to financially support the use of nurseries). The latest available statistics (from 2021) indicate that national nurseries can host a maximum of 28% of children, against the target of 45% set by the European Council in 2022 (Instituto Nazionale di Statistica 2023). The situation is even worse if we take territorial differences into account, with a large difference between northern and southern regions, where the numbers are much lower (around 10%). Overall, 33.4% of children under three years old attend nurseries in Italy (compared to the European average of 37.9%).

The potential value of robotic help increases in such contexts, at least from the caregivers' (especially mothers') point of view. Home robots could revolutionize the lives of primary caregivers (typically women) to whom robotic assistance could offer valuable time to pursue activities other than caregiving, such as work or education. Robots could "lift the burden of women's care work" (Parks 2010), although this would not necessarily be a value from a conservative government's point of view, if, or to the extent that, it endorses an ideology aiming to keep women socially subordinate, notably in education and professional life. Another socioeconomic consideration is whether this assistance would be available only for those who can afford it. Or is it also possible to offer assistance to families of modest economic means (who cannot afford expensive daycare or private human assistance)? It is beyond the scope of the present paper to analyze more deeply this type of sociopolitical and economic issues, but even so, it is important to consider socioeconomic factors in addressing the use of childcare robots and to the need to assess the (positive or negative) impact that the introduction of robotic childcare may have upon society.

6.4 Conclusion

We have here proposed a three-dimensional evaluation as a useful approach to assess childcare robots, with three factors that need to be considered: type, context, and extent. The evaluation of using robots in childcare will depend on the type of care it is intended for, in what context, and the extent to which it is used.

Focusing primarily on the child's perspective, in particular on requirements for healthy brain development in infants and children, we have argued for the relevance of the nature of the physical body of the child's caretaker, including the presence versus absence of a mind that notably permits (or not) mutual psychological relationships. We suggested that the satisfaction of some infants' needs (i.e., tactile stimulation, smell, eye contact) requires the kind of physical (i.e., bodily) constitution that is presently typical of humans. Robots may satisfy some infants' needs that depend only on executing some relevant functions (e.g., singing a lullaby), or for which the emulation of human features (e.g., facial expressions) is sufficient. In contrast, they are less able (if at all) to satisfy needs that are more deeply "physical," more precisely biological, in both their origin and satisfaction (e.g., emotional bonding mediated by physical touch with a warm-blooded body). It seems likely that both families and children could benefit from using some robotic devices, but if or when the robotic complement begins to approach an increasingly large and perhaps almost complete replacement of human caregivers in contexts where (presently specific) human aspects of care are more crucial, concerns arise. Relevant factors to consider are: the age of the child; the type of robot-child connection; the type of family, parent, or caregiver (age, education, socioeconomic status, etc.); the broader social and human environment beyond the family; and the cultural and sociopolitical structures in which the child develops. Technological and social inventions such as childcare robots do not occur in a political void but can have strong sociopolitical and economic impact, differently depending on which social context we are analyzing. A fuller assessment of the pros and cons of introducing robots in childcare will need to be interdisciplinary and involve psychological, social, and political sciences, including gender studies, in addition to the technical and scientific expertise.[1]

References

Abe, Kasumi, Masahiro Shiomi, Yachao Pei, Tingyi Zhang, Narumitsu Ikeda, and Takayuki Nagai. 2018. "ChiCaRo: Tele-Presence Robot for Interacting with Babies and Toddlers." *Advanced Robotics* 32 (4): 176–190. https://doi.org/10.1080/01691864.2018.1434014.

Altınok, Nazli, Harriet Over, and Malinda Carpenter. 2023. "Young Children Use Imitation Communicatively." *Journal of Experimental Child Psychology* 231 (July): article no. 105654. https://doi.org/10.1016/j.jecp.2023.105654.

Arroyo, Dante, Yuichi Ishiguro, and Fumihide Tanaka. 2017. "Design of a Home Telepresence Robot System for Supporting Childcare." In *Companion of the 2017 ACM Conference on Computer Supported Cooperative Work and Social Computing*, 131–134. New York: ACM Press. https://doi.org/10.1145/3022198.30263.

Bainbridge, Wilma A., Justin W. Hart, Elizabeth S. Kim, and Brian Scassellati. 2011. "The Benefits of Interactions with Physically Present Robots over Video-Displayed Agents." *International Journal of Social Robotics* 3 (1) (January): 41–52. https://doi.org/10.1007/s12369-010-0082-7.

[1] This research has received funding from the project Counterfactual Assessment and Valuation for Awareness Architecture—CAVAA (European Commission, EIC 101,071,178). We thank our colleagues at CRB for their comments at a higher seminar which helped us to improve the clarity of the text.

Bartocci, Marco, Lena L. Bergqvist, Hugo Lagercrantz, and K. J. S. Anand. 2006. "Pain Activates Cortical Areas in the Preterm Newborn Brain." *Pain* 122 (1) (May): 109–117. https://doi.org/10.1016/j.pain.2006.01.015.

Belpaeme, Tony, Paul Baxter, Robin Read, Rachel Wood, Heriberto Cuayáhuitl, Bernd Kiefer, Stefania Racioppa, et al. 2013. "Multimodal Child-Robot Interaction: Building Social Bonds." *Journal of Human-Robot Interaction* 1 (2) (January): 33–53. https://doi.org/10.5898/JHRI.1.2.Belpaeme.

Bornstein, Marc H. 2012. "Cultural Approaches to Parenting." *Parenting: Science and Practices* 12: 212–221. https://doi.org/10.1080/15295192.2012.683359

Breazeal, Cynthia. 2003. "Emotion and Sociable Humanoid Robots." *International Journal of Human-Computer Studies* 59 (1–2) (July): 119–155. https://doi.org/10.1016/S1071-5819(03)00018-1.

Cabibihan, John-John, Hifza Javed, Marcelo Ang, and Sharifah Mariam Aljunied. 2013. "Why Robots? A Survey on the Roles and Benefits of Social Robots in the Therapy of Children with Autism." *International Journal of Social Robotics* 5 (4) (November): 593–618. https://doi.org/10.1007/s12369-013-0202-2.

Cameron, E. L. 2018. "Olfactory Perception in Children." *World Journal Otorhinolaryngology-Head and Neck Surgery* 4 (1) (March): 57–66. https://doi.org/10.1016/j.wjorl.2018.02.002.

Çetinçelik, M., C. F. Rowland, and T. M. Snijders. 2020. "Do the Eyes Have It? A Systematic Review on the Role of Eye Gaze in Infant Language Development." *Frontiers in Psychology* 11: article no. 589096. https://doi.org/10.3389/fpsyg.2020.589096.

Changeux, Jean-Pierre. 2004. *The Physiology of Truth: Neuroscience and Human Knowledge.* Cambridge, MA: Belknap.

Changeux, Jean-Pierre. 2006. "The Ferrier Lecture 1998: The Molecular Biology of Consciousness Investigated with Genetically Modified Mice." *Philosophical Transactions of the Royal Society B: Biological Sciences* 361 (1476) (December 29): 2239–2259. https://doi.org/10.1098/rstb.2006.1832.

Clabaugh, Caitlyn E., David Becerra, Eric Deng, Gisele Ragusa, and Maja J. Matarić. 2018. "Month-Long, In-Home Case Study of a Socially Assistive Robot for Children with Autism Spectrum Disorder." In *Companion of the 2018 ACM/IEEE International Conference on Human-Robot Interaction*, 87–88. New York: ACM Press. https://doi.org/10.1145/3173386.317701.

David, Dayle, Pierre Thérouanne, and Isabelle Milhabet. 2022. "The Acceptability of Social Robots: A Scoping Review of the Recent Literature." *Computers in Human Behavior* 137 (December): article no. 107419. https://doi.org/10.1016/j.chb.2022.107419.

de Graaf, Maartje M. A., Somaya Ben Allouch, and Jan A. G. M. van Dijk. 2016. "Long-Term Evaluation of a Social Robot in Real Homes." *Interaction Studies* 17 (3): 461–490. https://doi.org/10.1075/is.17.3.08deg.

De Santis, Agostino, Bruno Siciliano, Alessandro De Luca, and Antonio Bicchi. 2008. "An Atlas of Physical Human-Robot Interaction." *Mechanism and Machine Theory* 43 (3) (March): 253–270. https://doi.org/10.1016/j.mechmachtheory.2007.03.003.

Donohue, Meghan Rose, Rebecca A. Williamson, and Erin C. Tully. 2020. "Toddlers Imitate Prosocial Demonstrations in Bystander but Not Transgressor Contexts." *Journal of Experimental Child Psychology* 192 (April): article no. 104776. https://doi.org/10.1016/j.jecp.2019.104776.

Dosso, Jill A., Ela Bandari, Aarti Malhotra, Gabriella K. Guerra, Jesse Hoey, François Michaud, Tony J. Prescott, and Julie M. Robillard. 2022a. "User Perspectives on Emotionally Aligned Social Robots for Older Adults and Persons Living with Dementia." *Journal of Rehabilitation and Assistive Technologies Engineering* 9. https://doi.org/10.1177/20556683221108364.

Dosso, Jill A., Ela Bandari, Aarti Malhotra, Jesse Hoey, Francois Michaud, Tony J. Prescott, and Julie M. Robillard. 2022b. "Towards Emotionally Aligned Social Robots for Dementia: Perspectives of Care Partners and Persons with Dementia." *Alzheimer's & Dementia* 18 (S2) (December): e059261. https://doi.org/10.1002/alz.059261.

Evers, Kathinka. 2015. "Can We Be Epigenetically Proactive?" In *Open Mind: Philosophy and the Mind Sciences in the 21st century*, eds. Thomas Metzinger and Jennifer M. Windt, 497–518. Cambridge, MA: MIT Press. https://doi.org/10.7551/mitpress/10603.003.0040.

Evers, Kathinka, and Jean-Pierre Changeux. 2016. "Proactive Epigenesis and Ethical Innovation: A Neuronal Hypothesis for the Genesis of Ethical Rules." *EMBO Reports* 17 (10) (October): 1361–1364. https://doi.org/10.15252/embr.201642783.

Eyssel, Friedericke, Dieta Kuchenbrandt, and Simon Bobinger. 2011. "Effects of Anticipated Human-Robot Interaction and Predictability of Robot Behavior on Perceptions of Anthropomorphism." In *HRI '11: Proceedings of the 6th International Conference on Human-Robot Interaction*, 61–68. New York: Association for Computing Machinery. https://doi.org/10.1145/1957656.1957673.

Falck-Ytter, Terje, Gustaf Gredebäck, and Claes von Hofsten. 2006. "Infants Predict Other People's Action Goals." *Nature Neuroscience* 9 (7) (July): 878–879. https://doi.org/10.1038/nn1729.

Farisco, Michele, Kathinka Evers, and Arleen Salles. 2020. "Towards Establishing Criteria for the Ethical Analysis of Artificial Intelligence." *Science and Engineering Ethics* 26: 2413–2425. https://doi.org/10.1007/s11948-020-00238-w.

Fridin, Marina, and Mark Belokopytov. 2014. "Acceptance of Socially Assistive Humanoid Robot by Preschool and Elementary School Teachers." *Computers in Human Behavior* 33 (April): 23–31. https://doi.org/10.1016/j.chb.2013.12.016.

Garcia, Sarah E., and Eric C. Tully. 2020. "Children's Recognition of Happy, Sad, and Angry Facial Expressions across Emotive Intensities." *Journal of Experimental Child Psychology* 197 (September): article no. 104881. https://doi.org/10.1016/j.jecp.2020.104881.

Georgas, James. 2003. "Family: Variations and Changes across Cultures." *Online Readings in Psychology and Culture* 6 (3). https://doi.org/10.9707/2307-0919.1061.

Heinrich, Carolyn J. 2014. "Parents' Employment and Children's Wellbeing." *Future of Children* 24 (1) (Spring): 121–146. https://doi.org/10.1353/foc.2014.0000.

Hertenstein, Matthew J. 2011. "Tactile Stimulation." In *Encyclopedia of Child Behavior and Development*, eds. Sam Goldstein and Jack A. Naglieri, 1469–1471. Boston: Springer. https://doi.org/10.1007/978-0-387-79061-9_2867.

Hsin, Amy, and Christina C. Felfe. 2014. "When Does Time Matter? Maternal Employment, Children's Time with Parents, and Child Development." *Demography* 51 (5) (October 1): 1867–1894. https://doi.org/10.1007/s13524-014-0334-5.

Ingebretsen Kucirkova, Natalia, and Elisabeth Stray Gausel. 2023. "Incorporating Smell into Children's Museums: Insights from a Case Study in Norway." *Curator* 66 (4) (October): 547–559. https://doi.org/10.1111/cura.12573.

Instituto Nazionale di Statistica. 2023. "Statistiche Report: Offerta di Nidi e Servizi Integrativi per la Prima Infanzia, Anno Edicativo 2021/2022." November 23. https://www.istat.it/wp-content/uploads/2023/11/REPORT-ASILI2021-2022.pdf.

Jo, Doori, Jae-gil Lee, and Kun Chang Lee. 2014. "Empirical Analysis of Changes in Human Creativity in People Who Work with Humanoid Robots and Their Avatars." In *Learning and Collaboration Technologies: Designing and Developing Novel Learning Experiences*, eds. Panayiotis Zaphiris and Andri Ioannou, 273–281. Cham: Springer. https://doi.org/10.1007/978-3-319-07482-5_26.

Kabacińska, Katarzyna, Tony J. Prescott, and Julie M. Robillard. 2021. "Socially Assistive Robots as Mental Health Interventions for Children: A Scoping Review." *International Journal of Social Robotics* 13 (5) (August): 919–935. https://doi.org/10.1007/s12369-020-00679-0.

Kahn, Peter H. Jr., Heather E. Gary, and Solace Shen. 2013. "Children's Social Relationships with Current and Near-Future Robots." *Child Development Perspectives* 7 (1) (March): 32–37. https://doi.org/10.1111/cdep.12011.

Katz, L. C., and C. J. Shatz. 1996. "Synaptic Activity and the Construction of Cortical Circuits." *Science* 274 (5290) (November 15): 1133–1138. https://doi.org/10.1126/science.274.5290.1133.

Khalulyan, Allie, Katie Byrd, Jonathan Tarbox, Alexandra Little, and Henrike Moll. 2021. "The Role of Eye Contact in Young Children's Judgments of Others' Visibility: A Comparison of Preschoolers with and without Autism Spectrum Disorder." *Journal of Communication Disorders* 89 (January-February): article no. 106075. https://doi.org/10.1016/j.jcomdis.2020.106075.

Kwak, Sonya, Jinyung Jung, Eunmee Shin, and Myung Suk Kim. 2008. "Design Guidelines for Childcare Robots with an Ethnographic Studies of Dual Income and Single Income." *Bulletin of Japanese Society for the Science of Design* 55 (2): 65–74. https://doi.org/10.11247/jssdj.55.65_2

Lagercrantz, Hugo. 2005. *I barnets hjärna.* Stockholm: Bonnier Fakta.

Lagercrantz, Hugo, and Jean-Pierre Changeux. 2009. "The Emergence of Human Consciousness: From Fetal to Neonatal Life." *Pediatric Research* 65 (3) (March): 255–260. https://doi.org/10.1203/PDR.0b013e3181973b0d.

Lansford, J. E. 2022. "Annual Research Review: Cross-Cultural Similarities and Differences in Parenting." *Journal of Child Psychology and Psychiatry* 63 (4) (April): 466–479. https://doi.org/10.1111/jcpp.13539.

Lee, Jieon, Daeho Lee, and Jae-gil Lee. 2022. "Can Robots Help Working Parents with Childcare? Optimizing Childcare Functions for Different Parenting Characteristics." *International Journal of Social Robotics* 14 (1) (January): 193–211. https://doi.org/10.1007/s12369-021-00784-8.

Li, Jamy. 2015. "The Benefit of Being Physically Present: A Survey of Experimental Works Comparing Copresent Robots, Telepresent Robots and Virtual Agents." *International Journal of Human-Computer Studies* 77 (May): 23–37. https://doi.org/10.1016/j.ijhcs.2015.01.001.

Lou, H. C., J. P. Changeux, and A. Rosenstand. 2017. "Towards a Cognitive Neuroscience of Self-Awareness." *Neuroscience & Biobehavioral Reviews* 83 (December): 765–773. https://doi.org/10.1016/j.neubiorev.2016.04.004.

Ministère de l'Éducation nationale. 2024. "L'école maternelle." Accessed October 2, 2024. https://www.education.gouv.fr/l-ecole-maternelle-11534.

Mwangi, Eunice, Emilia I. Barakova, Marta Diaz, Andreu Català Mallofre, and Matthias Rauterberg. 2017. "Gaze-Based Hints during Child-Robot Gameplay." In *Social Robotics: 9th International Conference, ICSR 2017, Tsukuba, Japan, November 22–24, 2017, Proceedings*, eds. Abderrahmane Kheddar et al., 413–422. Cham: Springer. https://doi.org/10.1007/978-3-319-70022-9_41.

Naneva, Stanislava, Marina Sarda Gou, Thomas L. Webb, and Tony J. Prescott. 2020. "A Systematic Review of Attitudes, Anxiety, Acceptance, and Trust towards Social Robots." *International Journal of Social Robotics* 12 (6) (December): 1179–1201. https://doi.org/10.1007/s12369-020-00659-4.

Nelson, Nicole L., and Catherine J. Mondloch. 2018. "Children's Visual Attention to Emotional Expressions Varies with Stimulus Movement." *Journal of Experimental Child Psychology* 172 (August): 13–24. https://doi.org/10.1016/j.jecp.2018.03.001.

Novianti, Ria, Suarman, and Nur Islami. 2023. "Parenting in Cultural Perspective: A Systematic Review of Paternal Role across Cultures." *Journal of Ethnic and Cultural Studies* 10 (1): 22–44. https://doi.org/10.29333/ejecs/1287.

Oonaka, Shinichi. 2013. Child-care robot and a method of controlling the robot. US Patent 8,376,803, filed March 25, 2005, and issued February 19, 2013.

Parks, Jennifer A. 2010. "Lifting the Burden of Women's Care Work: Should Robots Replace the 'Human Touch'?" *Hypatia* 25 (1) (Winter): 100–120. https://doi.org/10.1111/j.1527-2001.2009.01086.x.

Pelachaud, Catherine, Patrice Debré, Christine Noiville, Raja Chatila, and Jean-Gabriel Ganascia (Comité Ethique). 2024. COMETS Avis 2024–46 *Le phénomène d'attachement aux robots dits <<sociaux>>. Pour une vigilance de la recherche scientifique.* 2024–46, CNRS COMETS. hal–04692480.

Posner, Michael I., and Mary K. Rothbart. 2007. *Educating the Human Brain.* Washington, DC: American Psychological Association.

Sarda Gou, Marina, Thomas L. Webb, and Tony Prescott. 2021. "The Effect of Direct and Extended Contact on Attitudes towards Social Robots." *Heliyon* 7 (3) (March): e06418. https://doi.org/10.1016/j.heliyon.2021.e06418.

Shiomi, Masahiro, and Norihiro Hagita. 2017. "Social Acceptance toward a Childcare Support Robot System: Web-Based Cultural Differences Investigation and a Field Study in Japan." *Advanced Robotics* 31 (14): 727–738. https://doi.org/10.1080/01691864.2017.1345322.

Skolverket. 2024. "Statistik." Accessed October 2, 2024. https://www.skolverket.se/skolutveckling/statistic.

Tulving, Endel. 1983. *Elements of Episodic Memory.* New York: Oxford University Press.

Venture, Gentiane, Bipin Indurkhya, and Takamune Izui. 2017. "Dance with Me! Child-Robot Interaction in the Wild." In *Social Robotics: 9th International Conference, ICSR 2017, Tsukuba, Japan, November 22–24, 2017, Proceedings*, eds. Abderrahmane Kheddar et al., 375–382. Cham: Springer. https://doi.org/10.1007/978-3-319-70022-9_37.

Wang, Zhidan, Rebecca A. Williamson, and Andrew N. Meltzoff. 2015. "Imitation as a Mechanism in Cognitive Development: A Cross-Cultural Investigation of 4-Year-Old Children's Rule Learning." *Frontiers in Psychology* 6: article no. 562. https://doi.org/10.3389/fpsyg.2015.00562.

Wever, Mirjam C. M., Lisanne A. E. M. van Houtum, Loes H. C. Janssen, Wilma G. M. Wentholt, Iris M. Spruit, Marieke S. Tollenaar, Geert-Jan Will, and Bernet M. Elzinga. 2022. "Neural and Affective Responses to Prolonged Eye Contact with One's Own Adolescent Child and Unfamiliar Others." *NeuroImage* 260 (October 15): article no. 119463. https://doi.org/10.1016/j.neuroimage.2022.119463.

Wiesel, Torsten N., and David H. Hubel. 1963. "Effects of Visual Deprivation on Morphology and Physiology of Cells in the Cats Lateral Geniculate Body." *Journal of Neurophysiology* 26: 978–993.

Wilford, Sara. 2009. *Nurturing Young Children's Disposition to Learn.* St. Paul, MN: Redleaf.

Zanchettin, Andrea Maria, Luca Bascetta, and Paolo Rocco. 2013. "Acceptability of Robotic Manipulators in Shared Working Environments through Human-like Redundancy Resolution." *Applied Ergonomics* 44 (6) (November): 982–989. https://doi.org/10.1016/j.apergo.2013.03.028.

Kathinka Evers is Professor of Philosophy, Senior Researcher at the Centre for Research Ethics & Bioethics (CRB) at Uppsala University, Sweden, and Professor ad honoram at the *Universidad Central de Chile*, Santiago. She has been Invited Professor on the Chair Condorcet at École Normale Supérieure, Paris (2002); and at *Collège de France*, Paris (2006-7). From 2013-21, she was a member of the Science and Infrastructure Board of the European Human Brain Project (HBP), leading the Philosophy and Neuroethics research. Today, she co-leads philosophy research in Horizon 2020 projects Neurotwin and CAVAA. Her research focuses on philosophy of mind and brain, artificial intelligence, bioethics, and neuroethics.

Michele Farisco is part of the Centre for Research Ethics & Bioethics (CRB) at Uppsala University, Sweden, and Head of the Bioethics Unit at Biogem, Molecular Biology and Genetic Research Institute in Ariano Irpino (AV), Italy. His work has been widely developed at the intersection of different fields, especially philosophy, neuroscience, and AI, with the combination of theoretical and practical analyses. He has authored several books and many articles covering topics such as posthuman philosophy, ethical and legal implications of genetics and neuroscience (ELSI), consciousness, artificial intelligence, bioethics, and neuroethics.

Part II
Regenerative Medicine and Enhancement Technologies

Chapter 7
Navigating the Nuanced Ethical Landscape of Gene Therapy

Natalia Wewior

Abstract Since the discovery of the double helix structure of DNA, a cascade of research has made gene therapy a reality. In recent decades, the therapeutic applications of gene therapy have impacted individuals across the world. While gene therapy has merit, its promises are tempered by ethical considerations that warrant a thorough appraisal. In this chapter, I detail the implications of somatic gene therapy at the nexus of three fundamental themes, including (1) the intersection of health, disease, and the human condition; (2) global disparities and associated issues of access and uptake; and (3) the emphasis of and sensitivity to genetics. My goal is to elucidate the ethical considerations of gene therapy while adding context to their uniqueness, probability, and scope, and reframing them in the context of different ethical frameworks or principles. Accordingly, the purpose of this chapter is to share a balanced perspective of the morally salient considerations of gene therapy. The sound deployment of gene therapy further requires that multimodal safeguards are implemented and adhered to across stakeholder groups.

Keywords Gene therapy · Genomic medicine · Genetic disease · Social determinants of health

7.1 Introduction

We have entered a new era of medicine, one that had previously existed only in the realm of science fiction. Owing to decades of innovation and the tenacity of those in the field, the emergence of gene therapy has made it possible to modulate human health at the most granular and elemental level. The promises of gene therapy have prompted clinical trials and drug approvals across the world, many of which have transformed people's lives. We witnessed such a case firsthand when Ashanthi DeSilva, then four years old, became the first patient to successfully undergo gene

---

N. Wewior (✉)
Broad Institute, Cambridge, MA, USA
e-mail: nwewior@broadinstitute.org

M. C. Altman and D. Schwan (eds.), *Ethics and Medical Technology*, The International Library of Bioethics 113, https://doi.org/10.1007/978-3-031-94690-5_7

therapy for her severe combined immunodeficiency disease (SCID) (Stasiak 2001; Philippidis 2016).

While genomic medicine spans a spectrum of ends, approaches, and technologies, I specifically focus on gene therapy (GT) in this chapter. By definition, GT is a medical approach that uses genetic material for therapeutic applications—that is, to prevent, treat, or cure disease (American Society of Gene & Cell Therapy 2022; Cleveland Clinic 2023). At present, the US Food and Drug Administration (FDA) has approved twenty-three GT products for clinical use (US Food and Drug Administration 2024; American Society of Gene & Cell Therapy 2025; Hildreth 2025). These products, which are approved for use in the United States, constitute most of the thirty-three gene therapy products approved globally for clinical use, alongside thirty-five RNA products and seventy-two non-genetically modified cell therapies (American Society of Gene & Cell Therapy 2025).

The implications of GT range from profound social benefits to unintended and irremediable global harms. In many ways, the positive applications and outcomes associated with GT are boundless and have already been felt around the world. There are countless success stories of individuals, like Ashanthi, whose lives have been transformed and whose life expectancies have significantly increased because they received such treatments. Yet alongside this newfound hope, GT also raises pressing ethical concerns that cannot be understated. Its deployment and adoption demand careful consideration and critical reflection from all stakeholder groups.

When arriving at a crucial juncture, we must consider both the risks and benefits that inform the utility and governance of GT; GT is not all good or all bad. My goal here is to provide both nuance and clarity to the growing ethical dimensions of GT. I start by outlining the current landscape of GT and then describe the relevant ethical considerations, with a goal of reframing these issues in light of potential benefits while drawing on specific ethical frameworks.

The deployment of GT and other technologies does not happen in a vacuum, so we must confront the ethics of GT with respect to the current and evolving social climate, shifts in human values and behaviors, and the institutions that impact our daily lives. My intention is not to oversimplify, deter, or distract from the critical ethical considerations or substantial harms that could transpire, but rather to highlight their nuances in the context of their uniqueness, probability, and scope.

7.2 Defining Gene Therapy

GT is a distinct area of genomic medicine with a unique therapeutic mechanism. The application and administration of genomic medicine is, in ways, inherently risky because it leverages genomics. The majority of marketed drugs are small molecules that are designed to selectively interact with their molecular targets and activate or inhibit biological process (Li and Kang 2020; Southey and Brunavs 2023), though other drug modalities exist and are emerging, such as next generation peptides, cellular therapies, antibody drug conjugates, protein degraders, and other biologics

(Gurevich and Gurevich 2015; Blanco and Gardinier 2020; Müller et al. 2021). GT instead relies on the genetic makeup of the body as its mechanism. GT thus makes lasting changes that impact human health, reshape the human condition, and address the root of health problems (as opposed to merely managing symptoms or disease progression) (Pfizer 2025). By harnessing the power of genomics, GT exemplifies personalized medicine in practice.

Advancements in GT have refined our understanding of GT itself, as well as the technologies that fall under it. As its name implies, GT has historically been defined as either introducing a new or modified copy of a gene into the body, replacing a gene with a healthy copy, or inactivating a gene that is not functioning properly (Center for Biologics Evaluation and Research 2020). The mechanisms of GT have expanded to include gene (or genome) editing, which involves the deliberate manipulation of specific loci in the genome (Xu and Li 2020; Fridovich-Keil 2025). When conceptualizing gene therapy, there is a growing understanding that 98% of our genome is made up of non-coding regions that play an important role in the regulation of human disease, and those non-coding regions are being explored as potential GT targets. Alongside the evolution of the concept of GT is the debate about whether the definition of "gene" is confined to protein-coding regions or if it is inclusive of non-coding regions (Salzberg 2018; Green 2025). The former is the commonly accepted definition of GT, in which case I support a shift from using the term "gene therapy" to "genome therapy" (as well as "genome editing") to recognize the potential of non-coding regions as therapeutic targets. Nonetheless, I will call it gene therapy (GT) in this discussion because of its prevalence in the academic literature and in public usage.

GT can be administered in vivo or ex vivo. With in vivo approaches, targeted changes to the genetic material are made within the body of the patient. These approaches are generally most useful for treating internal organs such as hearts, brains, and lungs (Razi Soofiyani et al. 2013). With ex vivo approaches, cells are harvested from a person and modified outside of the body before being transplanted back into the body. These techniques are most commonly used to treat disorders or diseases affecting the blood or whose affected tissues and organs can be reached by blood cells (Razi Soofiyani et al. 2013). There are both viral and non-viral systems for delivering the genetic material into the body. One ethically important distinction is that gene therapy consists of both somatic and germline gene therapy. With somatic gene therapy, modifications to genetic makeup affect only the treated individual, whereas germline modifications are inherited by future generations.

The ethical considerations of GT ought to be both informed by and reflective of the current regulatory landscape, successes and limitations, and available information regarding ongoing clinical trials. Of the 2,117 GTs in development around the world, oncology and rare diseases remain the most commonly targeted therapeutic areas, with myeloma, acute myelogenous leukemia, non-Hodgkin lymphoma, B-cell lymphoma, and ovarian cancer prevailing as the top diseases for which GTs are being developed. Other therapeutic targets include additional oncological diseases, retinitis pigmentosa, muscular dystrophy, and thalassemia (American Society of Gene & Cell Therapy 2025). The United States parallels these global trends: of the twenty-three

GTs (including genetically modified cell therapies) approved for clinical use, seven are cancer immunotherapies (CAR T-cell therapies), one is a TCR T-cell therapy, and fifteen are "other" GTs (Hildreth 2025). Imlygic, the first GT approved in the US (in 2015), treats melanoma (American Society of Gene & Cell Therapy 2025). From 2025 on, the FDA anticipates approving ten to twenty cell and GT products annually, based on the pace of the current regulatory pipeline and success rates of previous GT products (Gottlieb 2019).

As we step into this new frontier of medicine, we must be acutely aware of where we are, where we are going, and what is at stake. I will focus on the ethical considerations of somatic GT, because germline GT occasions a distinct set of ethical concerns. Moreover, there are no germline GT products approved for clinical use in the United States, nor is federal funding allowed for research on its use. I will discuss GT and its associated ethical considerations in the context of its applications, deployment, and access, since global and national infrastructures—shaped by the pharmaceutical industry, socioeconomic inequities, insurance systems, and mistrust in medicine—inform these ethical concerns and their magnitude.

7.3 Ethical Implications and Their Nuanced Potentiality

Before exploring the ethical considerations of GT (organized across three central themes), it is critical to acknowledge the safety concerns. These issues merit a careful appraisal and discussion, and while they are ethically relevant, they will not be addressed below. Because unsafe GTs have potentially lethal consequences with immediate impact, safety concerns must be addressed before considering downstream ethical consequences. My exploration of the ethical considerations assumes that the safety concerns have been (or will be before the time of deployment) mitigated or reduced to the greatest extent and that the GT product has received regulatory approval.

7.3.1 The Intersection of Health, Disease, and the Human Condition

As described above, GT is defined most simply by its capacity to use genetic material to prevent, treat, or cure disease. Federal regulations and guidance reflect this motif, as GT products meet the definition of "biological product" in Sect. 351(i) of the Public Health Service (PHS) Act (42 U.S.C. 262[i]): "such products are applicable to the prevention, treatment, or cure of a disease or condition of human beings" (US Department of Health and Human Services 1993; Center for Biologics Evaluation and Research 2020). However, the therapeutic applications of GT are complicated by ongoing disagreement over how to define diseases, disorders, syndromes, and any and all human conditions that may not meet the normative definition of "good" or "normal" health. Despite the broad consensus that GT should be limited to therapeutic applications, scholars and researchers disagree about what qualifies as a disease, disorder, syndrome, or condition meriting therapeutic application, and about the implications of these classifications. The difficulty of this question brings us to an impasse in further elucidating the boundaries of GT.

So long as these conceptual boundaries remain blurred, GT may fuel the slippery slope to non-therapeutic enhancement. The term "non-therapeutic" here denotes any application that does not prevent, treat, or cure disease. Some potential targets appear plainly non-therapeutic, such as those that are related to aesthetic appearance. There are other potential GT targets, however, whose applications and utility may waver between conferring therapeutic relief or promoting a non-therapeutic, optimal, or improved state. Even if we succeeded at carefully distinguishing therapeutic targets from non-therapeutic enhancements, the reality is that what is therapeutic for one individual may be enhancing for another (Committee on Human Gene Editing 2017; Ansah 2022). GT interventions thus fall on a spectrum of treatment-prevention-enhancement, depending on their intended use (Committee on Human Gene Editing 2017). Even in the cases of targets such as skin color or short stature, which at first glance may seem plainly non-therapeutic, there may be affected individuals for whom GT would be therapeutic, such as those living with vitiligo or growth hormone deficiency (respectively) (Ansah 2022).

This grows increasingly complicated when non-therapeutic uses intersect with mental health conditions, and we ask whether GT treatment is justified on that basis. In other words, in cases where aesthetic appearance, intelligence, physical performance, and other comparable targets adversely affect mental health or manifest as mental illnesses, there is a question of whether such targets of GT are warranted on therapeutic grounds.

Along similar lines, if the applications of GT are more broadly intended to reduce suffering, increase human flourishing, and promote well-being, it is difficult to say what range of targets, therapeutic or not, are appropriate. That is, even beyond disease, additional reflection is needed to ascertain what our obligations are to humanity and whether such technologies ought to be implemented on the basis of increasing quality of life, beyond the scope of health and disease. It may seem paradoxical, however, that this pursuit of perfection or contentment may produce the opposite of its intended effect. By deeming particular phenotypes more worthy or desirable than others, societal pressures and expectations are worsened, further inducing an unsustainable quest for self-perfection and the erosion of mental health. When worthy or desirable phenotypes become more prevalent, those who do not conform to such standards are adversely affected, experiencing exacerbated social inequalities and inequities, as well as their negative associated outcomes.

The advent of any new technologies, therapeutics, procedures, or methods raises the question of whether we place the moral weight on their intended uses or their potential misuses and misapplications. There are deontological and virtue-based claims to be made that the intended uses of GT take precedence. These frameworks focus on the morality of actions and expression of virtues (respectively), and they place less emphasis on outcomes or results of actions. Through these lenses, the moral significance of GT is assigned to its intended use rather than its unintended uses or potential misuses. So long as GT intends to reduce the barriers to normatively "good" health instead of raising the glass ceiling through enhancements, GT ought to be appraised by its potential to confer therapeutic relief (Wewior 2022).

The potential for non-therapeutic enhancement exists for controversial therapies, such as medical aid in dying, but also for other applications, such as in vitro fertilization, stem cell therapies, and organ transplantations that benefit individuals globally. Additionally, and beyond the question of moral intent, the risks of misuse and misapplication are not unique to GT, nor have they been prohibitive in the approval and uptake of numerous other medical technologies. For example, drugs such as central nervous system stimulants and depressants, pain relievers, and cold and allergy medications are often misused. Such products can be obtained through medical tourism or used recreationally, outside of carefully regulated environments. By contrast, somatic gene therapy has been subject to the strictest regulation in its development and clinical trials, more so than any other form of therapy (Bayertz et al. 2008; Buedo et al. 2023). It is worth examining if or why GT ought to be held to a higher moral standard, and if a pragmatic ethical approach might support GT as long as the uses of GT are strictly regulated.

Another noteworthy point is that products are regularly used off-label and are even done so under the supervision of healthcare providers (Committee on Human Gene Editing 2017). One of the latest (and far-reaching) examples is semaglutide injections, which were developed to treat diabetes and which are being used off-label for weight loss. Beyond clinically indicated therapies, there exists a multitude of products (both pharmaceutical and non-pharmaceutical) whose intended applications are strictly enhancing, and they are not prohibited or condemned for that reason. The widespread adoption of neuromodulators that reduce signs of aging is another example, and one could even make the case for coffee (caffeine) and its intended effect on energy and alertness. Drawing these parallels is meant to raise the question: should GT, just because it can be used for non-therapeutic purposes, be considered any more morally problematic than existing and widely used products?

The blurred characterization of health, normalcy, and disease affect what we mean by enhancement, but they also complicate which conditions are pathologic and therapeutic targets for GT. There is an extensive body of literature on stigma and health-related experiences across multiple disease domains. Applying GT to particular phenotypic targets, such as disabilities, can suggest that the affected individuals deviate from a "healthy" norm or are "diseased," propagating stigma and its downstream implications (Parens and Asch 2003; Meagher et al. 2020). The labeling of such human conditions fuels harmful narratives that further erode social interaction and people's sense of identity (Link and Phelan 2001; Sankar et al. 2006). This is a particularly salient concern for the communities with deafness, blindness, and dwarfism. The utilization of GT for such human conditions could imply that the affected individuals have something in need of fixing or correction. The incidence of stigmatization, identity erosion, and othering will increase as those conditions become less prevalent.

So long as the boundaries of health, normalcy, and disease remain unclear, natural human variation may be framed as pathologic. Nonetheless, the endorsement and acceptance of non-GT stigmatized conditions may be useful in evaluating its moral soundness as a therapy. The end goal of GT is akin to those of existing therapies that are already widespread, such as ocular surgery for blindness, cochlear implants for deafness, and growth hormone therapy for dwarfism (Ansah 2022; Wewior 2022). Again, when considering the endorsement and uptake of interventions for such conditions, further discussion is warranted to discern whether GT is more morally problematic than other existing treatments.

Beyond deontological and virtue-based considerations, there may also be utilitarian and justice-based claims supporting GT: namely, restricting access to and uptake of GT from those who could benefit would overtly harm the affected individuals and exacerbate existing inequalities. Until the risks potentially posed by GT become realities, they are theoretical in nature. Focusing on these risks deflects from the tangible, quantifiable benefits of GT and can impede progress on advancements to which the affected individuals rightly deserve access.

7.3.2 Global Disparities and Issues in Access and Uptake

Both health and non-health disparities play a crucial role in appraising issues of access and uptake of GT. When novel technologies are introduced to the public, there are significant concerns over whether those technologies will be made accessible to vulnerable populations or only to those who are already advantaged. This is particularly evident when considering the incidence of certain genetic diseases (or more generally, diseases that could be modulated by GT) among marginalized groups. A quintessential example is sickle cell disease (SCD), a monogenic disease that affects about 100,000 individuals in the United States, 90% of whom are non-Hispanic Black or African American (US Centers for Disease Control and Prevention 2024). On a global scale, there are 515,000 babies born annually with SCD, 75% of whom are born in Africa (GBD 2021; Munung et al. 2023; Sickle Cell Disease Collaborators 2023). In addition to some monogenic diseases like SCD, minority groups may also be disproportionately affected by polygenic or multifactorial diseases, such as obesity and type-2 diabetes, in which genetics are a significant risk factor, making them potential GT targets (West et al. 2017). Marginalized groups face health disparities *and* higher cases of genetic diseases, which taken together demand moral attention.

First, different levels of access to genetic testing affect the uptake of GT and reinforce disparities across a multitude of disease types and marginalized groups. On a global scale, sequencing-based diagnostics and noninvasive prenatal testing are not routinely available in lower- and middle-income countries (LMICs) (Phillips et al. 2021; Bateman-House 2024). And in the United States, where genetic testing is available, several barriers complicate the diagnostic process, such as "clinical heterogeneity, incomplete utilization of gene testing, inconsistent coding practices, and general lack of physician awareness or expertise" (Gonzaludo et al. 2019, 1781).

Disparities in access to genetic testing, screening, and diagnostics result in less availability of GT.

When treatment becomes clinically indicated, the high price of GT is perhaps the most palpable barrier to access. Lenmeldy, a GT product approved by the FDA in March 2024 to treat metachromic leukodystrophy, set a world record with its wholesale cost of $4.25 million (Bateman-House 2024; Smith 2024). Such high costs are not sustainable even for advantaged individuals, so they present a dramatic barrier for people of low socioeconomic status and the uninsured. In addition to high costs of treatment, a feedback loop emerges in which individuals with genetic diseases incur increasing expenses and financial challenges, further compounding their hardships. Individuals with suspected genetic diseases experience a greater economic impact through amplified healthcare utilization compared to their counterparts with non-genetic diseases (Gonzaludo et al. 2019). Moreover, as novel GTs enter the public domain, financial challenges are exacerbated in part due to "extreme medication pricing being linked to (1) discriminatory insurance coverages (Gruber 2019), (2) onerous reimbursement payee issues (Naveed and Calderon 2021), and (3) severe copay burdens that create high rates of medication noninitiation and abandonment (Gleason et al. 2009; Doshi et al. 2017; Dusetzina et al. 2022)" (Subica 2023, 877). Compounding medical debt may further lead to the forgoing of medical treatment, mental health impacts, adverse health outcomes, and additional downstream effects that reinforce both health and non-health disparities.

Despite the exorbitant costs of commercially available GT, advocates for its use have suggested that the lifetime costs of disease management may exceed the cost of GT. The cost efficiency debate also does not factor in the improved quality of life, which may outweigh the financial costs and may be preferable on utilitarian grounds (Munung et al. 2023). GT is also not unique in having higher costs in its early stages. Like all medical technologies, GT has the potential to reduce its associated costs over time. As compared to ex vivo procedures that are costly and complex, in vivo approaches could reduce manufacturing prices (Bateman-House 2024; Olayiwola et al. 2024). This would benefit LMICs, whose drug costs are directly related to manufacturing costs (Cruz et al. 2022; Olayiwola et al. 2024). In due time, the lower costs and sequential access for vulnerable populations who would benefit from GTs most will likely lead to more just outcomes.

Beyond financial barriers, vulnerable populations experience gaps in accessing GT by means of commercially available GT products or active clinical trials. For example, although SCD is most prevalent in Africa, there are currently no commercially available GT products or clinical trials using GT in Africa. More broadly, despite many disease targets being identified as global health priorities for LMICs and those countries having poorer associated outcomes, the overwhelming majority of GT products and clinical trials are in high-income countries, where the disease targets are less common (Cornetta et al. 2018). In short, GT products and clinical trials are usually not available in the places where they are most needed.

Even if financial and geographic barriers were removed, the question of uptake would still remain. A multitude of barriers to uptake persist, and inclusivity in research is further hindered by mistrust in medicine and research, educational and language barriers, lower levels of genetic literacy, and a myriad of other factors (Bateman-House 2024; Olayiwola et al. 2024). The significant underrepresentation of minority groups in genomic research and GT clinical trials are not only exemplary of health disparities but also directly affect the efficacy and outcomes of GTs for those populations (Bateman-House 2024).

While the deployment of GT may exacerbate health inequalities and inequities, it also presents an opportunity to reduce them. The non-genetic determinants of health cannot be understated. Independent of genetic risk, social determinants often lead to worse outcomes, as is the case for African Americans in comparison to European Americans for chronic kidney disease and acute lymphoblastic leukemia in children (Pui et al. 2003; Peralta et al. 2016; West et al. 2017). However, the higher incidence of some monogenic and polygenic diseases in minority groups presents an opportunity for GT to be prioritized for affected populations, in accordance with theories of justice. Moreover, it is worth exploring whether GT is warranted as a means to reduce health inequalities and inequities given that the social determinants of health persist and are reinforced at the institutional level, rather than being mitigated through legislation and reform. I have argued elsewhere that there are procedurally just pathways that can inform the prioritization of disease targets based on the fact that both monogenic and polygenic diseases disproportionately affect minority groups, and by prioritizing their advancement, the groups most affected will experience the greatest benefit (Wewior 2022).

7.3.3 The Emphasis on and Sensitivity of Genetics

While the ethical considerations above are not unique to GT, they may be amplified in comparison to other therapies. The perceptions and attitudes about genetics as a field vary in positive or negative sentiment, are stratified across populations, and are based on a multitude of factors. Since it deals with the building blocks of life, the field of genetics is intrinsically contentious. Some people believe that using GT is akin to playing God and tampering with the very essence of humanity. This is a prominent concern in deontological ethics and is common across religions and cultures.

Advocating that we use genomic medicine for any and all human conditions reinforces the concept of genetic determinism, the idea that our phenotypes (i.e., our observable characteristics) are solely determined by our genetic makeup (Guthrie 2025). The implications of genetic determinism can harm people, regardless of whether they have a genetic disease (or disease that could be targeted by GT). The reduction of humanity to a genetic blueprint discounts the external forces that shape our identities and influence our life outcomes. At the individual level, genetic determinism may diminish people's sense of personal agency and self-control. At the population level, an emphasis on genetic makeup propagates discriminatory discourse that exacerbates the oppression of and violence toward already vulnerable populations (Robinson et al. 2024). Deterministic thinking also fuels eugenics, the pseudoscience that supports selective breeding to improve the genetic quality of the human race. Despite being debunked by scientists, the lingering scars of history sustain harmful narratives today. Moreover, deterministic thinking distracts institutions from the systemic contributors of discrimination, potentially hindering progress in remediating them.

In the context of disease, there are also both individual-level and population-level implications of GT. At the individual level, there are psychosocial implications of genetic diagnosis, such as fears about discrimination, strained relationships, and financial burden (Genetic Alliance 2010). A positive test or diagnosis for a genetic disease can reduce one's sense of self-control, adversely impact clinical management and lifestyle choices, and ultimately lead to poorer health outcomes (Sankar et al. 2006; Genetic Alliance 2010). These implications are conceivably worsened when genetic results are misinterpreted or inconclusive and when additional services, such as genetic counseling, are not available. At the population level, genetic determinism can lead to discounting the social determinants of health and other systemic drivers of disease.

At the same time, genetic framing may be helpful in the event of a genetic diagnosis for some affected individuals. Genetic framing may be beneficial for countering stigma (Easter 2012), mitigating personal blame, and increasing a sense of community (Sankar et al. 2006). The genetic basis of disease may also reduce uncertainty in disease pathology, increase understanding of the natural course of disease, and augment autonomy by empowering those affected individuals to use their knowledge and understanding to make more informed decisions about their health and lives more generally. Experiences are not uniform though, and they may vary by disease and disease type. In a study exploring the relationship between disease cause and felt stigma, the genetic or hereditary causes of disease were viewed more favorably by the deaf community and less favorably by individuals with breast cancer (Sankar et al. 2006). Participants with a genetic or hereditary basis for being deaf or hard of hearing generally viewed the cause positively, seeing it as "part of who I am," and citing stronger communication skills and family connection. Conversely, a genetic or hereditary basis of breast cancer was viewed negatively, with concerns related to increased risk to relatives, need for more medical management, and the anticipation of a diagnosis.

Although there is an association between GT and genetic determinism, it is important to distinguish between the two. The application of GT, and the identification of the genetic components of disease more broadly, simply acknowledge that there are genetic contributors, without implying that the genetic basis is a primary or chief cause. More research is needed to adequately elucidate the relationship between genetics and external factors, and to further promote the shift from genetic determinism to a more sophisticated paradigm. In the interim, a promising body of literature in epigenetics is providing insight into the biological markers of social determinants of health, such as gene expression and DNA methylation (West et al. 2017). The findings of epigenetic research run counter to the misleading narratives of genetic determinism by bridging genetics and the social determinants of health, in a way that fosters potential for GT, without the negative implications of genetic determinism.

There is an inherent sensitivity to genetic information that renders the operationalization of GT ethically fraught. Forgoing any deterministic undertone, genetic makeup is unique to each individual. The privacy and confidentiality of genetic information is important to uphold the principle of autonomy. Genetic information also transcends individuals and includes information about their biological relatives, which can compound concerns over privacy and confidentiality. As GT becomes more commonplace, the handling of and access to genetic information will undoubtedly increase, and with it questions of intended use as well as potential for abuse. There are negative implications at the individual level, such as genetic discrimination that is not protected by the Genetic Information Nondiscrimination Act (GINA). At the community or population level, and in the case that genetic information is made accessible to pharmaceutical companies or genetic databases, there are concerns about ownership and commercialization.

Despite these concerns, people are generally optimistic about the field of genetics and are aware of its personal utility (Clayton et al. 2018; LePoire et al. 2018; Pearce et al. 2024). The same is generally true for GT, and people are more favorable than not of GT as a promoter of health (Robillard et al. 2014; Delhove et al. 2020; Pearce et al. 2024). The perceptions, considerations, and concerns of the public must guide its deployment. On these grounds alone, suppressing GT would be contrary to respect for autonomy and justice.

7.4 Conclusion

In our lifetime, we have experienced many firsts of genomic medicine. As GT has developed, so have its ethical considerations, which are profound and all the more pressing in the context of evolving political, social, and economic climates, both nationally and globally. In truth, these changing landscapes may be more influential than any other factors. Accordingly, the ethics of GT ought to be an ongoing conversation with multiple stakeholders.

Overcoming the ethical hurdles is not simple or straightforward. Instead, morally salient considerations should be embedded in the fabric of regulatory, outreach, and advocacy initiatives. Regulatory initiatives may include use of the accelerated approval pathway (Berry et al. 2024), synthesis of regulatory requirements and frameworks across countries (Drago et al. 2021), and endorsement of expanded access (Kearns et al. 2021; Maryamchik et al. 2025). Public engagement at the micro level, such as community advisory boards, and at the macro level, such as the Global Gene Therapy Initiative (GGTI), exemplify cross-collaborations among stakeholders to diversify input (Olayiwola et al. 2024). The deployment of GT ought to be contingent on the implementation of and adherence to multimodal safeguards.

It is often said that biotechnology highlights moral problems rather than creating them (Fletcher 2008; Buedo et al. 2023). Whether GT will follow suit or veer down another path is not determined by the technology itself but by the individuals who employ it. It is our collective responsibility to deploy GT in service of humanity, with cases like Ashanthi serving as a beacon of hope.

References

American Society of Gene & Cell Therapy. 2022. "Gene Therapy Basics." Last modified October 31, 2022. https://patienteducation.asgct.org/gene-therapy-101/gene-therapy-basics.

American Society of Gene & Cell Therapy. 2025. "Gene, Cell, & RNA Therapy Landscape Report: Q4 2024 Quarterly Report." Accessed March 3, 2025. https://www.asgct.org/publications/landscape-report.

Ansah, Emmanuel Owusu. 2022. "Ethical Challenges and Controversies in the Practice and Advancement of Gene Therapy." *Advances in Cell and Gene Therapy* 2022 (1) (January): 1015996. https://doi.org/10.1155/2022/1015996.

Bateman-House, Alison. 2024. "Somatic Gene Therapy: Ethics and Access." *Annual Review of Genomics and Human Genetics* 25: 421–438. https://doi.org/10.1146/annurev-genom-021623-104458.

Bayertz, Kurt, Rainer Paslack, and Kurt W. Schmidt. 2008. "Summary of 'Gene Transfer into Human Somatic Cells. State of the Technology, Medical Risks, Social and Ethical Problems: A Report.'" *Human Gene Therapy* 5 (4) (April): 465–468. https://doi.org/10.1089/hum.1994.5.4-465.

Berry, Diane, Kate Donigan, Lisa Kahlman, James Long, Christina Markus, and Caitlin K. McCombs. 2024. "Optimizing Regulatory Frameworks for Gene Therapies in Rare Diseases: Challenges and Solutions." *Molecular Therapy: Methods & Clinical Development* 32 (4) (December 12): 101386. https://doi.org/10.1016/j.omtm.2024.101386.

Blanco, Maria-Jesus, and Kevin M. Gardinier. 2020. "New Chemical Modalities and Strategic Thinking in Early Drug Discovery." *ACS Medicinal Chemistry Letters* 11 (3) (March 12): 228–231. https://doi.org/10.1021/acsmedchemlett.9b00582.

Buedo, Paola, Alahi Bianchini, Katarzyna Klas, and Marcin Waligora. 2023. "Bioethics of Somatic Gene Therapy: What Do We Know So Far?" *Current Medical Research and Opinion* 39 (10): 1355–1365. https://doi.org/10.1080/03007995.2023.2257600.

Center for Biologics Evaluation and Research. 2020. "Human Gene Therapy for Rare Diseases: Guidance for Industry." January. https://www.fda.gov/media/113807/download.

Clayton, Ellen W., Colin M. Halverson, Nila A. Sathe, and Bradley A. Malin. 2018. "A Systematic Literature Review of Individuals' Perspectives on Privacy and Genetic Information in the United States." *PloS One* 13 (10): e0204417. https://doi.org/10.1371/journal.pone.0204417

Cleveland Clinic. 2023. "Gene Therapy." Last modified December 4, 2023. https://my.clevelandclinic.org/health/treatments/17984-gene-therapy.

Committee on Human Gene Editing: Scientific, Medical, and Ethical Considerations; National Academies of Sciences, Engineering, and Medicine. 2017. *Human Genome Editing: Science, Ethics, and Governance*. Washington, DC: National Academies. https://nap.nationalacademies.org/catalog/24623/human-genome-editing-science-ethics-and-governance.

Cornetta, Kenneth, Kirtika Patel, Christopher Mwaniki Wanjiku, and Naftali Busakhala. 2018. "Equitable Access to Gene Therapy: A Call to Action for the American Society of Gene and Cell Therapy." *Molecular Therapy* 26 (12) (December): 2715–2716. https://doi.org/10.1016/j.ymthe.2018.11.002.

Cruz, Luis J., Somayeh Rezaei, Frank Grosveld, Sjaak Philipsen, and Christina Eich. 2022. "Nanoparticles Targeting Hematopoietic Stem and Progenitor Cells: Multimodal Carriers for the Treatment of Hematological Diseases." *Frontiers in Genome Editing* 4: 1030285. https://doi.org/10.3389/fgeed.2022.1030285.

Delhove, Juliette, Ivana Osenk, Ivanka Prichard, and Martin Donnelley. 2020. "Public Acceptability of Gene Therapy and Gene Editing for Human Use: A Systematic Review." *Human Gene Therapy* 31 (1–2) (January): 20–46. https://doi.org/10.1089/hum.2019.197.

Doshi, Jalpa A., Pengxiang Li, Hairong Huo, Amy R. Pettit, and Katrina A. Armstrong. 2017. "Association of Patient Out-of-Pocket Costs with Prescription Abandonment and Delay in Fills of Novel Oral Anticancer Agents." *Journal of Clinical Oncology* 36 (5) (December 20): 476–482. https://doi.org/10.1200/JCO.2017.74.5091

Drago, Daniela, Betsy Foss-Campbell, Keith Wonnacott, David Barrett, and Adora Ndu. 2021. "Global Regulatory Progress in Delivering on the Promise of Gene Therapies for Unmet Medical Needs." *Molecular Therapy: Methods & Clinical Development* 21 (June 11): 524–529. https://doi.org/10.1016/j.omtm.2021.04.001.

Dusetzina, Stacie B., Haiden A. Huskamp, Russell L. Rothman, Laura C. Pinheiro, Andrew W. Roberts, Nilay D. Shah, et al. 2022. "Many Medicare Beneficiaries Do Not Fill High-Price Specialty Drug Prescriptions." *Health Affairs* 41 (4) (April): 487–496. https://doi.org/10.1377/hlthaff.2021.01742.

Easter, Michele M. 2012. "'Not All My Fault': Genetics, Stigma, and Personal Responsibility for Women with Eating Disorders." *Social Science and Medicine* 75 (8) (October): 1408–1416. https://doi.org/10.1016/j.socscimed.2012.05.042.

Fletcher, John C. 2008. "Evolution of Ethical Debate about Human Gene Therapy." *Human Gene Therapy* 1 (1) (Spring): 55–68. https://doi.org/10.1089/hum.1990.1.1-55.

Fridovich-Keil, Judith L. 2025. "Gene Editing." *Encyclopedia Britannica.* Last modified February 13, 2025. https://www.britannica.com/science/gene-editing.

GBD 2021 Sickle Cell Disease Collaborators. 2023. "Global, Regional, and National Prevalence and Mortality Burden of Sickle Cell Disease, 2000–2021: A Systematic Analysis from the Global Burden of Disease Study 2021." *Lancet Haematology* 10 (8) (August): E585–E599. https://doi.org/10.1016/S2352-3026(23)00118-7.

Genetic Alliance, the New England Public Health Genetics Education Collaborative. 2010. *Understanding Genetics: A New England Guide for Patients and Health Professionals.* Washington, DC: Genetic Alliance.

Gleason, Patrick P., Catherine I. Starner, Brent W. Gunderson, Jeremy A. Schafer, and H. Scott Sarran. 2009. "Association of Prescription Abandonment with Cost Share for High-Cost Specialty Pharmacy Medications." *Journal of Managed Care Pharmacy* 15 (8) (October): 648–658. https://doi.org/10.18553/jmcp.2009.15.8.648.

Gonzaludo, Nina, John W. Belmont, Vladimir G. Gainullin, and Ryan J. Taft. 2019. "Estimating the Burden and Economic Impact of Pediatric Genetic Disease." *Genetics in Medicine* 21 (8) (August): 1781–1789. https://doi.org/10.1038/s41436-018-0398-5.

Gottlieb, Scott. 2019. "Statement from FDA Commissioner Scott Gottlieb, M.D. and Peter Marks, M.D., Ph.D., Director of the Center for Biologics Evaluation and Research on New Policies to Advance Development of Safe and Effective Cell and Gene Therapies." US Food and Drug Administration. January 15. https://www.fda.gov/news-events/press-announcements/statement-fda-commissioner-scott-gottlieb-md-and-peter-marks-md-phd-director-center-biologics.

Green, Eric. 2025. "Gene." National Human Genome Research Institute. Last modified March 3, 2025. https://www.genome.gov/genetics-glossary/Gene.

Gruber, Jonathan. 2019. "The Genetic Revolution Highlights the Importance of Nondiscriminatory and Comprehensive Health Insurance Coverage." *American Journal of Bioethics* 19 (10): 10–11. https://doi.org/10.1080/15265161.2019.1644822.

Gurevich, E. V., and V. V. Gurevich. 2015. "Beyond Traditional Pharmacology: New Tools and Approaches." *British Journal of Pharmacology* 172 (13) (July): 3229–3241. https://doi.org/10.1111/bph.13066.

Guthrie, O'neil W. 2025. "Gene Therapy: An Historical Overview for Familial Hearing Loss." *International Journal of Molecular Sciences* 26 (4) (February 2): article no. 1469. https://doi.org/10.3390/ijms26041469.

Hildreth, Cate. 2025. "List of U.S. FDA Approved Cell and Gene Therapy Products (43)." BioInformant. January 21. https://bioinformant.com/u-s-fda-approved-cell-and-gene-therapies/.

Kearns, Lisa, Carolyn Riley Chapman, Kenneth I. Moch, Arthur L. Caplan, Tom Watson, Andrew McFadyen, Pat Furlong, and Alison Bateman-House. 2021. "Gene Therapy Companies Have an Ethical Obligation to Develop Expanded Access Policies." *Molecular Therapy* 29 (4) (April): 1367–1369. https://doi.org/10.1016/j.ymthe.2021.03.008.

LePoire, Erin, Baishakhi Basu, Lorelei Walker, and Deborah J. Bowen. 2018. "What Do People Think about Genetics? A Systematic Review." *Journal of Community Genetics* 10 (2) (April): 171–187. https://doi.org/10.1007/s12687-018-0394-0.

Link, Bruce G., and Jo C. Phelan. 2001. "Conceptualizing Stigma." *Annual Review of Sociology* 27: 363–385. https://doi.org/10.1146/annurev.soc.27.1.363.

Li, Qingxin, and Congbao Kang. 2020. "Mechanisms of Action for Small Molecules Revealed by Structural Biology in Drug Discovery." *International Journal of Molecular Sciences* 21 (15) (August 1): 5262. https://doi.org/10.3390/ijms21155262.

Maryamchik, Elena, Laertis Ikonomou, Beth E. Roxland, Felix Grignon, Bruce L. Levine, and Bambi J. Grilley. 2025. "International Society for Cell & Gene Therapy Expanded Access Working Group Position Paper: Key Considerations to Support Equitable and Ethical Expanded Access to Investigational Cell- and Gene-Based Interventions." *Cytotherapy*. https://doi.org/10.1016/j.jcyt.2025.01.016.

Meagher, Karen M., Megan A. Allyse, Zubin Master, and Richard R. Sharp. 2020. "Reexamining the Ethics of Human Germline Editing in the Wake of Scandal." *Mayo Clinic Proceedings* 95 (2) (February): 330–338. https://doi.org/10.1016/j.mayocp.2019.11.018.

Müller, Christa E., Finn K. Hansen, Michael Gütschow, Craig W. Lindsley, and Dennis Liotta. 2021. "New Drug Modalities in Medicinal Chemistry, Pharmacology, and Translational Science: Joint Virtual Special Issue by Journal of Medicinal Chemistry, ACS Medicinal Chemistry Letters, and ACS Pharmacology & Translational Science." *ACS Medicinal Chemistry Letters* 12 (10) (October 14): 1508–1509. https://doi.org/10.1021/acsmedchemlett.1c00476.

Munung, Nchangwi Syntia, Obiageli E. Nnodu, Patrick Ohiani Moru, Akpaka A. Kalu, Benido Impouma, Marsha J. Treadwell, and Ambroise Wonkam. 2023. "Looking Ahead: Ethical and Social Challenges of Somatic Gene Therapy for Sickle Cell Disease in Africa." *Gene Therapy* 31 (5–6) (May): 202–208. https://doi.org/10.1038/s41434-023-00429-7.

Naveed, Aimen, and Hillary Calderon. 2021. "Onasemnogene Abeparvovec (AVXS-101) for the Treatment of Spinal Muscular Atrophy." *Journal of Pediatric Pharmacology and Therapeutics* 26 (5): 437-444. https://doi.org/10.5863/1551-6776-26.5.437.

Olayiwola, Olabimpe, Adam Castillejo, Michael Louella, Moses Supercharger, Evelyn Harlow, Lynda Dee, et al. 2024. "Nothing about Us without Us: Advocacy and Engagement in Genetic Medicine." *Science Translational Medicine* 16 (746) (May 8): https://doi.org/10.1126/scitranslmed.adn2401.

Parens, Erik, and Adrienne Asch. 2003. "Disability Rights Critique of Prenatal Genetic Testing: Reflections and Recommendations." *Mental Retardation and Developmental Disabilities Research Reviews* 9 (1): 40–47. https://doi.org/10.1002/mrdd.10056.

Pearce, Angela, Lucas A. Mitchell, Stephanie Best, Mary-Anne Young, and Bronwyn Terrill. 2024. "Publics' Knowledge of, Attitude to and Motivation towards Health-Related Genomics: A Scoping Review." *European Journal of Human* Genetics 32 (7) (July): 747–758. https://doi.org/10.1038/s41431-024-01547-5.

Peralta, Carmen A., Kirsten Bibbins-Domingo, Eric Vittinghoff, Feng Lin, Myriam Fornage, Jeffrey B. Kopp, and Cheryl A. Winkler. 2016. "APOL1 Genotype and Race Differences in Incident Albuminuria and Renal Function Decline." *Journal of the American Society of Nephrology* 27 (3) (March): 887–893. https://doi.org/10.1681/ASN.2015020124.

Pfizer. 2025. "Gene Therapy: Genes as Medicine." Accessed March 3, 2025. https://www.pfizer.com/science/innovation/gene-therapy/genes-as-medicines.

Philippidis, Alex. 2016. "Making History with the 1990 Gene Therapy Trial." *GEN: Genetic Engineering and Biotechnology News*. March 10. https://www.genengnews.com/insights/making-history-with-the-1990-gene-therapy-trial/.

Phillips, Kathryn A., Michael P. Douglas, Sarah Wordsworth, James Buchanan, and Deborah A. Marshall. 2021. "Availability and Funding of Clinical Genomic Sequencing Globally." *BMJ Global Health* 6 (2) (February): e004415. https://doi.org/10.1136/bmjgh-2020-004415.

Pui, Ching-Hon, John T. Sandlund, Deqing Pei, Gaston K. Rivera, Scott C. Howard, Raul C. Ribeiro, et al. 2003. "Results of Therapy for Acute Lymphoblastic Leukemia in Black and White Children." *JAMA: Journal of the American Medical Association* 290 (15) (October 15): 2001–2007. https://doi.org/10.1001/jama.290.15.2001.

Razi Soofiyani, Saeideh, Behzad Baradaran, Farzaneh Lotfipour, Tohid Kazemi, and Leila Mohammadnejad. 2013. "Gene Therapy, Early Promises, Subsequent Problems, and Recent Breakthroughs." *Advanced Pharmaceutical Bulletin* 3 (2) (December): 249–255. https://doi.org/10.5681/apb.2013.041.

Robillard, Julie M., Dylan Roskams-Edris, Boris Kuzeljevic, and Judy Illes. 2014. "Prevailing Public Perceptions of the Ethics of Gene Therapy." *Human Gene Therapy* 25 (8) (August): 740–746. https://doi.org/10.1089/hum.2014.030.

Robinson, Gene E., Rina Bliss, and Matthew E. Hudson. 2024. "The Genomic Case against Genetic Determinism." *PLoS Biology* 22 (2) (February): e3002510. https://doi.org/10.1371/journal.pbio.3002510.

Salzberg, Steven L. 2018. "Open Questions: How Many Genes Do We Have?" *BMC Biology* 16: article no. 94. https://doi.org/10.1186/s12915-018-0564-x.

Sankar, Pamela, Mildred K. Cho, Paul Root Wolpe, and Cynthia Schairer. 2006. "What Is in a Cause? Exploring the Relationship between Genetic Cause and Felt Stigma." *Genetics in Medicine* 8 (1) (January): 33–42. https://doi.org/10.1097/01.gim.0000195894.67756.8b.

Smith, Gerry. 2024. "World's Most Expensive Drug Is Now $4.25 Million Gene Therapy." *Bloomberg*. March 20. https://www.bloomberg.com/news/articles/2024-03-20/world-s-most-expensive-drug-is-now-4-25-million-gene-therapy.

Southey, Michelle W. Y., and Michael Brunavs. 2023. "Introduction to Small Molecule Drug Discovery and Preclinical Development." *Frontiers in Drug Discovery* 3: 1314077. https://doi.org/10.3389/fddsv.2023.1314077.

Stasiak, Andrzej. 2001. "Gene Therapy." *EMBO Reports* 2 (3) (March 1): 180. https://doi.org/10.1093/embo-reports/kve059.

Subica, Andrew M. 2023. "CRISPR in Public Health: The Health Equity Implications and Role of Community in Gene-Editing Research and Applications." *American Journal of Public Health* 113 (8) (August): 874–882. https://doi.org/10.2105/AJPH.2023.307315.

US Centers for Disease Control and Prevention. 2024. "Data and Statistics on Sickle Cell Disease." May 22. https://www.cdc.gov/sickle-cell/data/index.html.

US Department of Health and Human Services. 1993. "Application of Current Statutory Authorities to Human Somatic Cell Therapy Products and Gene Therapy Products; Notice." *Federal Register* 58 (197) (October 14): 53248–53251. https://www.fda.gov/media/76647/download.

US Food and Drug Administration. 2024. "Approved Cellular and Gene Therapy Products." Last modified December 20, 2024. https://www.fda.gov/vaccines-blood-biologics/cellular-gene-therapy-products/approved-cellular-and-gene-therapy-products.

West, Kathleen Mcglone, Erika Blacksher, and Wylie Burke. 2017. "Genomics, Health Disparities, and Missed Opportunities for the Nation's Research Agenda." *JAMA: Journal of the American Medical Association* 317 (18) (May 9): 1831–1832. https://doi.org/10.1001/jama.2017.3096.

Wewior, Natalia. 2022. "Maximizing the Access and Uptake of Genome Editing as a Prevention and Treatment of Disease." Master's thesis, Johns Hopkins University. https://jscholarship.library.jhu.edu/server/api/core/bitstreams/c706efde-8479-436e-bd51-120a315f5223/content.

Xu, Yuanyuan, and Zhanjun Li. 2020. "CRISPR-Cas Systems: Overview, Innovations and Applications in Human Disease Research and Gene Therapy." *Computational and Structural Biotechnology Journal* 18: 2401–2415. https://doi.org/10.1016/j.csbj.2020.08.031.

Natalia Wewior is a Senior Compliance Specialist at the Broad Institute of MIT and Harvard, USA, working in the lab of Pardis Sabeti. Wewior oversees compliance with the regulations and policies that govern research procedures, and further supports the lab with navigating the ethical, legal, and social issues that are pertinent to pathogen genomics and international research. She holds a Master of Bioethics degree from the Johns Hopkins Bloomberg School of Public Health.

Chapter 8
The Targets Problem for Germline Genetic Interventions

Bryan Cwik

Abstract Any potential therapeutic use of germline genetic interventions seems to bring with it questions about which genetic variants are pathogenic and which are normal; what normal variation in the human genome is; how we fix reference sequences for important genes and how we measure individual variation against these sequences; and what traits we think warrant genetic intervention. There is, it seems, simply no way to think about germline genetic interventions without raising questions about which genes, which conditions, and which aims the technology should target. This chapter lays out and explores the targets problem for germline genetic interventions: the problem of determining which genes are justifiable targets of germline genetic interventions, and what criteria can be utilized in some future version of reproductive medicine that could include germline intervention to separate permissible from impermissible targets.

Keywords Gene editing · CRISPR · Genetics · Molecular therapy · Emerging technologies

8.1 Introduction

In the Summer of 2019, Denis Rebrikov, a Russian molecular biologist and geneticist, announced that he was enrolling individuals in a clinical trial to alter a gene in human embryos that can lead to congenital deafness (Cyranoski 2019). Rebrikov was interested in editing a mutation in the *GJB2* gene, and he had found individuals who themselves were deaf and carriers of the deafness causing *GJB2* allele, and who were interested in gene editing to prevent passing the allele on to any of their prospective children. The use of gene editing of germline cells to prevent hereditary deafness has been studied in murine models (for example, editing of the *TMC1* gene, sometimes called the "Beethoven gene," which is responsible for progressive hearing loss) (Urnov 2018), but germline genome editing is not currently an option for

B. Cwik (✉)
University of Florida, Gainesville, FL, USA
e-mail: cwikb@ufl.edu

M. C. Altman and D. Schwan (eds.), *Ethics and Medical Technology*, The International Library of Bioethics 113, https://doi.org/10.1007/978-3-031-94690-5_8

this aim. Russian authorities announced that they did not support Rebrikov's work, and instead fully endorsed the World Health Organization's position that germline genome editing should not (now) be used in human subjects. Rebrikov defended his plans to move forward with his experiment, though he said he would not transfer any edited embryos to begin a pregnancy unless he received approval from regulatory authorities (Cohen 2022; Mallapaty 2022).

The use of genetic interventions to target genes that lead to disabilities such as hereditary deafness has long been a subject of intense bioethical debate and controversy (Glover 2008; Darnovsky and Hasson 2020; Padden and Humphries 2020), and it illustrates a general dynamic in ethical issues about germline genetic interventions. Any potential use of this technology for clearly pathological conditions seems to carry with it the potential for use for other, less clearly pathological conditions. If the technology for altering the nuclear DNA of germline cells progresses to the point where you can make a change to the *SMN1* gene to prevent spinal muscular atrophy, or *MYBPC3* to prevent hypertrophic cardiomyopathy, then it would also allow you to make a change to *GJB2* to prevent congenital deafness. Any possible clinical use of germline genetic interventions forces us to consider which genes, which conditions, and for which aims the technology should or should not be used. The aim of this chapter is to lay out and explore an aspect of this general set of questions about germline genetic interventions, the *targets problem.*[1] Simply put, the targets problem is the problem of determining which genes are justifiable targets of germline genetic interventions, and what criteria can be utilized in some future version of reproductive medicine that could include germline intervention to separate permissible from impermissible targets.

I will discuss the prospects for therapeutic uses of germline genetic interventions in Sects. 8.2–8.3, and then argue in Sect. 8.4 that selection of targets for germline genetic interventions raises very serious issues about incorporation of future uses of germline interventions into reproductive medicine, before a brief conclusion in Sect. 8.5. Before I begin, I want to offer some observations about the stakes of the discussion and the terms and tone of the debate. My focus here is on medicine as it is practiced in well-developed health systems, specifically for individuals who have reliable access to a decent level of healthcare resources and can access reproductive medical care. But the most urgent (in all senses of the term) medical challenges of our time for the human family as a whole are the persistent inequalities in access to primary healthcare (for data, see World Health Organization 2023), the failure

---

[1] This chapter is part of set of papers on the different ethical issues involved with potential future clinical uses of germline genetic intervention (GGI) in reproductive medicine, and specifically is a sequel to my 2020 paper, "Revising, Correcting, and Transferring Genes" (Cwik 2020b), in which I argued for sorting ethical issues about GGI along four dimensions: (1) *targets* ("Which genes are actionable for GGI?"); (2) *goals* ("What aims are justifiable for uses of GGI?"); (3) *outcomes* ("What is the full suite of acceptable effects of using GGI, intended or unintended, near-, medium-, and long-term, biological, social, cultural, and political?"); and (4) *mechanisms* ("What are the specific techniques used to alter genes in germline cells and what are the issues with using these techniques?"). This chapter continues and further develops the line of argument in that paper by laying out and arguing for some of the very serious difficulties with selection of targets for GGI.

of responsible agents to meet even the most minimal demands of the human right to health for the worst-off members of the human family, and disparities in health that are a function of oppression both inter- and intra-nationally (Farmer et al. 2006; Hooper et al. 2020).

Germline genetic intervention receives far too much attention from medical ethicists, and the hyper-focus on this and other emerging medical technologies has had a distorting effect on bioethics (Fabi and Goldberg 2022). I am guilty of this, as almost all my written work over the past several years has been on this topic. Nevertheless, what to do about germline genetic interventions *is* a problem, and it will require sustained attention as research progresses if the technology gets closer to potential clinical use. But it is important to recognize this as exactly that—work on one set of issues, but work that is certainly not meant to distract from or downplay the moral urgency of the situation facing our most vulnerable fellow persons and the important work to be done on many other questions and issues raised by medicine and the state of the early twenty-first century world.

8.2 Prospects for Germline Gene Therapies

I will use "germline genetic intervention" (GGI) as shorthand for making changes to the genetic material of germline cells. This is a broad category of possible medical interventions, as it includes a variety of cell types (oocytes, sperm, zygotes, and precursor cells such as spermatogonial stem cells), editing of nuclear and mitochondrial DNA, and possibly even the generation of germline cells from somatic cells through in vitro gametogenesis (Notini et al. 2020). There are individual sets of issues for each of these different kinds of intervention, as well as general issues that seem to be raised by all.

My focus in this chapter is on therapeutic uses of GGI—uses of GGI to prevent disease in prospective persons. There is a significant amount of skepticism in the literature that there ever *could* be legitimate therapeutic uses of GGI. Some have argued that there is no medical need for GGI at all, and GGI really "treats" the "preference" for a "genetically-related child" (Andorno et al. 2020; Sparrow 2022), a point that, if taken to its logical conclusion, undercuts the rationale for pretty much all reproductive medicine. I have briefly addressed this elsewhere (Cwik 2022),[2] but a full discussion of this claim is outside the scope of this chapter. There are interesting philosophical questions about the ostensible value of genetic ties (Velleman 2005; Gheaus 2018), questions that are not only of theoretical interest but are poignant practical matters for individuals struggling with infertility. However, these issues are bracketed here, and the chapter assumes the current status quo in medicine, which is

---

[2] For discussion, see Segers (2023). Inmaculada de Melo Martin (2022) appeals to justice in arguing that, regardless of whether GGI has any therapeutic potential, we should instead use our limited resources for research on assisted reproductive technologies to improve interventions that would help the many more individuals dealing with infertility.

that infertility and heritable genetic disease are medical issues that can be addressed in reproductive medicine for those who wish to have children.

Much of the bioethics literature on GGI is about science fiction scenarios where changes to nuclear DNA via genome editing are made for purposes of biomedical enhancement—that is, to "confer advantageous traits not related to avoiding disease or preserving health" (Daley et al. 2019). Some bioethicists have argued that the underlying function of talking about therapeutic uses of GGI is to accustom people to the idea of using the technology for enhancement or eugenics (Darnovsky and Hasson 2020; Sparrow 2022). I will have nothing to say in this chapter about enhancement (except for a brief note in footnote 11), nor about the charge that work like this is part of an implicit strategy to build support for enhancement. This is not because enhancement is not an interesting topic, or because it is not relevant to discussion about GGI. On the contrary, hypotheticals about enhancement are interesting tools for thinking about anxieties about genetics and the various myths and legends about genetic determinism that persist in our culture. The problem addressed in this chapter is part of a family of ethical issues generated by potential future clinical applications of GGI in reproductive medicine, a topic which, as I have argued extensively elsewhere (Cwik 2019, 2021, 2022), has not received adequate attention in the biomedical ethics literature on GGI (relative to the amount of space devoted to enhancement).[3] Though I am not going to argue these points here, I consider the idea of using GGI (and any emerging biomedical technology that could offer hope for currently intractable conditions) for enhancement monstrous and a subversion of the moral mission of medicine. Any future use of GGI should be restricted only to legitimate medical applications—that is, to heal, treat, and prevent disease.

Most of the interest to date in GGI as a therapeutic tool is in editing of pathogenic genes (that is, a genetic variant that causes or raises the risk of disease) in nuclear or mitochondrial DNA that are causes of rare disorders (Turocy et al. 2021). Though the instance of any one of these diseases is small, the total burden of this sort of disease worldwide is quite substantial (Wolf et al. 2019; Turocy et al. 2021; Stark and Scott 2023) and is a fairly large contributor to the global burden of disease, generating at least a prima facie case for research and development of GGI.[4] For potential future therapeutic interventions, CRISPR (an acronym for Clustered Regularly Interspaced Short Palindromic Repeats) is the technique that usually gets the most attention, though it is not the only way to edit germline cells. CRISPR can be used to disable genes, alter their function (and so alter whole biochemical pathways in organisms), and work with other techniques to introduce novel genetic material (Wang and Doudna 2023). CRISPR is not, however, the last word in gene editing; there are serious technical difficulties with CRISPR (Turocy et al. 2021; Liang et al. 2023; Pacesa et al. 2024) and there are other novel techniques in development. It is important not to assume that "CRISPR-based germline genome editing" and

---

[3] There are notable exceptions: for instance, see Palacios-González (2017), Cavaliere (2018), Ranisch (2020), Evans (2021), de Melo Martin (2022), and Segers (2023), among others.

[4] Some think these points constitute more than just a prima facie case. For example, see Gyngell et al. (2019).

"germline genetic interventions" mean the same thing. CRISPR is one technique for genetic intervention, and germline genome editing is one strategy, but GGI is a broader category than just use of CRISPR on the nuclear DNA of germline cells.

Research into the technology is, at this stage, very preliminary, and there is simply not enough known to answer many of the questions about what the potential clinical utility of GGI would or could be. For instance, for germline genome editing (editing of nuclear DNA), most of the research to date has been "proof of concept" studies (that is, experiments to show that it is possible to alter pathogenic genotypes in germline cells) (Ma et al. 2017; Lea and Niakan 2019; Wolf et al. 2019; Turocy et al. 2021) or has focused on understanding the precise biochemical processes involved with editing of (and especially repair of induced lesions on) DNA in germline cells (Liang et al. 2023). Work on mitochondrial replacement therapies (MRT), in which pathogenic mitochondrial DNA is removed from an oocyte and is replaced with non-pathogenic donor mitochondrial DNA from another individual's oocyte, is somewhat more advanced (Herbert and Turnbull 2018), and there have been live births from embryos following mitochondrial replacement (Zhang et al. 2017).[5] However, it is still a matter of serious discussion as to whether MRT is ready to move beyond the investigational stage, and there are significant questions about which conditions are the right targets for future research on the technique (Russell et al. 2020). There is a great need for research here, not just for translational aims but also for purposes of understanding a set of crucial questions about human development (Lea and Niakan 2019; Rugg-Gunn et al. 2023). An argument could be made that developing this understanding is an important *cognitive goal* of this area of biomedical research, and that dealing with the set of issues involved with basic research on GGI constitutes the biggest ethical challenge at the moment.[6]

Another method for dealing with monogenic disorders is somatic cell gene editing, which involves the editing of non-germline cells in existing individuals (as opposed to editing germline cells to affect the properties of future people). One example is making changes to hematopoietic stem cells to treat hemoglobinopathies such as sickle cell anemia (Daley 2024). Somatic gene editing-based therapies have had some enormous successes in recent years, after decades of mixed success (Doudna 2020; Ledford 2022; Wang and Doudna 2023; Daley 2024), and there is a great deal of interest and optimism in the near- to medium-term clinical potential of such interventions (Wang and Doudna 2023). An immediate question here is why GGI would offer any therapeutic advantage over somatic gene editing-based interventions. If it is possible to use somatic gene editing to deal with the same issues, then why

[5] There have also been at least two individuals born from embryos in which CRISPR was used to alter nuclear DNA (that is, gene editing), twin girls born from a pregnancy initiated as part of the infamous He Jiankui "experiment." Unlike MRT, however, there is no discussion about whether germline genome editing should be used to create pregnancies, and there is instead a strong consensus to the contrary. He's "experiment" was almost universally condemned, widely considered a total failure, and landed He Jiankui a serious punishment and time in jail. On the He Jiankui case, see Greely (2021).

[6] On the idea of cognitive goals of medicine, see Boorse (2016) and Broadbent (2019, chs. 2–3).

opt for GGI, given the high risk, potential for negative social impacts, and ethically fraught nature of GGI (Lander et al. 2019)?

There are some potential reasons to think that GGI could offer some therapeutic benefit over somatic gene editing-based interventions for monogenic disorders. GGI could potentially eliminate a pathogenic genotype from a family line permanently, ensuring that future individuals will not need gene therapy or reproductive medical interventions (Lea and Niakan 2019; Turocy et al. 2021). Somatic gene editing interventions that deal with specific monogenic diseases and target specific cell types have small target populations, whereas a GGI-based intervention could potentially be usable for any monogenic disorder. If you can edit in one cell (a fertilized zygote) a pathogenic genotype (say, a mutated *HBB* gene that causes sickle cell anemia), you could in principle use the same platform for targeting any genotype (say, an allele of *SMN1* that causes spinal muscular atrophy), as (1) you are only making a change to the nuclear DNA of a single cell (as opposed to scores of cells that must be edited, in the case of somatic gene editing), and (2) you can use the same delivery mechanism, since you are only dealing with a single cell type (fertilized zygotes, as opposed to somatic gene editing-based therapies, which must be tailored to different types of cells depending on the goal of the intervention) (Wolf et al. 2019; Turocy et al. 2021).[7] Additionally, many conditions start causing damage in utero or after birth before they are detected and could be treated with a somatic gene therapy, which means that presumably GGI would be a better method to prevent this damage (Turocy et al. 2021).

However, as noted above, the precise mechanics of the biochemical processes involved with editing human germline cells are still not completely understood. On the whole, GGI is still in the early stages of translational research and is far from becoming a part of the portfolio of assisted reproductive technologies.[8] Beyond this, there are substantial ethical questions about research, such as questions about the use of embryos in GGI research (Turocy et al. 2021), questions about how clinical trials for GGI could be ethically done (Cwik 2017, 2020a), and more. For the present, it is unclear if GGI has any clinical future, but research up to this point has raised interest in whether there are translational pathways for GGI (Ranisch et al. 2023).[9]

---

[7] This only scratches the surface of the difficulties with somatic gene editing. There are, for instance, a host of issues about delivery of editors in somatic gene editing (Wang and Doudna 2023; Daley 2024) and immunogenicity (Srivastava 2020). This is not the place to go through all the difficulties with somatic gene editing-based interventions. For our purposes, it is important to note that somatic gene editing is not a proven and safe thing, whereas GGI is the opposite; rather, there are still serious technical and safety concerns with somatic gene editing.

[8] Again, with the possible exception of MRT. On ethical issues with the clinical use of MRT, see Adashi and Cohen (2016) and Palacios-González (2017).

[9] Evans (2021) characterizes some of the recent bioethical literature on GGI as thinking about a post-somatic/germline world—thinking about how to draw barriers between justifiable and unjustifiable uses in a world where some germline uses are permissible. This chapter is firmly situated within this trend in the literature.

8.3 Germline Genetic Interventions as Assisted Reproductive Technology

In addition to issues about technical feasibility, there are significant questions about whether GGI offers any therapeutic benefit not captured by other existing assisted reproductive technologies (ARTs). For example, for two progenitors who are both carriers of a recessive pathogenic genotype and who want to ensure a pregnancy with an embryo free from the genotype, preimplantation genetic diagnosis (PGD) (in which embryos are screened for the genotype before transfer, and only those free of it are implanted to create a pregnancy) would have the same outcome as germline genome editing. There is some disagreement about how many patients would not have PGD as an option (Viotti et al. 2019; Turocy et al. 2021), but it is by any measure small, and smaller than the total population of individuals who access ART. And there are, of course, other options for becoming a parent for individuals in this sort of predicament—surrogacy, or creating an embryo with a donated oocyte or donated sperm, or adoption. What benefit, then, does GGI offer at all?

The presence of these alternatives has led some to argue that GGI has no therapeutic potential, because it offers nothing that existing ARTs and other options do not already capture (Lander et al. 2019; Botkin 2020). PGD, in particular, seems to cover much if not all of the same ground (Viotti et al. 2019). However, GGI may have potential benefits over PGD. First, there are individuals for whom PGD would either not work or would be difficult. There are situations where both individuals are not just carriers but have a pathological trait and are homozygous for the relevant genotype (such as two individuals with sickle cell disease). As Jeffrey Botkin notes, for two progenitors who are heterozygous for a recessive pathogenic genotype, by standard Mendelian arithmetic most created embryos in an in vitro fertilization (IVF) cycle would be free of the disease-causing genotype (Botkin 2020). But if there are two progenitors who are both homozygous for the genotype (which would mean they themselves have the disease), PGD would not work. The number of these individuals could increase in the future as somatic gene editing-based interventions allow individuals with serious congenital disorders to live longer and healthier lives (Lander et al. 2019). Although these situations are exceptions—in most cases, PGD alone is likely to be sufficient (Lander et al. 2019; Botkin 2020)—there is still a set of individuals for whom PGD will not be sufficient with their chosen partner.

Second, given baseline difficulties with PGD and IVF, these techniques would not be sufficient in cases where other factors reduce the odds of success (Steffann et al. 2018; Lea and Niakan 2019; Ranisch 2020). Complicating factors affecting success of transfer of embryos for individuals, factors affecting ability for some individuals to produce sufficient oocytes to ensure a large enough batch of potentially transferable embryos, and factors affecting success and risks of oocyte retrieval procedures all may make PGD difficult. Establishing a pregnancy with IVF typically takes several cycles, which then requires a large enough batch such that PGD alone would allow you a sufficient set of transferable embryos. In such cases, using GGI to increase the number of available embryos (*if*—and it's a big if—GGI is effective enough to accomplish this) by correcting pathogenic genotypes in the process of fertilization may increase the chances of a successful pregnancy. It is unclear as of now whether these issues are best dealt with via GGI or the focus of research should be on improving IVF to make it a less clunky process (Lander et al. 2019; Viotti et al. 2019; Botkin 2020; de Melo Martin 2022). Without continued research into GGI, it is difficult to know whether this hypothetical scenario (using GGI + IVF to increase chances of having a successful pregnancy) is a realistic possibility (and improving success rates for IVF and PGD is something that should probably be an aim of research anyway, regardless of any considerations about GGI).

Finally, there are ethical and legal issues with the process of PGD (Cavaliere 2018; Lea and Niakan 2019). There may, for instance, be individuals who have strong religious or other ethical objections to PGD, given that the process creates some embryos that may never be transferred. A hypothetical ultra-efficient process of using GGI along with IVF and PGD to create one embryo at a time for transfer—something that would only be possible given many improvements to IVF and PGD, and a very efficient GGI process—could be a way for such individuals to avail themselves of ART to conceive a child free of any pathological trait. How many such individuals there are or would be—how many individuals who are carriers of a recessive trait or have a partner who has a dominant pathological genotype *and* have strong religious or ethical objections to PGD or live in locales with laws restricting embryo selection in PGD *and* would not have objections to use of a hyper-efficient IVF + PGD + GGI process—is pretty much impossible to find out, but is almost certainly going to be small.

Add these scenarios together, and you begin to see a portrait of a potential future for therapeutic uses of GGI in which GGI is part of a portfolio of different ARTs and functions as a kind of "last mile" intervention for those whom PGD and IVF alone would not be sufficient. Any one of these interventions in the portfolio will capture some portion of the patient population; the existence of all of them will increase the total number of individuals covered by available options. This is a modest future for therapeutic uses of GGI indeed. All of this, however, is speculative and depends on whether GGI really does end up functionally equivalent, in terms of clinical outcomes, to PGD, something that is impossible to know unless and until research into GGI progresses to the point where actual clinical applications begin to take shape. There are several foreseeable future paths: GGI may be so safe, accurate, efficient, and cheap that it can be combined with several ARTs in a variety of clinical settings and would then offer a clear improvement over PGD. Alternatively, it may be so risky that it would only be justifiable in the rarest of cases. It may also end up that, although GGI becomes technically feasible, its risk/benefit profile rules it out of clinical use altogether. And it also may be the case that demand for GGI is quite small—that in the remainder of cases not covered by existing ARTs, individuals would rather opt for adoption or surrogacy or gamete donation. The only way to begin to get answers to these questions is continued research into therapeutic uses of GGI.

8.4 The Targets Problem

Suppose that we end up with a GGI-based intervention that functions as a platform and so can be used on different genes, can make efficient and accurate alterations to those genes, and can be used on many different conditions. This would be pretty close to the ideal of gene editors to have a platform that can be used to make bespoke therapies as medical need dictates (Urnov 2021). One set of questions we need to ask about this intervention would be what genes would be actionable *targets*, and what *goals* and *outcomes* would be justifiable, for this intervention (Cwik 2020b). Some genotypes and outcomes seem to have fairly clear-cut clinical utility; other targets likewise seem to have no clinical utility (for example, any use of GGI to select traits for aesthetic purposes, such as to choose blue-eyed children). Even if such applications were permissible (a highly dubious prospect overall, and one that, as I said above, I believe should be impermissible as it involves a non-therapeutic use of GGI), we would at best classify these as having "personal utility" (Grosse and Khoury 2006), like direct-to-consumer genetic testing for genes such as *OR2M7*.[10] But there are other targets that are not so clear cut, such as the use of *GJB2* to prevent hereditary deafness. How do we differentiate good from bad targets and outcomes?

One way to tackle this problem is to analogize it to the general issue of actionability in medical genetics. There are already available criteria for defining specific genes of actionable targets for testing and therapeutic intervention. The American College of Medical Genetics and Genomics (ACMG) maintains a regularly updated list of "gene-phenotype pairs for opportunistic screening to facilitate the identification and/or management of risks for selected genetic disorders through established interventions" (Miller et al. 2023). The concept of actionability is complex (Chin-Yee and Plutynski 2023), but there may be some initial progress to be made on this question by seeing how far existing criteria could extend to deal with selection of targets for GGI. One possible starting point could be to adopt the general standard for genetic testing and screening in pediatrics that restricts these to early onset conditions for which intervention can make a clear difference (Ross et al. 2013). As noted above, if the condition is early onset then a neonatal or early life somatic gene therapy may be a less optimal strategy, as damage could already start accruing by the time the condition is detected and the intervention administered, possibly making it a good candidate for GGI.

There are, however, some elements of the targets problem that cannot be dealt with in this manner. To get at just how difficult these will be, consider some of the language used in the recent joint report by the US National Academies of Science and the UK Royal Society. According to Recommendation 4 in this report: "Initial uses of heritable human genome editing (HHGE) [that is, editing of nuclear DNA in germline cells] … should be limited to circumstances that meet the following criteria:

---

[10] A single nucleotide polymorphism in *OR2M7* is one of 871 genetic variants believed to be implicated in whether an individual can smell the distinctive "asparagus pee" odor to their urine after eating asparagus; see Markt et al. (2016) (note the statistics pun in the title of their paper).

- The use of HHGE is limited to *serious monogenic diseases* … [defined as] one that causes severe morbidity or premature death;
- The use of HHGE is limited to changing *a pathogenic genetic variant* … to *a sequence that is common in the relevant population* …
- No embryos without the disease-causing genotype will be subject to the process of genome editing and transfer … and
- … the use of HHGE is limited to situations in which prospective parents (i) have no option for having a genetically-related child that does not have the *serious monogenic disease*…or (ii) have extremely poor options." (National Academy of Medicine, National Academy of Sciences, and the Royal Society 2020, 9–10; emphasis added throughout).

Recommendation 4 invokes three concepts—"serious monogenic disorder," "pathogenic genetic variant," and "sequence that is common in the relevant population"—which have three features in common: (1) they are not, as stated, clear; (2) it is difficult to see how they could be made clear in a way that allows them to function as intended; and (3) even if they could be made clear, these notions are contestable.

To start, the language of "serious" genetic disorders is problematic (Kleiderman et al. 2019). In this report, "serious" is defined in terms of "severe morbidity and premature death." Infantile Tay-Sachs fits this bill, and selection of blue eye color clearly does not. But many monogenic conditions with severe morbidity are not necessarily connected to premature death; thanks to the drug nusinersen, spinal muscular atrophy type 1 (SMA-1) no longer must result in premature death (Gyngell et al. 2020), though SMA-1 is usually classified as a condition that results in severe morbidity even with pharmaceutical treatment. "Severe morbidity" here is not a clear standard. Does it refer to severity of outcome, or severity of symptoms and suffering? Some monogenic disorders that have severe outcomes do not have severe symptoms or result in a great deal of suffering. For example, hypertrophic cardiomyopathy, a condition caused by a mutation in the *MYBPC3* gene, can have mild or even no symptoms, though individuals with the condition have a much higher risk of cardiovascular events and may have (but not in all cases) a higher risk of premature death, depending on how the condition manifests (Ma et al. 2017). By this standard, then, it is not clear whether either SMA-1 or hypertrophic cardiomyopathy would be clear-cut candidates for GGI. Maybe that is the way it should be—perhaps our criterion for "serious monogenic disease" should be quite restrictive. Even if so, that requires argument and is not something that can be stipulated via definition of "serious monogenic disorder."

The case that framed this chapter—use of GGI to prevent hereditary deafness—shows how difficult it will be to use "pathogenic genetic variant" as a standard here. Is a mutation in *GJB2* that leads to deafness a "pathogenic" (that is, one that causes or raises the risk of disease) variant? That depends on whether hereditary deafness is "pathological" (as opposed to, say, a variation on human physiology) or is "pathological" in the right way. We could opt here for an inclusive application of this criterion—perhaps there are lots of pathogenic genetic variants, but not every pathogenic variant is a target for GGI (the variant would have to result in, say, a "serious monogenic disorder"). There are many genetic variants associated with myopia (Wojciechowski and Hysi 2013). These are pathogenic, in that myopia is a disorder that justifies medical interventions (glasses, contact lenses, laser eye surgery), but myopia would, under even very permissive criteria, likely fall short of a justifiable target for GGI.[11] We could say *GJB2* is pathogenic but that congenital deafness is not a "serious monogenic disorder," so *GJB2* is not a justifiable target. This looks arbitrary. Again, there are conditions that do not result in both severe morbidity and premature death that look like they are at least possible candidates for GGI, and the claim that mutations in *GJB2* do not result in severe morbidity requires an argument as to why lacking hearing is not "severe morbidity."[12]

The "monogenic" qualifier in the criterion of "serious monogenic disorder" is also a problem. One reason why we might want to restrict gene editing to single genes is because this could limit the damage we could do with gene editing, at least temporarily (Cwik 2019). Suppose advances in gene editing research open the door one day to a GGI-based intervention for multifactorial gene editing, allowing for the targeting of multiple loci in multiple genes at once. In this case, would we hold that individuals with, for instance, pathogenic variants in a suite of tumor suppressor genes possess "pathogenic genetic variants" but are not candidates for GGI because any cancers they develop would not be monogenic disorders? If we drop the "monogenic" qualifier, this opens the door to asking whether many complex traits caused by multiple genes are "serious" diseases in a way that could be uncomfortable—propensity for schizophrenia, for instance, like propensity for early onset cancers is (believed to be) connected to possession of a suite of pathogenic variants (Sullivan 2005), and schizophrenia is certainly a condition that can often result in severe morbidity and premature death (from secondary effects of the illness). And finally, "sequence that is common in the relevant population" does not fare any better either. Though it might seem straightforward, the criterion implicitly invokes the idea that there is such a thing as a normal human genome and that we can fix the baseline for this in terms of what is common—that is, in terms of raw prevalence. Plenty of variants that are pathogenic are fairly common (the genetic bases of myopia, for instance), and so there is no necessary connection between "common" and "non-pathogenic" that would allow us to restrict changing a "pathogenic" variant only to a "common" one in all cases.

The point is not to excessively critique the authors of the above-discussed report and its Recommendation 4. The point is that what seems like a clear and sensible way to get a provisional framework for the use of GGI ends up raising substantial concerns.

[11] However, on a maximally unrestricted criterion, it would not. If GGI was permissible for *any* pathogenic condition—myopia, flat feet, and so on—then merely defining something as "pathogenic" makes it a target for GGI. We can call this the *Gattaca* criterion, after Andrew Niccol's now classic science fiction film, in which this maximally permissive criterion becomes *de rigeur* in reproductive medicine. *Gattaca* (the movie) is a conclusive argument for why a maximally unrestricted criterion is unacceptable.

[12] There are other reasons why genetic variants that lead to congenital deafness are not straightforwardly pathogenic, such as the social impacts on deaf individuals; for discussion, see Padden and Humphries (2020).

Recommendation 4 raises questions about which genetic variants are pathogenic and which are normal; what normal variation in the human genome is; how we fix reference sequences for important genes and how we measure individual variation against these sequences; and what traits we think warrant genetic intervention.[13]

It is worth noting here that there is an implicit naturalism about genetic disease that is behind the sort of approach in Recommendation 4. Delimiting a scope for medical intervention via a derivation from what is "normal" (defined as what is a species-typical and adaptive character) and what is "pathological" (defined as a maladaptive departure from normal variation) has long been the strategy of naturalist positions in the philosophy of medicine.[14] Christopher Boorse, who laid out the most influential such position in contemporary philosophy of medicine, was very explicit about this aim of his view:

> We must avoid confusing empirical questions with deep normative issues about the goals of human life and the role of health professionals in achieving them. The trouble with calling physical or mental or moral excellence health is that it tends to unite under one term a value-neutral notion, freedom from disease, with the most controversial of all prescriptions—the recipe for an ideal human being. (Boorse 1977, 572)[15]

For Boorse, the definitions of "health" and "disease" can be settled empirically by appeal to normal functioning, which could be fixed in terms of frequencies of characters in the human population coupled with an adaptationist account of what these characters contributed to survival and reproductive advantage. On his view, this could help limit medical interventions by placing traits or conditions that we merely disapproved of outside the scope of medicine.

Boorsean naturalism has been the subject of significant criticism and debate (Ereshefsky 2009; Boorse 2014). But when it comes to GGI, it is easy to see the attractions: if we can get a well-defined, empirically fixable set of criteria for justifiable targets of GGI (for instance, by setting these targets in terms of "severe morbidity and premature death," defined in Boorsean naturalist terms, or "a sequence that is common in the relevant population," defined in terms of raw prevalence), then we can successfully circumscribe the set of conditions and targets for which GGI would be appropriate in a way that (hopefully) restricts the scope of justifiable applications of the interventions (and rules out biomedical enhancement for free). But if

[13] It should be clear that these questions are not just questions about GGI but come up in many different areas of medical genetics, such as debates about what genes to include in standard screening panels. These may well be some of the biggest questions about genetics in medicine, but they are raised in a particularly intense way by thinking about selection of targets for GGI.

[14] Kleiderman et al. (2019) also note a connection between strategies for delimiting the scope of therapeutic applications for gene editing via a definition of "serious genetic disorder" to naturalist (they use the term "objectivist") theories of health and disease.

[15] Describing Boorse's position as a naturalist view is controversial. Broadbent (2019, 96–97), for example, argues that under common understandings of naturalism, Boorse's view ends up making health a non-natural property. Varga (2020) also argues that Boorse's position cannot ground a naturalist position about health and disease. Whether or not Boorse succeeds in laying out a plausible naturalism, Boorse (2014) is clear that he views his theory as a naturalist account. Interestingly enough, Boorse (2016) himself is skeptical about whether a proper goal and scope for medical intervention can be defined.

we cannot do this, then we are left with the discomfiting possibility that empirically grounded (and so, presumably, fact-based, consensus-generating, not contestable) concepts cannot be the sole basis for choosing targets for GGI.

Addressing this problem will be a major challenge for regulation of GGI, should GGI ever become a legitimate clinical possibility. At this stage the level of difficulty of the problem is unclear, as the nature of the targets problem depends a great deal on how the technology develops. At the end of § 3, we noted a few different possibilities for GGI—that it becomes so cheap, effective, and accessible that it is widely available in reproductive medicine, or that it is so cumbersome that it will only be used in the direst circumstances (if it is ever used at all). The targets problem is most acute in the first set of circumstances. If the technology is unusable except in rare cases where there are few or no other options, or if it ends up with no clinical benefits over existing ARTs like PGD, or if the risk/benefit profile of the technology rules out uses for, say, pathological but common conditions or conditions such as congenital deafness, then the set of justifiable targets for GGI will be naturally small and there will be little issue. Given the current state of research, it is a real possibility that the central question about selection of targets is about weighing which rare genetic disorders are worth the risks and expense of GGI. It may be the case that, instead of having to narrow the list of targets of GGI to avoid various dystopian science fiction scenarios, we have to choose from an already narrow list of which targets justify use of GGI. Or to put it differently, it may be the case that we do not have to worry about how to restrict use of GGI to "serious monogenic disorders" or the like, but rather that we must worry about what clinical benefits would justify its use at all.

8.5 Conclusion

But if GGI progresses to the point where clinical use for a variety of conditions is a real possibility, the targets problem will become more acute, and this means getting not just some clarity on issues about which conditions warrant GGI or which genotypes are justifiable targets for GGI, but clarity on these issues that can be *usable* in regulating the use of the technology. Drawing fine-grained red lines around specific uses of GGI, permitting some and forbidding others, looks, on its face, like an almost impossibly difficult institutional design problem. How to draw usable and enforceable red lines around unjustifiable uses of platform technologies—technologies that are widely applicable and maximally versatile, such that introducing them for one use automatically introduces them for others (artificial intelligence is the current go-to example)—has a claim to be one of the biggest regulatory and policy problems of our time (Kaebnick et al. 2016; Cwik 2021).

Novel biomedical technologies do not emerge in a vacuum, and what pathways (if any) GGI will take will depend on economic, political, demographic, and cultural factors at play in the world of the mid-twenty-first century in ways that are impossible to responsibly speculate on from our current vantage. Worldwide policy responses to the possibility of the technology have varied widely (Baylis et al. 2020). There are some ethical questions about GGI that cannot be adequately addressed unless and until research and an overall global policy landscape begins to take shape. Besides ethical questions about clinical use, other drivers of law and policy (not to mention politics and culture) may result in a policy landscape that is unfavorable or forbidding for GGI. It is not hard to imagine a future where religious, political, cultural, or social objections to research that involves human germline cells, use of ARTs such as PGD and germline genome editing, and large parts of reproductive medicine generally (even including IVF) become severely restricted to the point of irrelevance or even illegality. Nevertheless, there is a strong general sentiment—behind both the interest in the topic in the bioethics literature and responses like holding international summits and crafting policy frameworks—that GGI is too potentially disruptive and consequential to adopt a "wait-and-see" approach. Whether this itself is the right move—whether we can try to ease the landing of disruptive emerging technologies by engaging in ethical discussion ahead of time—is a significant question in its own right about many technologies other than GGI (Kaebnick et al. 2016; Mathews et al. 2022). Should a great deal of technical progress and the right set of factors come to pass, we could get to the point in the not-terribly-distant future where it is sensible to begin considering next steps, beyond basic research, for GGI into the clinic. In that scenario, the targets problem will be a crucial part of examining whether (and if so, how) GGI could be used responsibly with clinical benefit in reproductive medicine.[16]

8.6 Disclosure of Interests

The author is a member of the Scientific Advisory Board for the Oregon Health and Science University Center for Embryonic Cell and Gene Therapy. The author is a pro bono member and does not receive an honorarium for their service.

[16] The ideas and arguments in this chapter have had many different lives over the past four years. Versions of this chapter were presented at a Stanford University Law and Biosciences Workshop in February 2024; the 6th Reproductive Ethics Conference at University of Texas Medical Branch-Galveston in January 2022; and an Oregon Bioethics and Humanities Colloquium at the Oregon Health and Science University Center for Ethics in December 2021 (the latter two were remote due to the COVID-19 pandemic). Thanks to audiences at these talks for their comments and questions, and thanks to Hank Greely and Bonginkosi Shozi for inviting me to Stanford and Tyler Tate for inviting me to OHSU. Thanks also to several anonymous referees, for their many helpful comments and remarks.

References

Adashi, Eli Y., and I. Glenn Cohen. 2016. "Going Germline: Mitochondrial Replacement as a Guide to Genome Editing." *Cell* 164 (6) (February 25): 832–835. https://doi.org/10.1016/j.cell.2016.02.018.

Andorno, Roberto, Françoise Baylis, Marcy Darnovsky, Donna Dickenson, Hille Haker, Katie Hasson, et al. 2020. "Geneva Statement on Heritable Human Genome Editing: The Need for Course Correction." *Trends in Biotechnology* 38 (4) (April): 351–354. https://doi.org/10.1016/j.tibtech.2019.12.022.

Baylis, Françoise, Marcy Darnovsky, Katie Hasson, and Timothy M. Krahn. 2020. "Human Germline and Heritable Genome Editing: The Global Policy Landscape." *CRISPR Journal* 3 (5) (October): 365–377. https://doi.org/10.1089/crispr.2020.0082.

Boorse, Christopher. 1977. "Health as a Theoretical Concept." *Philosophy of Science* 44 (4) (December): 542–573.

Boorse, Christopher. 2014. "A Second Rebuttal on Health." *Journal of Medicine and Philosophy* 39 (6) (December): 683–724. https://doi.org/10.1093/jmp/jhu035.

Boorse, Christopher. 2016. "Goals of Medicine." In *Naturalism in the Philosophy of Health: Issues and Implications*, ed. Élodie Giroux, 145–177. Cham: Springer. https://doi.org/10.1007/978-3-319-29091-1_9.

Botkin, Jeffrey R. 2020. "The Case for Banning Heritable Genome Editing." *Genetics in Medicine* 22 (3) (March): 487–489. https://doi.org/10.1038/s41436-019-0696-6.

Broadbent, Alex. 2019. *Philosophy of Medicine*. New York: Oxford University Press.

Cavaliere, Giulia. 2018. "Genome Editing and Assisted Reproduction: Curing Embryos, Society, or Prospective Parents?" *Medicine, Health Care, and Philosophy* 21 (2) (June): 215–225. https://doi.org/10.1007/s11019-017-9793-y.

Chin-Yee, Benjamin, and Anya Plutynski. 2023. "Concepts of Actionability in Precision Oncology." *Philosophy of Science* epub: 1–12. https://doi.org/10.1017/psa.2023.115.

Cohen, Jon. 2022. "Where Does Embryo Editing Stand Now?" *Science* 375 (6587) (March 25): 1328–1329. https://doi.org/10.1126/science.abq1707.

Cwik, Bryan. 2017. "Designing Ethical Trials of Germline Gene Editing." *New England Journal of Medicine* 377 (20) (November 16): 1911–1913. https://doi.org/10.1056/NEJMp1711000.

Cwik, Bryan. 2019. "Moving Beyond 'Therapy' and 'Enhancement' in the Ethics of Gene Editing." *Cambridge Quarterly of Healthcare Ethics* 28 (4) (October): 695–707. https://doi.org/10.1017/S0963180119000641.

Cwik, Bryan. 2020a. "Intergenerational Monitoring in Clinical Trials of Germline Gene Editing." *Journal of Medical Ethics* 46 (3) (March): 183–187. https://doi.org/10.1136/medethics-2019-105620.

Cwik, Bryan. 2020b. "Revising, Correcting, and Transferring Genes." *American Journal of Bioethics* 20 (8): 7–18. https://doi.org/10.1080/15265161.2020.1783024.

Cwik, Bryan. 2021. "Gene Editing: How Can You Ask 'Whether' If You Don't Know 'How'?" *Hastings Center Report* 51 (3) (May–June): 13–17. https://doi.org/10.1002/hast.1256.

Cwik, Bryan. 2022. "Trojan Horses, Clinical Utility, and Parfitian Puzzles." *American Journal of Bioethics* 22 (9): 16–18. https://doi.org/10.1080/15265161.2022.2105434.

Cyranoski, David. 2019. "Russian 'CRISPR-Baby' Scientist Has Started Editing Genes in Human Eggs with Goal of Altering Deaf Gene." *Nature* 574 (7779) (October 24): 465–466. https://doi.org/10.1038/d41586-019-03018-0.

Daley, George Q. 2024. "Welcoming the Era of Gene Editing in Medicine." *New England Journal of Medicine* 390 (18) (May 9): 1642–1645. https://doi.org/10.1056/NEJMp2314279.

Daley, George Q., Robin Lovell-Badge, and Julie Steffann. 2019. "After the Storm—a Responsible Path for Genome Editing." *New England Journal of Medicine* 380 (10) (March 7): 897–899. https://doi.org/10.1056/NEJMp1900504.

Darnovsky, Marcy, and Katie Hasson. 2020. "CRISPR's Twisted Tales: Clarifying Misconceptions about Heritable Genome Editing." *Perspectives in Biology and Medicine* 63 (1) (Winter): 155–176. https://doi.org/10.1353/pbm.2020.0012.

de Melo Martin, Inmaculada. 2022. "Reproductive Embryo Editing: Attending to Justice." *Hastings Center Report* 52 (4) (July–August): 26–33. https://doi.org/10.1002/hast.1406.

Doudna, Jennifer A. 2020. "The Promise and Challenge of Therapeutic Genome Editing." *Nature* 578 (7794) (February 13): 229–236. https://doi.org/10.1038/s41586-020-1978-5.

Ereshefsky, Marc. 2009. "Defining 'Health' and 'Disease.'" *Studies in History and Philosophy of Biological and Biomedical Sciences* 40 (3) (September): 221–227. https://doi.org/10.1016/j.shpsc.2009.06.005.

Evans, John H. 2021. "Setting Ethical Limits on Human Gene Editing after the Fall of the Somatic/Germline Barrier." *Proceedings of the National Academy of Sciences* 118 (22) (June 1): e2004837117. https://doi.org/10.1073/pnas.2004837117.

Fabi, Rachel, and Daniel S. Goldberg. 2022. "Bioethics, (Funding) Priorities, and the Perpetuation of Injustice." *American Journal of Bioethics* 22 (1): 6–13. https://doi.org/10.1080/15265161.2020.1867934.

Farmer, Paul E., Bruce Nizeye, Sara Stulac, and Salmaan Keshavjee. 2006. "Structural Violence and Clinical Medicine." *PLoS Medicine* 3 (10) (October): e449. https://doi.org/10.1371/journal.pmed.0030449.

Gheaus, Anca. 2018. "Biological Parenthood: Gestational, Not Genetic." *Australasian Journal of Philosophy* 96 (2): 225–240. https://doi.org/10.1080/00048402.2017.1354389.

Glover, Jonathan. 2008. *Choosing Children: Genes, Disability, and Design*. Oxford: Clarendon.

Greely, Henry T. 2021. *CRISPR People: The Science and Ethics of Editing Humans*. Cambridge, MA: MIT Press.

Grosse, Scott D., and Muin J. Khoury. 2006. "What Is the Clinical Utility of Genetic Testing?" *Genetics in Medicine* 8 (7) (July): 448–450. https://doi.org/10.1097/01.gim.0000227935.26763.c6.

Gyngell, Christopher, Hillary Bowman-Smart, and Julian Savulescu. 2019. "Moral Reasons to Edit the Human Genome: Picking Up from the Nuffield Report." *Journal of Medical Ethics* 45 (8) (August): 514–523. https://doi.org/10.1136/medethics-2018-105084.

Gyngell, Christopher, Zornitza Stark, and Julian Savulescu. 2020. "Drugs, Genes and Screens: The Ethics of Preventing and Treating Spinal Muscular Atrophy." *Bioethics* 34 (5) (June): 493–501. https://doi.org/10.1111/bioe.12695.

Herbert, Mary, and Doug Turnbull. 2018. "Progress in Mitochondrial Replacement Therapies." *Nature Reviews Molecular Cell Biology* 19 (2) (February): 71–72. https://doi.org/10.1038/nrm.2018.3.

Hooper, Monica Webb, Anna María Nápoles, and Eliseo J. Pérez-Stable. 2020. "COVID-19 and Racial/Ethnic Disparities." *JAMA: Journal of the American Medical Association* 323 (24) (May 11): 2466–2467. https://doi.org/10.1001/jama.2020.8598.

Kaebnick, Gregory, Elizabeth Heitman, James P. Collins, Jason A. Delborne, Wayne G. Landis, Keegan Sawyer, Lisa A. Taneyhill, and David E. Winickoff. 2016. "Precaution and Governance of Emerging Technologies." *Science* 354 (6313) (November 11): 710–711. https://doi.org/10.1126/science.aah5125.

Kleiderman, Erika, Vardit Ravitsky, and Bartha M. Knoppers. 2019. "The 'Serious' Factor in Germline Modification." *Journal of Medical Ethics* 45 (8) (August): 508–513. https://doi.org/10.1136/medethics-2019-105436.

Lander, Eric, Françoise Baylis, Feng Zheng, Emmanuelle Charpentier, Paul Berg, Catherine Bourgain, et al. 2019. "Adopt a Moratorium on Heritable Genome Editing." *Nature* 567 (7747) (March 14): 165–168. https://doi.org/10.1038/d41586-019-00726-5.

Lea, Rebecca A., and Kathy K. Niakan. 2019. "Human Germline Genome Editing." *Nature Cell Biology* 21 (12) (December): 1479–1489. https://doi.org/10.1038/s41556-019-0424-0.

Ledford, Heidi. 2022. "Gene Therapy's Comeback: How Scientists Are Trying to Make It Safer." *Nature* 606 (7914) (June 16): 443–444. https://doi.org/10.1038/d41586-022-01518-0.

Liang, Dan, Aleksei Mikhalchenko, Hong Ma, Nuria Marti Gutierrez, Tailai Chen, Yeonmi Lee, et al. 2023. "Limitations of Gene Editing Assessments in Human Preimplantation Embryos." *Nature Communications* 14 (1) (March 7): article no. 1219. https://doi.org/10.1038/s41467-023-36820-6.

Ma, Hong, Nuria Marti-Gutierrez, Sang-Wook Park, Jun Wu, Yeonmi Lee, Keiichiro Suzuki, et al. 2017. "Correction of a Pathogenic Gene Mutation in Human Embryos." *Nature* 548 (7668) (August 24): 413–419. https://doi.org/10.1038/nature23305.

Mallapaty, Smriti. 2022. "How to Protect the First 'CRISPR Babies' Prompts Ethical Debate." *Nature* 603 (7900) (March 10): 213–214. https://doi.org/10.1038/d41586-022-00512-w.

Markt, Sarah C., Elizabeth Nuttall, Constance Turman, Jennifer Sinnott, Eric B. Rimm, Ethan Ecsedy, et al. 2016. "Sniffing Out Significant 'Pee Values': Genome Wide Association Study of Asparagus Anosmia." *BMJ* 355: i6071. https://doi.org/10.1136/bmj.i6071.

Mathews, Debra J. H., Celynne A. Balatbat, and Victor J. Dzau. 2022. "Governance of Emerging Technologies in Health and Medicine—Creating a New Framework." *New England Journal of Medicine* 386 (23) (June 9): 2239–2242. https://doi.org/10.1056/NEJMms2200907.

Miller, David T., Kristy Lee, Noura S. Abel-Housn, Laura M. Amendola, Kyle Brothers, Wendy K. Chung, et al. 2023. "ACMG SF v3.2 List for Reporting of Secondary Findings in Clinical Exome and Genome Sequencing: A Policy Statement of the American College of Medical Genetics and Genomics (ACMG)." *Genetics in Medicine* 25 (8) (August): 100866. https://doi.org/10.1016/j.gim.2023.100866.

National Academy of Medicine, National Academy of Sciences, and the Royal Society. 2020. *Heritable Human Genome Editing*. Washington, DC: National Academies. https://nap.nationalacademies.org/catalog/25665/heritable-human-genome-editing.

Notini, Lauren, Christopher Gyngell, and Julian Savulescu. 2020. "Drawing the Line on In Vitro Gametogenesis." *Bioethics* 34 (1) (January): 123–134. https://doi.org/10.1111/bioe.12679.

Pacesa, Martin, Oana Pelea, and Martin Jinek. 2024. "Past, Present, and Future of CRISPR Genome Editing Technologies." *Cell* 187 (5) (February 29): 1076–1100. https://doi.org/10.1016/j.cell.2024.01.042.

Padden, Carol, and Jacqueline Humphries. 2020. "Who Goes First? Deaf People and CRISPR Germline Editing." *Perspectives in Biology and Medicine* 63 (1) (Winter): 54–65. https://doi.org/10.1353/pbm.2020.0004.

Palacios-González, César. 2017. "Are There Moral Differences between Maternal Spindle Transfer and Pronuclear Transfer?" *Medicine, Health Care and Philosophy* 20 (4) (December): 503–511. https://doi.org/10.1007/s11019-017-9772-3.

Ranisch, Robert. 2020. "Germline Genome Editing versus Preimplantation Genetic Diagnosis: Is There a Case in Favor of Germline Interventions?" *Bioethics* 34 (1) (January): 60–69. https://doi.org/10.1111/bioe.12635.

Ranisch, Robert, Katharina Trettenbach, and Gardar Arnason. 2023. "Initial Heritable Genome Editing: Mapping a Responsible Pathway from Basic Research to the Clinic." *Medicine, Health Care, and Philosophy* 26 (1) (March): 21–35. https://doi.org/10.1007/s11019-022-10115-x.

Ross, Laine Friedman, Howard M. Saal, Karen L. David, and Rebecca R. Anderson. 2013. "Technical Report: Ethical and Policy Issues in Genetic Testing and Screening of Children." *Genetics in Medicine* 15 (3) (March): 234–245. https://doi.org/10.1038/gim.2012.176.

Rugg-Gunn, Peter J., Naomi Moris, and Patrick P. L. Tam. 2023. "Technical Challenges of Studying Early Human Development." *Development* 150 (11) (June): dev201797. https://doi.org/10.1242/dev.201797.

Russell, Oliver M., Gráinne S. Gorman, Robert M. Lightowlers, and Doug M. Turnbull. 2020. "Mitochondrial Diseases: Hope for the Future." *Cell* 181 (1) (April 2): 168–188. https://doi.org/10.1016/j.cell.2020.02.051.

Segers, Seppe. 2023. "Heritable Genome Editing: Ethical Aspects of a Developing Domain." *Human Reproduction* 38 (11) (November): 2055–2261. https://doi.org/10.1093/humrep/dead167.

Sparrow, Robert. 2022. "Human Germline Genome Editing: On the Nature of Our Reasons to Genome Edit." *American Journal of Bioethics* 22 (9): 4–15. https://doi.org/10.1080/15265161.2021.1907480.

Srivastava, Arun. 2020. "AAV Vectors: Are They Safe?" *Human Gene Therapy* 31 (13–14) (July): 697–699. https://doi.org/10.1089/hum.2020.187.

Stark, Zornitza, and Richard H. Scott. 2023. "Genomic Newborn Screening for Rare Diseases." *Nature Reviews Genetics* 24 (11) (November): 755–766. https://doi.org/10.1038/s41576-023-00621-w.

Steffann, Julie, Pierre Jouannet, Jean-Paul Bonnefont, Hervé Chneiweiss, and Nelly Frydman. 2018. "Could Failure in Preimplantation Genetic Diagnosis Justify Editing the Human Embryo Genome?" *Cell Stem Cell* 22 (4) (April 5): 481–482. https://doi.org/10.1016/j.stem.2018.01.004.

Sullivan, Patrick F. 2005. "The Genetics of Schizophrenia." *PLoS Medicine* 2 (7) (July): e212. https://doi.org/10.1371/journal.pmed.0020212.

Turocy, Jenna, Eli Y. Adashi, and Dieter Egli. 2021. "Heritable Human Genome Editing: Research Progress, Ethical Considerations, and Hurdles to Clinical Practice." *Cell* 184 (6) (March 18): 1561–1574. https://doi.org/10.1016/j.cell.2021.02.036.

Urnov, Fydor. 2018. "An Ode to Gene Edits That Prevent Deafness." *Nature* 553 (7687) (January 11): 162–163. https://doi.org/10.1038/d41586-017-08645-z.

Urnov, Fydor. 2021. "Imagine CRISPR Cures." *Molecular Therapy* 29 (11) (November 3): 3103–3106. https://doi.org/10.1016/j.ymthe.2021.10.019.

Varga, Samogy. 2020. "Epistemic Authority, Philosophical Explication, and the Bio-statistical Theory of Disease." *Erkenntnis* 85 (4) (August): 937–956. https://doi.org/10.1007/s10670-018-0058-9.

Velleman, J. David. 2005. "Family History." *Philosophical Papers* 34 (3): 357–378. https://doi.org/10.1080/05568640509485163.

Viotti, Manuel, Andrea R. Victor, Darren K. Griffin, Jason S. Groob, Alan J. Brake, Christo G. Zouves, and Frank L. Barnes. 2019. "Estimating Demand for Germline Genome Editing: An *In Vitro* Fertilization Clinic Perspective." *CRISPR Journal* 2 (5) (October): 304–315. https://doi.org/10.1089/crispr.2019.0044.

Wang, Joy Y., and Jennifer A. Doudna. 2023. "CRISPR Technology: A Decade of Genome Editing Is Only the Beginning." *Science* 379 (6629) (January 20): eadd8643. https://doi.org/10.1126/science.add8643.

Wojciechowski, Robert, and Pirro G. Hysi. 2013. "Focusing In on the Complex Genetics of Myopia." *PLoS Genetics* 9 (4) (April): e1003442. https://doi.org/10.1371/journal.pgen.1003442.

Wolf, Don P., Paul A. Mitalipov, and Shoukhrat M. Mitalipov. 2019. "Principles of and Strategies for Germline Gene Therapy." *Nature Medicine* 25 (6) (June): 890–897. https://doi.org/10.1038/s41591-019-0473-8.

World Health Organization. 2023. "Primary Health Care." November 15. https://www.who.int/news-room/fact-sheets/detail/primary-health-care.

Zhang, John, Hui Liu, Shiyu Luo, Zhuo Lu, Alejandro Chávez-Badiola, Zitao Liu, et al. 2017. "Live Birth Derived from Oocyte Spindle Transfer to Prevent Mitochondrial Disease." *Reproductive BioMedicine Online* 34 (4) (April): 361–368. https://doi.org/10.1016/j.rbmo.2017.01.013.

Bryan Cwik is Associate Professor of Bioethics, Law, and Medical Professionalism in the Department of Community Health and Family Medicine and the School of Physician Assistant Studies at the University of Florida College of Medicine, and a member of the University of Florida Genetics Institute, USA. For 2025-2028, he is a Glenn and Deborah Renwick Fellow in AI Ethics in the University of Florida Engineering Leadership Institute. He primarily works on emerging technologies and their applications in different areas of medicine.

Chapter 9
Enhancing Injustice: Justice and the Ethics of Human Genetic Enhancement

Ryan Tonkens

Abstract This chapter focuses on justice-based considerations that emerge in the debate about the ethics of human genetic enhancement, including the potential for genetic enhancement to impact the moral equality of persons, concerns about the fair distribution of the benefits of genetic enhancement, and ways in which genetic enhancement could be used that are unjustly discriminatory. It is argued that the genetic enhancement enterprise (GEE) will fail to meet some minimal requirements for being just, especially for those who are the least well-off in society, but that other values (such as liberty and well-being) may prevent it from being morally unacceptable. However, the GEE may become severely unjust (and thereby morally reprehensible) if: (1) it does not help to remedy existing injustices, if it can help to do so; (2) it amplifies existing inequalities, for example, by changing the requirements for participation in the dominant cooperative framework in manner that is exclusionary rather than inclusive; (3) it creates new injustice(s) that cannot be adequately addressed via fair and effective policy; and (4) it fails to adequately protect those who choose not to participate in the GEE from being unable to access resources for satisfying their basic needs.

Keywords Genetic discrimination · Genetic enhancement · Human genome editing · Justice

9.1 Introduction

In some countries, the gene editing technology CRISPR/Cas-9 is already being used to treat genetic disease in humans. For example, in 2023 the United Kingdom's Medicines and Healthcare products Regulatory Agency approved a new treatment for sickle cell disease, called exagamglogene autotemcel (or Casgevy). The United States Food and Drug Administration also approved this treatment in January 2024, as

R. Tonkens (✉)
Lakehead University, Thunder Bay, ON, Canada
e-mail: rtonkens@lakeheadu.ca

M. C. Altman and D. Schwan (eds.), *Ethics and Medical Technology*, The International Library of Bioethics 113, https://doi.org/10.1007/978-3-031-94690-5_9

did Health Canada in September 2024. In principle, the same gene editing technology can be used for the genetic enhancement of humans—that is, to modify human genetic material to bring about augmented traits or capabilities, yielding genetic predispositions beyond "normal" or "species-typical" functioning (e.g., Daniels 1985)—even going beyond what is currently humanly possible. The purpose of this chapter is to critically engage with the ethics of human genetic enhancement, focusing on justice-related concerns that emerge in that context.

Many of the ethical issues will have different answers depending on the particular theory of justice that one subscribes to. For example, Allen Buchanan et al. (2000) argue that conclusions about whether we ought to use genetic technology and whether the state ought to make genetic technology available to citizens will be different depending on whether we endorse a brute-luck egalitarian view or a social structural view of equal opportunity. Moreover, there are different varieties of egalitarianism beyond these two accounts (e.g., all-luck egalitarianism), as well as non-egalitarian theories of justice, such as libertarianism and prioritarianism.

For the purpose of this chapter, I adopt a wide understanding of justice that includes two general elements: equality (i.e., the equal treatment of moral equals, including protection from unjust discrimination) and fairness (i.e., fair distribution of resources and opportunities, including access to the means for satisfying basic needs). Evaluating whether specific genetic enhancements are just and whether a particular manifestation of the genetic enhancement enterprise (hereafter GEE) is just will be based on, at minimum, their being consistent with equality and fairness. A similar understanding of justice is endorsed by the World Health Organization (WHO) Expert Advisory Committee on Developing Global Standards for Governance and Oversight of Human Genome Editing (2021), exemplified in several of the ethical principles and values that should inform decision-making about genome editing (including genetic enhancement), including:

- Social justice: "A commitment to develop human genome editing in ways that: (i) promote human health, collective well-being and the common good; (ii) look after the needs of communities experiencing greater health burdens; (iii) reduce socioeconomic inequality; and (iv) avoid discrimination"; and
- Equal moral worth: "A commitment to recognize and treat all people as having equal moral worth and their interests as deserving of equal moral consideration, with a particular need to recognize and protect the interests of persons with disabilities and of future generations" (World Health Organization 2021, 14).

It is worth noting that, while the WHO committee captures the elements of justice proposed above (equality, fairness, and non-discrimination), some of the corresponding normative prescriptions that the committee proposes are open for debate. For example, one element of justice that is *assumed* by the WHO's definition of the principle of "social justice" is "a commitment to develop human genome editing in ways that … reduce socioeconomic inequality" (14).[1] While I am sympathetic to

[1] It is better to cast a wider net with the "principle of social justice" than *socioeconomic* injustices alone, to include political and historical injustices, for example.

the goal of using genetic enhancements to help reduce inequality, it is unfortunate that the WHO committee makes this claim without argument or explanation. Important questions emerge about the extent to which the GEE needs to reduce existing socioeconomic inequalities, as opposed to not perpetuating them, and also whether *each* genetic enhancement needs to do so. Moreover, it is *assumed* that genetic edits can be used in ways that reduce socioeconomic inequalities (about which I say more below). Similarly, some will disagree with the WHO committee that the interests of future generations of humans ought to be provided with *equal* moral consideration, let alone a "particular need to recognize and protect the interests … of future generations" (14).

In Sect. 9.2, I provide an overview of some of the main components of the ethics of human genetic enhancement, including some key points of consensus as well as unsettled issues subject to ongoing debate. In Sect. 9.3, I raise important ethical and philosophical questions about the relationship between embarking on the GEE ethically and responsibly and the fact that inequalities and injustices already exist within society. I then critically engage with some of the most important justice-based concerns that emerge in the context of human genetic enhancement, focusing on the moral equality of persons (Sect. 9.4), access to genetic enhancement technology and the distribution of the benefits of that technology (Sect. 9.5), and unjust genetic discrimination (Sect. 9.6).

9.2 The Debate on the Ethics of Genetic Enhancement

Philosophers have been writing about the potential impacts of genetic technology since at least the final decades of the twentieth century. Long before the ability to successfully edit DNA, technology emerged that allowed for the generation of information about the genetic constitution of individuals and populations (i.e., genetic information), and a lot of attention was given to ethical questions about how such information should be used (Dickenson 2004), including access by health and life insurance organizations, or by employers as part of the hiring process (Kitcher 1997). As the field of assisted human reproduction developed and became more sophisticated, related ethical questions emerged there as well. For example, should genetic information generated via prenatal genetic diagnosis (PGD) technology inform the decision of which embryos to transfer based on sex-linked disease?

Some general conclusions that have been reached within the academic debate on the ethics of human genetic enhancement are worth highlighting. First, genetic enhancement needs to be safe (and effective) in order for it to be morally acceptable (Harris 2010; Lander et al. 2019). Indeed, the general case in favor of human genetic enhancement appeals to the immense potential benefits of the technology, once it is developed to a point where it is safe and effective. Genetic enhancements have the potential to provide benefits to individuals—for example, benefits they accrue from being stronger and smarter—as well as benefits to the human species—for example, delaying cell degeneration, higher intelligence that can be used for trying to resolve the world's most pressing problems, and altered skin pigment for enhanced resistance to radiation.

Second, in order for genetic enhancement to be morally acceptable, the deplorable aspects of historical, non-liberal eugenics programs need to be avoided, including undue infringement on the liberties of citizens, such as the right to pursue one's own family-building goals without undue intrusion from, or barriers imposed by, the state. If the genetic enhancement enterprise is pursued, then it ought to be liberal rather than non-liberal (Agar 1998, 2008).

While there is agreement that non-liberal eugenics is morally deplorable, there continues to be discussion about what role the state ought to play in orchestrating and monitoring the GEE—for example, devoting public and private resources to the research and development of genetic enhancement technology, and "allowing individuals and organizations the freedom to choose to develop or use such technology" (Buchanan 2011a, 178).[2] Some have noted that the state will have a strong interest in promoting some kinds of genetic enhancement in citizens, especially those enhancements that promise to help boost productivity, such as augmented memory capacity (Buchanan 2011b) and physical and psychological stamina. Moreover, some have argued that there is a moral obligation to boost overall well-being (Savulescu 2001). The extent to which the state may promote or require genetic enhancements without becoming unacceptably non-liberal remains an important and unsettled issue.

A third general conclusion to emerge from the current debate is that there are no features of enhancement that objectively distinguish it from genetic treatment (i.e., therapeutic interventions aiming at treating or curing disease or disability, or the restoration of "normal" or human species-typical functioning). One implication of this is that it may not be possible to categorically condone genetic treatment while also categorically rejecting genetic enhancement (Baylis 2019). Genetic interventions lie on a continuum across treatment/enhancement, and many interventions are both therapeutic *and* enhancing, such as genetically editing the process that leads to human cell degeneration (aging) and boosting immune system functioning.

In addition to a widespread rejection of the treatment/enhancement distinction, there is general agreement (though not consensus) that attempts to distinguish *genetic* enhancement from other kinds of human enhancements are untenable. Humans have been enhancing their capabilities for a very long time and through various means, such as literacy, intergenerational sharing of knowledge, pharmaceuticals, smartphones, and agriculture; and there is no principled difference between non-genetic enhancements and genetic enhancements, especially somatic interventions (non-heritable genetic modifications, performed on somatic cells, i.e., all cells in the human body

---

[2] This understanding of the genetic enhancement enterprise is inspired by Buchanan's (2011b) definition of the "enhancement enterprise." However, I do not follow Buchanan in also including in this definition (1) "the creation of a vigorous and informed public debate about the benefits and risks" of the technologies, or (2) "developing effective and morally sensitive policies and institutions for coping with the challenges of enhancement" (178). The genetic enhancement enterprise can (and perhaps will) manifest in ways that do not involve meaningful public engagement, and/or effective and morally sensitive policies and institutions, so it is a mistake to include these elements within the definition of the GEE.

that are not reproductive cells) as opposed to germline interventions (heritable genetic modifications, performed on reproductive cells). When considering whether a particular human enhancement is morally acceptable, then, we do well not to reject genetic enhancements out of hand just because they are *genetic* enhancements.

It is worth noting that germline genetic interventions have attracted more controversy and aversion compared to somatic interventions. For example, Eric Lander et al. (2019) have called for a (non-permanent) moratorium on germline applications of genome editing, especially for enhancement purposes (as opposed to what they call "corrective" purposes). Quoting from the statement by the Organizing Committee for the first International Summit on Human Gene Editing, the central reasons behind this are about resolving "'the relevant safety and efficacy issues,'" and seeking "'broad societal consensus about the appropriateness of the proposed application'" of gene-editing technology to the human germline (Lander et al. 2019, 166; Baltimore et al. 2015). Moreover, the WHO committee and others raise concerns about the fact that future generations of humans are not able to provide consent to germline genetic interventions, although there is the potential for them to be harmed by such decisions (inherited off-target mutations, genetic mosaicism, etc.). Others disagree with these concerns, and they present strong arguments in favor of allowing germline gene editing, especially for prophylactic or therapeutic purposes, citing the immense potential therapeutic and research benefits of safe germline genetic editing (Gyngell et al. 2017).

Lastly, there is also widespread rejection of "anti-enhancement" views (Buchanan 2011b, 13)—that is, views that hold that genetic enhancement is morally unacceptable across the board, or that there is something inherently morally unacceptable about genetic enhancement. One such anti-enhancement view worth mentioning here is the view of Jürgen Habermas (2003), who offers a thoughtful and unique critique of genetic enhancement, but one that does not also rule out therapeutic applications of genome editing (see also Sandel 2007).

Habermas raises ethical concerns about how the genetically enhanced person may come to understand the degree to which they are in control of their own life-course and which projects to take on. If people who are genetically enhanced by their parents come to see the ingrained intentions of their parents as guiding who they are supposed to be and the life-course they are predetermined to choose, then, according to Habermas, this could have negative psychological and emotional impacts on the enhanced person, resulting in a compromised ethical self-understanding of themselves as being the sole author of their life-course. According to Habermas, if this were to occur, then it would compromise the experience of people as having authoritative control of their own life-courses, which is a prerequisite for liberty and the foundation of human dignity.

While I believe that Habermas's view is largely misunderstood,[3] it also relies on a substantial empirical claim, about the actual experience of the genetically enhanced

---

[3] Even where critics admit that Habermas's view is challenging to interpret or claim that it is ambiguous, they do not always consider interpretations that are more charitable to Habermas. Buchanan, for example, reasons that Habermas is claiming that the genetically enhanced person either is "incapable of regarding themselves as free" or "that they would not be free" (2011b,

person and their ethical self-understanding. This empirical claim will remain untested and unanswered unless such genetically enhanced people are created. Moreover, Habermas's concern is attached to *prenatal* genetic enhancements and does not obviously transfer to post-natal, self-caused genetic enhancements. Yet, if such genetic enhancements become possible in the future, those people who are making their own choices about whether to be genetically enhanced may not be susceptible, at all or to the same degree, to the psychological and emotional harms at the heart of Habermas's view, for it would be their own intentions now ingrained in their genetic makeup, rather than the intentions of their parents.

9.3 Unjust Societies Embarking on the Genetic Enhancement Enterprise

When a country embarks on the GEE, it is likely that there will already be some inequities and injustices existing within that country, and thus the country would not be meeting the (ideal) standards of justice. While there will be some variability across different countries, it is likely that some (perhaps many) people within the society are the targets of unfair treatment by the state or its institutions. For example, they are targets of systemic racism or other forms of unjust discrimination, and/or they are not receiving fair opportunities to access resources for satisfying their basic needs. Disappointingly, in Canada (where I am writing) there are many examples of injustices to draw on, including inequality in wages paid to women and men, inequality in access to clean drinking water (see, e.g., Philibert et al. 2020), and systemic racism in healthcare delivery, which in many cases leads to the avoidable death of vulnerable patients (McCallum and Perry 2018). Moreover, specific groups have been the targets of historical injustices, many of which persist today. For example, Indigenous Peoples suffer from unjust imperial and colonial activities such as industrial and residential schooling (Talaga 2024), unjust laws (e.g., Canada's Indian Act [R.S.C., 1985, c. I-5]—which remains in force today), and a failure of the federal government to adequately meet its commitments to truth and reconciliation initiatives (Truth and Reconciliation Commission of Canada 2015).

An important philosophical question is about how a society that is already unjust in some ways, but which nevertheless purports to value social justice (i.e., equality, fairness, and non-discrimination), ought to approach the prospect of research and development of human genome editing technologies, including genetic enhancement technologies, and the project of embarking on the genetic enhancement enterprise more generally:

> *Should resources be devoted to the research and development of human genetic enhancement technologies (and the corresponding governance and monitoring of*

---

5). On my reading of Habermas, the crucial claim is that the enhanced person *may* not perceive themselves as the sole author of their life-course, given the parental intentions etched into their edited genome—even though they *are* free, and are *capable* of regarding themselves as such.

the genetic enhancement enterprise) given that social injustice exists within that country?

Importantly, this question is relevant even *if* the GEE will not exacerbate existing injustices or create new ones. The choice to pursue a GEE amidst unresolved yet resolvable injustices within society says something about the character of that society, and those in power ought to be held accountable for justifying the decision to embark on the GEE under those circumstances.

Many contributors to the debate on the ethics of genetic enhancement believe that genetic enhancement technology has the potential to be used in ways that address and reduce existing injustices. The WHO's principle of social justice discussed earlier echoes this, by requiring that applications of genome editing reduce social inequalities. So, one possible answer to the above question, and a potentially significant reason in favor of developing (some types of) genetic enhancement, is that doing so can be used to help remedy existing injustices.

It is an empirical question whether genetic enhancements can be used to address, reduce, and eliminate existing injustices, and the extent to which they *will* do so, if they can. Such empirical questions cannot be satisfactorily answered without actually researching and developing genetic enhancement, and so this answer to the above question is currently only speculative. Moreover, as there are other ways to address, reduce, and eliminate existing injustices without requiring the research and development of genetic enhancement technologies, this reason in favor of developing genetic enhancement technologies has the additional burden of needing to demonstrate that genetic enhancements are equal to or superior to such existing alternatives for reducing the particular injustice.

Inequalities attached to some types of human enhancements that are currently available (to some) can provide an important baseline when considering justice-related concerns regarding genetic enhancements. For example, literacy is a human enhancement that has benefited many people, and has perhaps even benefited the human species overall, yet it has also shifted the basic expectations for being able to participate in the dominant cooperative framework; people who are illiterate have limited ability to fully participate. That such enhancements exist in the context of unjust social arrangements ought to give us pause and deserves close scrutiny.

It is worth dwelling on this idea, as it is perhaps the most plausible answer to the above question available to those who endorse embarking on the genetic enhancement enterprise. Is it possible for specific genetic enhancements to reduce existing injustices? Whether a genetic enhancement can help to combat an existing injustice depends on what the injustice is. Therefore, in order to answer this question, we first need to know about the nature and source of the specific injustice that genetic enhancement is purportedly reducing or eliminating.

Can genetic enhancement alleviate injustices having to do with unequal or lack of access to clean drinking water? Perhaps the human genome could be modified in such a way that humans would not require as much hydration as they currently do to survive. Or perhaps humans could be made to tolerate higher concentrations of mercury in their bodies without corresponding health complications. Such applications of genetic enhancement would seem to lessen the harmful burden of being the victim of the injustice of having no access to, or unequal access to, clear drinking water. For some, reduced or eliminated harm may be sufficient to conclude that the injustice is thereby reduced or eliminated. However, this again raises the importance of having a nuanced understanding of the nature and source of the injustice, for it may be that contaminated drinking water is *a symptom of* injustice, rather than the injustice itself—part of this will depend on an understanding of the reasons *why* clean drinking water is not available for a particular person or group of people. Moreover, this raises the additional complication of needing to evaluate the moral acceptability of using genetic enhancement to reduce existing injustice, beyond whether it *can* reduce injustice—in this case, a moral evaluation of the act of addressing existing injustices by modifying the genetic constitution of the victims of such injustices, rather than by modifying the underlying background conditions creating the injustices.

A different example is the prospect of using genetic enhancements to assist with making people less racist (or xenophobic, transphobic, etc.), and so contribute to reducing the pervasiveness of racism in healthcare delivery and other areas of social and political life (on "moral enhancement," see Douglas 2008). This application of genetic enhancement would have the benefit of not requiring victims of injustice to modify themselves in order to be treated as moral equals.

As these examples demonstrate, it seems possible that genetic enhancements could be used to address, reduce, or eliminate some types of existing injustice, either through reducing the harms associated with the injustice or through modifying certain elements that contribute to unjust behavior, and thereby increase the likelihood of preventing such unjust behavior in the future. However, such potential for reducing social injustice is connected to complex physiological processes and genetic traits, such as xenophobia, humility, a sense of restorative justice, etc. The requisite scientific understanding and technological sophistication to modify these traits is not available at this time. Moreover, even if it was, such modifications are unlikely to reduce injustices in the near-term future, if uptake is slow and since there are other (non-genetic) factors contributing to racism (xenophobia, transphobia, etc.) being pervasive in society. Therefore, at best, the potential for genetic enhancements to eliminate or reduce social injustice is not available in the near-term, so this answer to the above question is not a compelling one (at this time).[4]

Critics may respond by suggesting that the prospect of research and development of genetic enhancement technology and of the GEE more generally do not need to address this concern about *existing* social injustices. There is freedom to innovate, alongside the importance of advancing scientific knowledge. Furthermore, it is unrealistic to expect that research and development of genetic enhancement will halt altogether, despite any social justice concerns; if necessary, some will go underground or seek private funding. Moreover, genetic enhancement is not the first new human enterprise to come about in the face of existing social injustices. Therefore, the

---

[4] My point here is about *genetic* enhancements in particular. Other kinds of human enhancement could potentially address or reduce existing social inequalities and injustices.

existence of social injustice is not only an insufficient reason to enact a moratorium on genetic enhancement. Attempting to do so is unrealistic and futile.

This response is not convincing. For one thing, the appeal to tradition does not show that the pursuit of genetic enhancement under conditions of existing social injustice is just or morally acceptable, even if it is true that other developments have occurred amidst preexisting injustice. If justice has historically been subverted in favor of scientific progress, liberties to innovate, and the quest for human betterment, this does not entail that justice cannot or should not be prioritized. Moreover, even if it is true that there are some liberties at stake, like the freedom to innovate, surely this ought to be balanced with other important values, such as social justice, when they come into conflict. The key issue is about how much weight different values (social justice, well-being, autonomy, market ideals such as profit-maximization, etc.) ought to be given in the decision-making about whether to pursue new initiatives amidst existing social injustices.

Buchanan offers a conditional argument to support the pursuit of the GEE amidst social injustices: *if* the risk has been worth taking with past developments, then "it's hard to see that it would be any different with biomedical enhancements—at least those that are likely to yield significant social benefit" (2011a, 131). Note that Buchanan does not consider who gets the privilege to decide whether the risk has been worth taking. When considering such positions, it is important to keep in mind that choices are being made about the perspective from which to analyze the potential benefits and harms of genetic enhancement. It is unlikely that professional academic philosophers will be at serious risk of being left behind in the advent of a GEE within their society, and it is unlikely that they will not have reasonable access to resources and opportunities. Conversely, for people who are already unable to participate in the dominant cooperative framework (e.g., people who are illiterate and people living in poverty), the risk of developing technologies such as genetic enhancement may not be acceptable or "worth taking," given that such people will likely not benefit from such technologies, even if they do have access to them (Tonkens 2021). This is especially true if the GEE and the availability of genetic enhancements do not address illiteracy or the harms of not being able to participate in the dominant, literate society. Indeed, if the widespread use of genetic enhancement made it such that some people are not able to participate in the dominant cooperative framework, either because they are not provided with reasonable opportunity to participate already, or because the framework has changed in such a way that now excludes them, then this is a serious concern.

9.4 Moral Equality of (Post)persons

There is a longstanding moral presumption that, as a matter of justice, all entities with the same moral status ought to be afforded with the same moral acknowledgment (e.g., through rights and legal protections), unless they do something which forfeits such protection. Some have argued that genetic enhancement technology could make it possible to alter humanity to such an extent that the result would be the creation of "posthumans," i.e., "beings with vastly greater capacities than present human beings have" (Bostrom 2003, 493). The idea most relevant for our purposes here is about what such "radical" enhancement might mean for the moral equality of persons, in case posthumans develop *augmented* capacities standardly attributed to personhood, such as the capacity for self-awareness and for communication with others, rationality, and self-determination, or they develop other capacities that can impact personhood, such that some or all posthumans may also be post*persons*, i.e., "beings with a higher [moral] status than that of persons" (Buchanan 2011b, 30). In such a future, persons and postpersons may not be moral equals, despite some overlap in their traits and characteristics. Because postpersons and persons may not have the same moral status—perhaps like the difference some believe to exist between "normal" adult humans, polar bears, and human fetuses—then one concern is that, if postpersons come to view persons as less than moral equals, postpersons may come to mistreat persons in some ways, as so often displayed in the treatment of entities with lower moral status by those with higher moral status.

Buchanan (2011b) explores the possible implications of the existence of postpersons by reference to whether it is possible for postpersons to have a "higher" moral status compared to persons. In considering this question, we have the opportunity to revisit longstanding assumptions about whether moral status is best conceptualized hierarchically (some higher, some lower) or non-hierarchically (as merely different). If moral status is meant to include something like protections afforded from being mistreated by others and corresponding moral obligations to treat others in certain ways, then having different protections/obligations does not by itself indicate a hierarchy of moral statuses. For example, postpersons with extended lives may have different moral obligations to far-future generations of humans because they have the potential to be alive when those far-future people come into existence, compared to the obligations of persons toward far-future people. Or imagine that postpersons are capable of engaging with material reality beyond four dimensions, whereas persons are not. Postpersons may then have obligations to respect three-dimensional space and time (and subsequent dimensions) in ways that persons do not, because persons cannot perceive beyond four dimensions.

One implication of this is that the assumption of moral equality of persons can fail to hold even if postpersons do not have a higher moral status compared to persons; all that is needed is that the moral status between the two is not the same (i.e., not equal).[5] Yet, it is not necessarily unfair for persons and postpersons to be treated differently if they do have different moral status. Importantly, one point that Buchanan does not consider is that it may not be up to *persons* to decide how postpersons come to understand their obligations toward persons (and other entities)—just like it is not up

[5] One of the reasons why the ethics of genetic enhancement is complex is because of the plurality of values and beliefs at play, including different views on moral status and personhood. To limit the discussion about personhood to Western philosophical perspectives on moral status is very narrow. There are many perspectives on moral status beyond this, some of which afford all species with equal moral status, and personhood is attributed far beyond "normal" adult human beings to include, e.g., nonhuman animals, trees, and rivers. For example, see Kimmerer (2013).

to octopuses to decide how human persons come to understand their responsibilities and obligations toward octopuses—and so it may be that discussion of such issues by mere persons is bound to be irrelevant.

9.5 Leaving No Person Behind: Distributive Justice and Genetic Enhancement

One of the most prominent justice-related issues in the context of the ethics of genetic enhancement is about fair access to the technology, more specifically access to its benefits. Early work on the ethics of genetic enhancement warned that the technology is likely to be expensive, at least initially, possibly only affordable to those who are wealthy, and less accessible or inaccessible to less affluent people (Mehlman and Botkin 1998). If genetic enhancements are expensive, then they will not be available to people living in poverty, unless those genetic enhancements are provided through public healthcare systems or made more affordable through state subsidies. If there is unequal access to safe and effective genetic enhancements, then those who have access (rich, affluent people) will have disproportionate (unfair) access to the benefits of the technology. At an individual level, this will make the enhanced person more competitive in the relevant aspects of life, such as employment, positions awarded based on merit, and mate selection. This would compound any existing competitive advantage(s) that the person already has. At a more general level, this may maintain or even exacerbate injustices grounded in inequalities between the rich and the poor.

Earlier I suggested that the claim that genetic enhancement will help to reduce existing social injustices is currently an unsubstantiated sentiment. Unfortunately, the prospect of genetic enhancement contributing to the maintenance or exacerbation of existing inequalities is a more likely eventuality, amplified in proportion to the sophistication of the technology and the kinds of genetic traits and characteristics that can be targeted successfully. The more that genes can be edited in ways that yield competitive advantages for enhanced individuals, the more those without access to enhancements will be left further behind—unless legal or political intervention offsets such disadvantages and marginalization.

Having access to genetic enhancement technology does not necessarily mean that the genetic alterations will lead to actual benefits. For example, being genetically predisposed to have augmented intelligence does not mean that the person will necessarily end up more intelligent, because they may not have access to other resources and opportunities to develop intelligence, such as nutritious food and education (Prince 2024). Notice that providing state subsidization for genetic enhancement to people living in poverty may be perceived as hypocritical, perhaps even insulting. This is because, in order for such enhancements to be actualized, social and environmental conditions need to allow for this, and such social and environmental prerequisites may not be in place for people living in poverty. Moreover, the genetic enhancements themselves are likely not going to have poverty-eliminating capabilities. Therefore, state subsidization of genetic enhancement for people living in poverty (and others) will likely be a waste of money unless other social benefits and protections are provided.

There have been some interesting proposals about how to distribute access to genetic enhancement technology under worst-case conditions where it is (initially) very expensive and not subsidized. Buchanan (2011b), for example, acknowledges that there will likely be inequality in access to biomedical enhancements, and he proposes that we distribute the technology as fast as possible and also create new institutions to govern the development of enhancements and to promote responsible, ethical innovation. Another example is the prioritarian argument presented by Alberto Giubilini and Francesca Minerva, "to subsidize enhancements for those who are worse off as a consequence of the social lottery (and possibly of the natural lottery without necessarily being disabled), and prohibit enhancements for those who are born in favorable social and economic circumstances (and possibly with favorable genetic endowments)" (2019, 346).

If the GEE is going to be pursued, then it is important to develop theoretically sturdy and practical proposals for fairly distributing the benefits of genetic enhancement technology. Despite any merits of Buchanan's and Giubilini & Minerva's proposals, one significant limitation of these views is that they assume everyone will use genetic enhancement technology, if only the technology is available and affordable. Making the benefits of gene editing technology available as quickly as possible, and prioritizing the subsidization of enhancements for those who are the least well-off, does not assist those who choose not to use genetic enhancements. Indeed, one important limitation of the debate on the ethics of genetic enhancement is that it does not currently address issues that will arise when safe, effective, and affordable gene editing is widely available, and some people choose not to use it and will be susceptible to harms resulting from that choice (e.g., being relatively uncompetitive for accessing social positions and accolades, compared to people who are genetically enhanced). Even if the technology is fairly distributed and the technology is accessible to all who want to use it, concerns about fairness and injustice linger, including questions about what (if any) protections and accommodations are owed to people who choose not to participate in the GEE. To my knowledge, these questions are not being raised within the ethical debate on genetic enhancement. They will require further attention if the GEE is embarked upon.

9.6 Non-discrimination

9.6.1 Inclusion, Disability, and the Expressivist Argument

An important critique of human gene editing is the disability critique, including the expressivist argument (Asch 1999). Decisions about which genetic conditions, traits, and characteristics to target are grounded in a particular socio-political and historical context, and such decisions are value-laden. State and institutional endorsement of a particular application of gene editing, as well as the act of individuals choosing to use that technology for that purpose, suggests endorsement of the same value(s), and expresses that the target condition, trait, or characteristic ought to be extracted and modified, or destroyed. When the condition, trait, or characteristic being targeted is a disability, this suggests that people who are disabled are less valuable compared to people who are not disabled. The existence of technology designed to avoid the creation of new people who are disabled *expresses that*, if given the choice, it is better to prevent people with those disabilities from coming into existence in favor of people without such disabilities. The expressivist argument entails that particular applications of gene editing thereby express discriminatory attitudes, attitudes which often imply that people who are disabled are not morally equal to people who are not disabled. Moreover, at root of the development and use of gene editing technology to eradicate disability lies a widespread yet misplaced belief that the lives of people who are disabled are not worth living (or not as worth living), and that such people necessarily have reduced or minimal quality of life.

It is important to consider the potential for the GEE to manifest in ways that are ableist. However, the expressivist argument has limitations in the context of the development and use of genetic *enhancement*. First, one may choose not to create new human life with a specific impairment without expressing anything derogatory, devaluing, or discriminatory about people who have the impairment one seeks to avoid. For example, decisions about reproductive mate selection have direct impacts on what kind of people (offspring) are created, yet such decisions need not express anything about people who are disabled—or about anyone else for that matter. Similarly, people may choose to have children who are disabled (see, e.g., Kaposy 2018), and this choice does not necessarily imply that people who are disabled are more valuable than people who are not disabled in that way. Second, if it is possible to use the same technology to create people *with* impairment or disability, then there is nothing inherent with the technology such that it devalues people with such impairment or disabilities. Many technologies can be used in ways that are unfair or discriminatory without being inherently unfair or discriminatory. Third, the expressivist argument is more pronounced in the context of people making choices for others (future children) about whether or not to be born with a disability. Yet, if one decides for oneself that they would prefer to not be disabled, then that does not necessarily attract the same concern compared to family builders or the state promoting ableism; it is a personal preference about how they would like their life to be, for them and according to them. Lastly, it is not clear the extent to which the disability critique will be relevant to the debate on genetic *enhancement* in the future, especially by the time that safe, effective, and affordable genetic enhancements are available. This is so for two reasons: (1) for reasons elucidated earlier, therapeutic applications of gene editing are more likely to occur first (preceding widespread genetic enhancement), which will impact the way(s) in which the disability critique manifests in practice, as well as the shape of socio-political and institutional response to the expressivist concerns in practice. There is reason to think that, once safe and effective genetic enhancement has become a real possibility, the disability critique may have taken on new forms, influenced as it may be by the experiences of individuals and institutions as genetic treatments become available and more widely consumed within a particular society; and (2) the focus of therapeutic applications of gene editing is on establishing "normal health functioning" and restoring health to some baseline, whereas enhancements are meant to go beyond normal or species-typical functioning. Thus, unless the orientation of the disability critique changes such that it considers otherwise normal or species-typical functioning to count as "disability," then the relevance and force of the disability critique seems less applicable and poignant when directed at genetic enhancement, as opposed to genetic treatment.

9.6.2 *Discrimination against Those Who Are Not Genetically Enhanced*

In a future where genetic enhancement technology is available, it is possible that genetically enhanced people will discriminate against, dominate, or oppress people who are not genetically enhanced (or have been enhanced with earlier, inferior iterations of enhancements [Sparrow 2019]) because non-enhanced people are perceived to be inferior ("the unenhanced") (Annas 2010). From the other direction, people who are not genetically enhanced may commit unjust discrimination toward people who are genetically enhanced if, for example, they are portrayed as "freaks" or "cheaters."

One important issue that has gone unrecognized in the debate on the ethics of enhancement is that ensuring access to safe and effective enhancements, including their diffusion to all groups of people within society, does not mean that people will choose to use them. Thus, independent of whether the problem of distributive justice is resolved, pronounced issues of discrimination arise. There is the potential for a more significant degree of harmful discrimination toward people who are not genetically enhanced when the technology is reasonably accessible to them, compared to when they are not enhanced because they do not have affordable access to the technology.

In general, discrimination is the unfair treatment of people based on actual or perceived features that are arbitrary and irrelevant to the context. For example, skin color is irrelevant to the capacity to care for children, so people should have an equal opportunity to access assisted human reproduction and adoption regardless of their skin color. Genetic discrimination is the "differential treatment of individuals based on actual, perceived or presumed genetic differences" (Otlowski et al. 2012).

One type of genetic discrimination is when information about a person's genetic predispositions is used as the basis for differential treatment, compared to those who do not have those genetic predispositions. One example of this is charging people with an (inherited) harmful variant of BRCA-1/-2 higher premiums for health insurance coverage, because people with this variant are statistically more likely to develop certain kinds of cancers (e.g., ovarian and breast cancer), even though many people with mutated BRCA-1/-2 do not actually develop cancer.

Concerns about this type of genetic discrimination are longstanding (Buchanan et al. 2000) and are associated with differential treatment of individuals based on information about aspects of themselves that are out of their control. I label this kind of genetic discrimination "inexorable," to emphasize that the person whose genetic information it is could not change anything about their genetic constitution; in this case, the genetic lottery has fixed the person's genes.

Prior to the advent of genome editing, the person with a harmful variant of BRCA-1/-2 could not have controlled having this mutation and the corresponding risk for developing certain cancers. Philip Kitcher (1997) urges us to take measures to guard against creating a new genetic underclass—what he calls the "new pariahs"—precisely because such people (the genetic unlucky) will have, or will be perceived as having, "bad genes," and there is nothing that they can do to change their genetic bad luck.

Because it allows people the possibility of "correcting for" or enhancing undesirable genetic mutations, the availability of human genome editing technology brings with it the possibility for a new strand of genetic discrimination:

> *Malleable Genetic Discrimination*: People who choose not to participate in the gene editing enterprise may be harmed because of this choice not to participate. In a place where safe, effective, and affordable gene editing is available, every person will either be genetically edited or genetically unedited, and this information about an individual's genetic modification status can be used in ways that are fair or ways that are unfair. In this case, the genetic information that is being used as the basis of unjustified differential treatment is not information about genetic predispositions but about the person's status as someone who has/has not been a consumer of gene editing technology. That is, it is information about their choice to use/not to use safe, effective, and affordable gene editing technology to try to control disease onset or to prevent disease, or even for purposes of genetic enhancement.

The genetically unedited will be at risk of genetic discrimination, of being treated differently because of their unedited genetic constitution, because it was their choice not to use gene editing technology, and therefore it was their choice to forgo the potential benefits, including any corresponding impact on their ability to access resources and opportunities, or even to participate in the dominant cooperative framework. In such cases, the foundation of the genetic discrimination is that the person's genetic constitution *is* something under their control, but they have chosen not to assert control.

I label this type of genetic discrimination "malleable" to emphasize that the person could have altered their genetic composition—and here we are assuming, for the sake of argument, that it could have been done in a manner that is safe, effective, and affordable. Genetic discrimination of this sort is the unfair differential treatment of a person because of their status as genetically unedited *by choice*. Such people are distinct from Kitcher's genetically unlucky—although they could end up being part of the class of "new pariahs"—since their genetic constitution is something that they could change but have chosen not to.[6]

Many have argued for protections for the genetically unlucky, and some such protections have emerged over time. One example is Canada's Genetic Non-discrimination Act (S.C. 2017, c. 3), which explicitly protects people who have no control over their genome from being the targets of (inexorable) genetic discrimination in the context of health insurance and other related services. There is a moral imperative to implement similar protections for people who knowingly and willingly forgo safe, effective, and affordable gene editing technology.

9.7 Conclusion

Even if it turns out to be possible to use genetic enhancements to reduce or eliminate existing social injustice(s), it is likely not to be possible in the near-term future, in part because it will depend on a deeper, more sophisticated understanding of polygenetic traits. Moreover, currently, the mainstream academic debate largely fails to adequately consider the perspectives and (likely) lived experiences of the least well-off, including what it will be like for them to either not have access to the benefits of genetic enhancement technology, or else to feel pressure to participate in the GEE because it is one of the only "opportunities" they have to compete for the resources necessary for satisfying their basic needs. These issues do not arise to the same degree (or at all) for people who do have access to genetic enhancements, or else who do not require genetic enhancements in order to be able to participate in the dominant cooperative framework. While those in control of the design and regulation of the GEE may seek to make the benefits widely available, and to do so as quickly as possible, those already experiencing injustice and those living in poverty will likely not be comforted by these good intentions alone. Important lessons may be available through examining human enhancements already pervasive in society, such as literacy and affordable access to postsecondary education.

Concerns about injustice become more pronounced and impactful to the extent that the GEE changes the dominant cooperative framework, since those who lack access to genetic enhancements will then be even more susceptible to being left behind. And even if the benefits of genetic enhancement technology do become easily accessible to everyone within society, important justice concerns would remain, including concerns about protections, accommodations, and perhaps remedial compensation for people who have had no control over the GEE coming into existence within their society and who choose not to use genetic enhancements for themselves or their children.

---

[6] In the context of genetic information and health or life insurance, this new concern being raised is more like someone's status as a cigarette smoker (something detrimental to their health and something within the person's control), rather than like having a diagnosis for a polygenetic disease that cannot be genetically edited away or that one cannot reasonably afford to genetically edit away.

A GEE that fails to properly respect the moral equality of persons, is unfair in the distribution of the benefits of genetic enhancement technology, and/or is discriminatory, is unjust. For societies that are committed to valuing justice, concerns raised in this chapter may be enough already to conclude that the GEE is morally unacceptable, at least at this time (and for a particular society). However, philosophically this will depend on answering additional questions about how to rank the value of social justice relative to other values, such as liberty and well-being, which are central values underpinning the views of prominent supporters of human genetic enhancement.

I contend that, in the context of the ethics of human genetic enhancement, the importance of prioritizing or giving weight to other values aside from social justice diminishes—and becomes morally irresponsible or reprehensible—to the extent that basic injustice is compounded by other factors that render the GEE *severely* unjust. The unjust GEE will be severely unjust if, in addition to failing to meet the basic tenets of justice described above, it also:

1. can, but does not, help to address or reduce existing social injustices, especially for the least well-off (and perhaps those benefiting the least from the GEE, depending on who those people are);
2. amplifies existing inequalities, for example, by changing the requirements for participation in the dominant cooperative framework in a manner that is exclusionary rather than inclusive;
3. creates new inequality or injustice(s) (e.g., unjust discriminatory treatment of persons by postpersons, or genetic enhancement certificates being required in order for someone to have access to certain positions or resources within society), especially if the new injustice(s) cannot be adequately addressed via fair and effective public policy, or can be so addressed but are not; and/or
4. is created/continues to operate within a socio-political context that fails to adequately protect those who choose not to participate in the GEE from being unable to access resources and opportunities for satisfying their basic needs, regardless of whether the GEE changes the dominant cooperative framework.

There could of course be other ways for the GEE to be severely unjust not listed above.

While it is possible for the GEE to be developed and implemented in a manner that is just, it is likely that the GEE will be unjust in some respects. An all-things-considered moral evaluation of such an unjust GEE will depend on how much value is placed on social justice relative to other values. Crucially, in order to avoid an unjust GEE from becoming severely unjust and therefore morally reprehensible, abundant resources will need to be devoted to the close monitoring and steering of the GEE, as well as careful stewardship from many people in positions of power within society. How a country responds to emerging injustices within that country will vary. However, it seems reasonable to suggest that slow government response to currently existing injustices likely foreshadows slow response to new or emerging injustices connected to the genetic enhancement enterprise. So, in order to avoid an unjust GEE turning into a severely unjust GEE, governments and their institutions will need to make genuine commitments to this goal and follow through on such commitments in practice and over time.

Some people may benefit from the GEE, especially if they have access to genetic enhancements and the requisite socioeconomic and environmental background conditions for those alterations to be manifested, and they choose to participate in the GEE. Others will not benefit from the GEE much or at all. For those people who get left behind in the wake of the GEE, it may be that their experience of injustice will be what is augmented or "enhanced," if nothing else. It is hard to imagine that the overall benefits of the GEE could outweigh the harms associated with being left behind or excluded from participation in the dominant cooperative framework, especially when many of the harms are a result of existing injustices, and others are the result of severe injustices unaddressed or spawned by the GEE itself.

References

Agar, Nicholas. 1998. "Liberal Eugenics." *Public Affairs Quarterly* 12 (2) (April): 137–155. https://www.jstor.org/stable/40441188.

Agar, Nicholas. 2008. *Liberal Eugenics: In Defence of Human Enhancement*. Malden, MA: Blackwell.

Annas, George J. 2010. *Worst Case Bioethics: Death, Disaster, and Public Health*. Oxford: Oxford University Press.

Asch, Adrienne. 1999. "Prenatal Diagnosis and Selective Abortion: A Challenge to Practice and Policy." *American Journal of Public Health* 89 (11) (November): 1649–1657. https://doi.org/10.2105/AJPH.89.11.1649.

Baltimore, David, Françoise Baylis, Paul Berg, George Q. Daley, Jennifer A. Doudna, Eric S. Lander, et al. 2015. "On Human Gene Editing: International Summit Statement." International Summit on Human Gene Editing. December 3. https://www.nationalacademies.org/news/2015/12/on-human-gene-editing-international-summit-statement.

Baylis, Françoise. 2019. *Altered Inheritance: CRISPR and the Ethics of Human Genome Editing*. Cambridge, MA: Harvard University Press.

Bostrom, Nick. 2003. "Human Genetic Enhancements: A Transhumanist Perspective." *Journal of Value Inquiry* 37 (4) (December): 493–506. https://doi.org/10.1023/B:INQU.0000019037.67783.d5.

Buchanan, Allen. 2011a. *Better Than Human: The Promise and Perils of Enhancing Ourselves*. Oxford: Oxford University Press.

Buchanan, Allen. 2011b. *Beyond Humanity? The Ethics of Biomedical Enhancement*. Oxford: Oxford University Press.

Buchanan, Allen, Dan W. Brock, Norman Daniels, and Daniel Wikler. 2000. *From Chance to Choice: Genetics and Justice*. Cambridge: Cambridge University Press.

Daniels, Norman. 1985. *Just Health Care*. Cambridge: Cambridge University Press.

Dickenson, Donna. 2004. "Consent, Commodification and Benefit-Sharing in Genetic Research." *Developing World Bioethics* 4 (2) (December): 109–124. https://doi.org/10.1111/j.1471-8731.2004.00087.x.

Douglas, Thomas. 2008. "Moral Enhancement." *Journal of Applied Philosophy* 25 (3) (August): 228–245. https://doi.org/10.1111/j.1468-5930.2008.00412.x.

Giubilini, Alberto, and Francesca Minerva. 2019. "Enhancing Equality." *Journal of Medicine and Philosophy* 44 (3) (June): 335–354. https://doi.org/10.1093/jmp/jhz002.

Gyngell, Christopher, Thomas Douglas, and Julian Savulescu. 2017. "The Ethics of Germline Gene Editing." *Journal of Applied Philosophy* 34 (4) (August): 498–513. https://doi.org/10.1111/japp.12249.

Habermas, Jürgen. 2003. *The Future of Human Nature*. Cambridge: Polity.
Harris, John. 2010. *Enhancing Evolution: The Ethical Case for Making Better People*. Princeton, NJ: Princeton University Press.
Kaposy, Chris. 2018. *Choosing Down Syndrome: Ethics and New Prenatal Testing Technologies*. Cambridge, MA: MIT Press.
Kimmerer, Robin Wall. 2013. *Braiding Sweetgrass: Indigenous Wisdom, Scientific Knowledge, and the Teachings of Plants*. Minneapolis, MN: Milkweed Editions.
Kitcher, Philip. 1997. *The Lives to Come*. New York: Simon and Schuster.
Lander, Eric S., Françoise Baylis, Feng Zhang, Emmanuelle Charpentier, Paul Berg, Catherine Bourgain, et al. 2019. "Adopt a Moratorium on Heritable Genome Editing." *Nature* 567 (7747) (March 14): 165–168. https://doi.org/10.1038/d41586-019-00726-5.
McCallum, Mary Jane Logan, and Adele Perry. 2018. *Structures of Indifference: An Indigenous Life and Death in a Canadian City*. Winnipeg: University of Manitoba Press.
Mehlman, Maxwell J., and Jeffrey R. Botkin. 1998. *Access to the Genome: The Challenge to Equality*. Washington, DC: Georgetown University Press.
Otlowski, Margaret, Sandra Taylor, and Yvonne Bombard. 2012. "Genetic Discrimination: International Perspectives." *Annual Review of Genomics and Human Genetics* 13: 433–454. https://doi.org/10.1146/annurev-genom-090711-163800.
Philibert, Aline, Myriam Fillion, and Donna Mergler. 2020. "Mercury Exposure and Premature Mortality in the Grassy Narrows First Nation Community: A Retrospective Longitudinal Study." *Lancet Planetary Health* 4 (4) (April): e141–e148. https://doi.org/10.1016/S2542-5196(20)30057-7.
Prince, Sinead. 2024. "Gene-Environment Interaction: Why Genetic Enhancement Might Never Be Distributed Fairly." *Journal of Medical Ethics* 50 (4) (April): 272–277. https://doi.org/10.1136/jme-2023-109101.
Sandel, Michael J. 2007. *The Case against Perfection: Ethics in the Age of Genetic Engineering*. Cambridge, MA: Harvard University Press.
Savulescu, Julian. 2001. "Procreative Beneficence: Why We Should Select the Best Children." *Bioethics* 15 (5–6) (October): 413–426. https://doi.org/10.1111/1467-8519.00251.
Sparrow, Robert. 2019. "Yesterday's Child: How Gene Editing for Enhancement Will Produce Obsolescence—and Why It Matters." *American Journal of Bioethics* 19 (7): 6–15. https://doi.org/10.1080/15265161.2019.1618943.
Talaga, Tanya. 2024. *The Knowing*. New York: HarperCollins.
Tonkens, Ryan. 2021. "Vulnerable Groups and the Hollow Promise of Benefit from Human Gene Editing." *Bioethics* 35 (6) (July): 574–580. https://doi.org/10.1111/bioe.12882.
Truth and Reconciliation Commission of Canada. 2015. *Calls to Action*. https://www2.gov.bc.ca/assets/gov/british-columbians-our-governments/indigenous-people/aboriginal-peoples-documents/calls_to_action_english2.pdf.
World Health Organization Expert Advisory Committee on Developing Global Standards for Governance and Oversight of Human Genome Editing. 2021. *Human Genome Editing: A Framework for Governance*. Geneva: World Health Organization. https://www.who.int/publications/i/item/9789240030060.

Ryan Tonkens is a bioethicist at Lakehead University's Centre for Health Care Ethics, Associate Professor in Bioethics and Philosophy at NOSM University, and instructor in the Department of Philosophy at Lakehead University in Thunder Bay, Canada. Tonkens has published in many areas of bioethics, including the ethics of gene editing (e.g., "Vulnerable Groups and the Hollow Promise of Benefit from Human Gene Editing" [2021]), the ethics of kidney selling (e.g., "Effective Altruists Ought to Be Allowed to Sell Their Kidneys" [2018]), and the ethics of uterus transplantation (e.g., "Gatekeeping Uterus Transplants: A Proposal for Eligibility Criteria and the Fair Allocation of Wombs" [2024]).

Chapter 10
Enhancing the Responsible Conduct and Innovation of Stem Cell Research through the Lens of Responsibilization

Lars Assen

Abstract Stem cell (SC) researchers should play an ethical role in furthering responsible conduct and innovation in their work. This chapter considers how this ethical role could be realized through the lens of *responsibilization.* Responsibilization involves how researchers are equipped in terms of knowledge, skills, and resources to take responsibility for the ethical implications of their work. Therefore, this chapter discusses the need for SC researchers to expand their understanding of the ethical dimension of their research. It calls for policy changes to ensure that responsible research aligns with societal values, organizational support, and education of virtue-based integrity training. Moreover, moral sensitivity and reasoning should be fostered by educating researchers on the notions of hard and soft impacts, and through moral imagination. Although this overview of ethical challenges is not exhaustive, the proposed blueprint for responsibilization can aid organizations and SC researchers in identifying additional ethical implications and accompanying responsibilities.

Keywords Stem cells · Responsible research and innovation (RRI) · Responsibilization · Responsibility

10.1 Introduction

Within the fields of stem cell (SC) research and regenerative medicine (RM), the myth of Prometheus has been a popular story to connect Greek mythology to these respective areas of research (Schneider 2004; Power and Rasko 2008; Bouros and Laurent 2013). According to the myth, Prometheus gifted humanity fire, a "technology" that had been only reserved for Greek gods. Angered by Prometheus's betrayal, the supreme god Zeus punished him (Dougherty 2006). This punishment has often been the focal point of the myth in the context of SC and RM research: Prometheus

L. Assen (✉)
Section of Knowledge, Transformation, and Society (KiTeS), University of Twente, Enschede, The Netherlands
e-mail: lars.assen@utwente.nl

M. C. Altman and D. Schwan (eds.), *Ethics and Medical Technology*, The International Library of Bioethics 113, https://doi.org/10.1007/978-3-031-94690-5_10

was doomed to be chained to a rock for eternity. Each day an eagle pecks his liver and eats it. Every night, Prometheus's liver regrows and the next day the same cycle repeats itself for eternity. Specifically, this regeneration of the liver stands out in the context of SC and RM research, as the liver has a natural regenerative capacity—albeit not as regenerative as Prometheus's liver (Power and Rasko 2008)—and symbolizes what those researchers hope to accomplish. As such, the myth of Prometheus is used as a trope. However, when we turn our attention to other parts of the myth, it could offer more meaningful insights for the field of SC research.

Let us first address the name Prometheus, which translates to "forethought," thinking through consequences before acting. While the myth centers around the gifting of fire to humanity, Prometheus did not merely gift the fire. Rather, Prometheus taught humanity the knowledge and techniques to use fire, thereby providing the ability to use it responsibly (Grene 1940; Dougherty 2006). For example, a fire could be used responsibly to warm people and to forge metal. Alternatively, fire could be used immorally by intentionally creating physical destruction or harm when proper forethought has been omitted. Because in ancient Greek literature fire often is a metaphor for technology in a broader sense (Dougherty 2006), this idea of ensuring that people have the right forethought to responsibly use technology could inspire SC research and conduct, such as understanding how to ethically source stem cells, how to work with them, as well as considering potential consequences of research decisions and outcomes for patients and society. As such, the focus is not only on the research conduct but also on how innovations could best be integrated into society. By thinking through such elements, it could illuminate which responsibilities are important and who is or could be responsible.

The idea of forethought and specifically anticipation is prominent in the field of Responsible Research and Innovation (RRI) and Ethical, Legal, and Social Aspects/Implications studies (ELSA/ELSI) (e.g., Owen et al. 2012; Lindner et al. 2016; Kuhlmann et al. 2019; Politi and Grinbaum 2020). In these fields, there have been discussions about how research could be conducted more responsibly and with more integrity, and how the goals and wishes of society could be aligned with research goals, thereby trying to circumvent the Collingridge dilemma (Jongsma and Bredenoord 2020). The dilemma is that early in the research on and creation of a new technology, possible negative impacts can be difficult to predict and as a result can prevent possible technological and scientific breakthroughs; while at later stages impacts are more easily identified, but intervening too late might have no effect in steering the development into an ethically or socially desirable direction (Collingridge 1980).

Several approaches have been proposed for how ethicists or social scientists could avoid this dilemma, such as Constructive Technology Assessment, embedded ethics, ethics parallel research, and up- or mid-stream analysis (Fisher et al. 2006; Boenink 2013; Rip and Robinson 2013; Jongsma and Bredenoord 2020). What these approaches all share is that ethicists are conducting their ethical analysis, early in the research process, often in collaboration with researchers. The collaboration has been described as a *conditio sine qua non* (Politi and Grinbaum 2020). This means that the collaboration between biomedical researchers and ethicists is important for the ethical improvement of biomedical research and that the insights gained from those collaborations cannot be retrieved elsewhere. Interestingly, these approaches often focus on the role that ethicists play in this collaboration while largely ignoring the role of researchers.

Simultaneously, it has been noted that researchers have a unique position due to their professional knowledge and insights: they could share knowledge, ideas, and visions with ethicists (see Grunwald 2013); reflect on research processes; and include different perspectives (see Jongsma and Bredenoord 2020). Thus, SC researchers could play a significant role in advancing the responsible conduct and innovation of SC research. Investigating such a possible role could improve existing ideas about collaboration and could clarify which knowledge, attitudes, and skills stakeholders should have to take (co-)responsibility for the ethical implications of their research.

This chapter aims to describe how SC researchers could take (co-)responsibility for the ethical implications of SC research and innovations. While different ethical challenges will be addressed, this chapter will not discuss all ethical challenges related to SC research, but rather offers an idea for responsible conduct and innovation in the SC field. Moreover, this chapter will address issues that are not necessarily unique to the field of SC research.

First, I will discuss the notion of *responsibilization* as a theoretical background for how SC researchers and other stakeholders should be equipped to take responsibility. This is a perspective that synthesizes existing and new ideas about how to improve the responsible conduct and translation of SC research, by making the SC researcher central in this process. Second, I will define the ethical scope of SC research in terms of responsible conduct and innovation. Thereafter, I will address how governance, organizational arrangements, and education and training could play a role in *responsibilizing* SC researchers.

10.2 Responsibility and Responsibilization

Hans Jonas (1979) has previously discussed the difficulties surrounding responsibility in biomedical research. He introduced "*the problem of many hands*": when multiple people are working on research or technologies, it is difficult to assess who may have acted blameworthy and thus to hold someone responsible for what went wrong (see also Waelbers 2009). It also affects whether we could hold someone morally responsible, as this is based upon uncoercive acts and whether actors could have foreseen the consequences of their actions (Swierstra and Jelsma 2005).

The problem of many hands involves the difficulty of holding individual SC researchers accountable or liable. As such, the problem impedes the assignment of moral responsibility. This, however, does not imply that SC researchers cannot take responsibility. SC researchers could still be motivated to take forward-looking responsibility and try to recognize and anticipate the ethical implications of their research. To realize this forward-looking dimension, the notion of responsibilization could be helpful.

The term responsibilization was used by sociologists to describe, among others, policy changes that increase personal responsibility in healthcare. The origins of the idea of responsibilization can be found in the works of Michel Foucault on how self-determination should be actualized, focusing on how people should take responsibility for their freedom and lives (Rose 1993; Brown 2021). Nicolas Rose (1993, 2013) used the term to describe issues of healthcare and personal responsibility. On this view, reponsibilization is the neoliberal idea that the state should encourage citizens to manage their health by setting a system in place where people would be able to take on that responsibility. On this account, to responsibilize is to shift responsibility from the state to the individual for their health outcomes. This specific idea of responsibilizing citizens in the context of health has been judged to be overwhelming and encumbering for citizens, especially vulnerable citizens (Wetenschappelijke Raad voor het Regeringsbeleid 2017).

Newer interpretations of responsibilization in different contexts are more fruitful. For example, in governance debates and the field of RRI, the underlying idea is to align policy goals with the attitudes, skills, and knowledge of individual actors, thereby employing a weaker notion of responsbilization (Lindner et al. 2016). As such, responsibilization is "disconnected" from citizenship and is understood in the context of professions and professionals, where there is a focus on how professionals can be enabled to take responsibility rather than merely being bestowed with responsibility. It is understood as "the governance of (self-)stimulating actors to care for their duties of being anticipatory, reflexive, responsive, etc. by drawing on a clear understanding of their responsibilities and un-coerced application of values. This stimulating governance can take the form of facilitating, equipping and rewarding of actors to take their responsibilities seriously" (Walhout et al. 2016, 51). The question now is how this general idea of responsibilization could be applied to the field of SC research and therapy. An ethical scope could offer moral direction, and thus an idea of which ethical challenges should be addressed, which responsibilities are related to those challenges, and what kind of "equipment" is needed to take on that responsibility.

10.3 Ethical Scope

To assess what responsibilization should target, I will discuss the ethical implications of SC research, such as societal impacts, and the actual conduct of research, including research integrity. I will examine these challenges in light of how SC researchers commonly perceive the ethical dimensions of their work.

The field of SC research has an abundant history of ethical challenges and implications. Human embryonic stem cells (hESCs) have often been the subject of ethical controversy, as questions have been raised regarding the sourcing of those cells and the moral status of embryos and those cells (Robertson 2001; de Wert and Mummery 2003; Hyun 2010). Induced pluripotent stem cells (iPSCs) have circumvented some of the ethical objections to this research (King and Perrin

2014). However, other ethical issues have risen to prominence, including the physical side effects of possible SC interventions; ownership, privacy, informed consent issues surrounding the storage of human tissue in biobanks; documenting the provenance of SCs; and the decrease of animal suffering when organoids could be used in research (Hyun 2010; Isasi et al. 2014; King and Perrin 2014; Andrews et al. 2015; MacPherson and Kimmelman 2019). More indirect ethical implications have also been recognized, including hype about stem cell research, creating social and global justice, the burden of normality, ensuring societal perspectives, responsibilities surrounding recontacting biobank donors regarding new genetic discoveries relevant to their health, and shifting perceptions of health and disease (Kamenova and Caulfield 2015; Ellison 2016; Assen et al. 2021; Sugarman et al. 2023). Ironically, the question of the moral status that iPSCs originally avoided has become relevant again in their applications, now that stem cell-based embryo models (SCB-EMs) and chimeras are possible (Hyun 2022).

Concerning research integrity, prominent fraudulent cases have taken place in the context of SC research. For example, South Korean SC researcher Hwang Woo-Suk committed fraud by falsifying findings (Hong 2008), and Italian SC researcher and surgeon Paolo Macchiarini claimed to have proof for his stem cell-covered tracheas but instead fabricated animal studies and misled patients about the efficacy of his surgeries, even leading to several unnecessary deaths (Day 2019). While these cases are clear-cut wrongdoings, research integrity in SC research is threatened by the need to publish and, more specifically, the need to publish positive results (Assen et al. 2022), which is also found in other fields of biomedicine (Tijdink et al. 2014). Moreover—and similar to other fields of research—research integrity is at stake due to questionable research practices (Mejlgaard et al. 2020) and the introduction of new technologies in the laboratory. For example, early career researchers sometimes have a better understanding of new technology in the laboratory than their supervisors. When early career researchers expect their supervisors to correct possible mistakes, but a supervisor does not have the knowledge or skills to do so with the new technology, this can lead to a gap in responsibility (Assen et al. 2022). This highlights the fact that, in order to comply with research integrity codes, researchers need to understand which factors could affect their research conduct.

SC researchers' and other biomedical researchers' perceptions of the ethical implications of their work have been surveyed in different qualitative studies (Longstaff et al. 2009; Niemansburg et al. 2015; Alahmad et al. 2020; Assen et al. 2022). These studies often suggest that SC researchers focus on issues regarding research integrity, research ethics, and the financial costs of research. Different studies have shown that SC researchers tend to focus on research integrity; research ethics, including the use of animals and informed consent procedures; and the costs of research (Longstaff et al. 2009; Alahmad et al. 2020; Assen et al. 2022). While these issues are important to consider, other socio-ethical implications of SC research are rarely recognized, if at all, such as issues related to SC tourism and SC clinics, social justice, and ensuring that cell lines are diverse (Knoppers and Isasi 2010; Ellison 2016); the inclusion of public perspectives (PytlikZillig and Tomkins 2011; Boon et al. 2022;

Carter et al. 2023); and how SC interventions could also be distributed to lower- and middle-income countries (Ellison 2016).

These ethical perceptions have consequences for the responsibilization of SC researchers. When SC researchers need to address ethical challenges and share concerns, visions and ideas with ethicists, it would be helpful to share all the relevant information. As discussed earlier, SC researchers often do not have a complete understanding of the ethical dimensions of their research and, as a result, may not recognize which information is relevant. While ethicists often have a broader understanding of the ethical dimensions, they may lack an understanding of new technologies and therefore may miss relevant information as well. This could lead to limitations in what SC researchers consider to be important information concerning what is ethically relevant in their work. While collaborating with ethicists may uncover the relevant information, this will likely be less efficient. Furthermore, ethical implications are not always apparent and do not cease to exist when ethicists are not present. To promote positive outcomes and prevent or mitigate negative ethical implications, the responsibilization of SC researchers should make them more morally sensitive to the ethical implications of their work and better able to recognize potential ethical problems.

10.4 Governance Dimension

Governance, such as legislation, regulation, policy, and guidelines, has a role in realizing the responsible conduct and innovation of SC research, since it realizes specific research possibilities and protects the needs and values of animals, research participants, and society. While governments play a crucial role, organizations such as the World Health Organization (WHO) and the International Society for Stem Cell Research (ISSCR) can serve a mediating role to further the protection of citizens and possibilities to advance SC research. However, unresponsive governance can complicate responsible innovation because it may limit research possibilities through legislation that is based on old norms. In turn, this can produce value conflicts between societal health benefits and the protection of human tissue (Isasi et al. 2022). These governance issues are represented in cases of regulatory brokerage and in cases of unresponsive governance, such as regulatory arbitrage.

Regulatory brokerage, in which a specific country develops legislation to gain competitive advantages over other countries, could lead to unwanted effects (Sipp and Sleeboom-Faulkner 2019). An example of regulatory brokerage can be found in Japan, where regulation has been changed in favor of introducing regenerative medicine faster. Here, Japanese insurance companies and patients effectively subsidize international companies that are attracted by the legislation (Sleeboom-Faulkner 2019). This legislation does not necessarily improve the position of patients in Japan, as these interventions are often expensive and may serve to negatively affect the financial sustainability of Japan's healthcare system (McCabe and Sipp 2016). Additionally, in these cases it is unclear what the efficacy and long-term safety of tissue-engineered interventions are before they enter the market. Rather, such interventions are primarily tested for safety in the short term during small clinical trials. While this could potentially bring promising interventions sooner to patients and as such promote SC research, it may also lead to unwanted long-term effects and ineffective treatments at the expense of the health of patients and the financial sustainability of the healthcare system (Chan 2017).

Situations of regulatory arbitrage happen when there is a lack of legislation or regulation (Assen et al. 2021). These situations could have detrimental effects on research participants and patients, as well as on the image of SC research and therapy. An example of such regulatory arbitrage can be found in the existence of SC clinics. Although in the United States only hemopoietic SC therapies to cure specific blood production disorders are FDA approved, there are many "stem cell clinics" in the US and in other countries that offer unproven SC interventions for other conditions. Often these clinics make claims that are not grounded in scientific evidence from clinical trials. Unfortunately, these SC interventions have led to severe harm and even cases of death (Bauer et al. 2018; Gopalan et al. 2021). Presently, SC clinics and accompanying tourism are still prevalent, though it has been argued that the WHO could play a mediating role in developing proposals for regulatory approaches that should be adopted by member states (Master et al. 2021).

Similarly, the ISSCR could play a pivotal role in advancing research possibilities with, among others, SCB-EMs, as these are bound by the "fourteen-day rule" of embryo cultivation. This rule dictates that human embryos created for laboratory research are only allowed to develop for fourteen days after fertilization. Because SCB-EM research could, in theory, have more potential when those models are validated in the weeks following the fourteen-day limitation, the ISSCR could propose specific protocols and norms to consider the cultivation of SCB-EMs on a case-to-case basis (Lovell-Badge et al. 2021). While the ISSCR does not directly affect national policies and regulations, its guidelines do stimulate stakeholders and policymakers to start public conversations about the fourteen-day rule relating to SCB-EMs (Lovell-Badge et al. 2021; Fabbri et al. 2023). Because societal alignment is necessary for the responsible conduct of SC research, such public engagement and deliberation would serve as a step forward for integrating SC research into society, highlighting potential responsibilities for SC researchers to engage with the public and policymakers (Fabbri et al. 2023). Additionally, the proposed relaxation for the fourteen-day rule could serve as well as a blueprint for discussions about other SC-based applications such as chimeras and cerebral organoids with more complicated structures (see Sawai et al. 2019).

10.5 Organizational Dimension

With regard to responsibilization, organizations—such as research institutes, universities, departments, and research groups—could equip researchers with more administrative and practical support, a positive work culture, additional time, and possibilities for training and education related to responsibilization. Such changes would likely have a positive effect on compliance with legal requirements and ethical norms of responsible research. This could also be promoted through organizational arrangements to eliminate possibilities and incentives to transgress research integrity codes. For instance, many researchers experience pressure to produce positive results and publish articles in high-ranking journals, as they are often assessed on their h-indices (Bouter 2015; Mejlgaard et al. 2020). Implementing ideas from initiatives related to "recognition and rewards programs" could help to mitigate such pressure, such as assessing researchers differently, or letting peers judge the quality of each other's research (Mejlgaard et al. 2020). Additionally, publication pressure may be mitigated by assessing researchers not solely on publication records but on collaboration with other researchers and patients, public engagement, and teaching and outreach activities (Universiteiten van Nederland 2019; Kramer and Bosman 2024). From a responsibilization perspective, it may be useful to recognize and reward researchers for identifying and anticipating the socio-ethical implications of their research. Of course, depending on the profile of the researcher, it may still be useful to include publication records as part of or the main assessment.

Organizational arrangements could also unburden SC researchers. To this end, work pressure could be alleviated and opportunities could be created to spend time on other responsibilities. Examples of such arrangements are administrative offices that support writing ethics approvals for animal studies and clinical trials, and communications offices that aid in organizing interactions, such as dissemination activities, among collaborators, patients, and the general public (Haven et al. 2020; Assen et al. 2022).

Moreover, organizations might also support a workplace climate that advances the responsible conduct of research and innovation. These changes could be realized by creating trust between researchers and divisions within research institutes, encouraging data openness, and clarifying performance expectations (Haven et al. 2020). Moreover, paying attention to positive role models and qualitative supervision helps to create such a culture, since the behavior and supervision of late-career researchers affect how early-career researchers behave in the laboratory (see Nejati and Shafaei 2018). This also highlights the need for organizations to offer workshops, training, or courses for researchers to become good role models and supervisors.

Lastly, universities, departments, and research groups could play a role in the distribution of responsibilities and overseeing those responsibilities. While it is unlikely that every SC researcher wants and can dedicate a lot of time to the identification and anticipation of ethical implications and to public engagement activities, it will be helpful to responsibilize every SC researcher to some extent, considering the existing workload and personal motivations. Therefore, organizations should identify researchers who are motivated to play a role in these responsibilities. To this end, those organizations should equip researchers with additional knowledge, skills, and time to ensure that researchers have the right capacities to fulfill those responsibilities (Gianni 2021). In addition, by ensuring that responsibilities are explicated and delegated, they could prevent possible gaps in responsibility (Nollkaemper 2018). The kind of training and education that organizations could offer will be discussed in the following section.

10.6 Educational Dimension

Since education is an essential dimension for the responsibilization of SC researchers, skills and knowledge can be developed and attitudes or changes in attitude could be prompted to improve the responsible conduct and translation of SC research. As discussed, qualitative studies suggest that many SC researchers consider research integrity and research ethics to be an important dimension of their research. While these issues still persist, it has been argued—specifically in light of responsible research and innovation initiatives—that SC research has other socio-ethical implications as well. As SC researchers have a role in identifying and anticipating of the ethical implications of their research, their understanding of the ethical dimensions of their work should ideally be broadened. To realize an increased responsibilized SC researcher, it is important to focus on education that enhances their moral sensitivity, or the ability to recognize what is morally salient (see Clarkeburn et al. 2002; Antes et al. 2009; Watts et al. 2017); and moral reasoning, or the ability to scrutinize different moral decisions and actions (Gerrits et al. 2023). For example, educational strategies that focus on discussing relevant ethical concepts and moral implications of morally charged scenarios and transferring insights from these discussions to other situations could enhance moral sensitivity. Moreover, roleplaying exercises could hone perspective-taking and, as such, aid the development of moral sensitivity, by identifying what is morally relevant in a situation, and moral reasoning, by evaluating the different perspectives (Gerrits et al. 2023).

To foster research integrity, teaching about codes and rules could be helpful as a normative baseline. However, a rule-based focus has limitations because such guidelines can be overwhelming, are often only updated infrequently, focus on the negative consequences of not following them, and often still need additional ethical reflection to apply a norm to the specific research situation (Pennock 2015; Pennock and O'Rourke 2017; Peels et al. 2019). While not a true panacea, a virtue-based approach could help to overcome some of these difficulties (Pennock 2015; Pennock and O'Rourke 2017).

In virtue ethics, a virtue is known for being both an attitude and an action. Thus, one can only be truly virtuous by being convinced that specific virtues are important and having the courage to act according to these virtues. For example, SC researchers could strive to internalize the intellectual virtue of "scientific curiosity."

When someone is curious about how phenomena could be explained scientifically, a researcher would be truly interested in creating an understanding of the research topic—for instance, by testing a hypothesis (Pennock and O'Rourke 2017). This curiosity could then only be maintained and realized in the attitude and relevant actions corresponding to scientific curiosity, such as using valid and relevant scientific methodology, working meticulously, and not acting in a way that conflicts with that virtue (e.g., data fabrication and falsification). Fully mastering virtues will often be difficult in an educational setting. Therefore, education should focus on how researchers can become virtuous, which involves a basic understanding of virtue ethics, how virtues could be cultivated through practice, and how role models play a role in identifying virtues and virtuous behavior. This approach would also focus on cultivating the practical wisdom required for research integrity (Goddiksen and Gjerris 2022), and create an awareness of how this form of integrity is affected by circumstantial changes (like the introduction of new technologies) and how a work climate affects their behavior positively or negatively. In a broader sense, prompting researchers to become virtuous could contribute to identifying responsibilities and the attitude to act upon them.

Another potential way to enhance the moral sensitivity of SC researchers is to clarify the distinction between hard and soft impacts. This distinction was proposed in the literature surrounding the ethics and philosophy of technology (Swierstra and te Molder 2012; Swierstra 2015), and it could be used as a heuristic tool to distinguish between two different types of ethical impacts that could both be interpreted negatively and positively (Assen et al. 2021). The hard impacts could best be understood as direct physical, causal effects of technology or research that are measurable or quantifiable. For SC research, these involve side effects of new interventions, therapeutic value, costs, and risk. These are often the types of ethical implications that SC researchers consider to be part of the ethical dimension of their research.

By contrast, soft impacts are the indirect and nonphysical effects of SC research or technology (see Swierstra and te Molder 2012). As such, they impact social structures and psychological aspects such as experiences, moral values, perceptions, and actions (van der Burg 2009). These impacts are not always as clear as hard impacts since whether the impact is positive or negative may vary depending on the context. Hard and soft impacts are also important for the responsible innovation of SC research, where the distinction can help researchers to understand how societal goals could be undermined due to the direct and indirect ethical effects of their research (see van der Burg 2009). When offered in an educational setting, the distinction between hard and soft impacts may serve as a heuristic tool to make researchers aware of the broader ethical dimensions of their research. It can also aid researchers in discussing the ethical dimension of their work with each other and with ethicists (Assen et al. 2021).

In addition, the development of moral imagination might help to further improve the moral sensitivity and moral reasoning of SC researchers (see Coeckelbergh 2006; Gerrits et al. 2023). In general, moral imagination involves a process through which ethical reflections on specific situations are stimulated through the use of narratives, metaphors, and images (Johnson 1993). The underlying idea is that moral sensitivity and reasoning are improved by learning how moral concepts can be interpreted in new situations, perspective-taking, and foreseeing what type of moral consequences certain actions or decisions have. To this end, teaching might include exercises inspired by roleplaying, writing and analyzing scenarios or narratives, and rewriting scenarios from diverse perspectives that include scientific, sociopolitical, and economic factors (Gerrits et al. 2023). Consequentially, cultivating moral imagination can help researchers consider relevant stakeholders and how to include relevant perspectives in ethical reflection.

10.7 Concluding Remarks and Outlook

SC researchers have unique insights into SC research due to their experience and knowledge. To further the responsible conduct and innovation of SC research through the collaboration with ethicists, SC researchers must be responsibilized on three levels:

1. Robust and responsive legislation is needed to protect research participants and patients from harm and to aid researchers in conducting research that could benefit society.
2. The organizational dimension helps to unburden researchers through (administrative) support to comply with legislation, creates working conditions that positively motivate research groups to foster research integrity, delegates responsibilities, and offers educational and training opportunities for individual researchers.
3. The educational dimension helps individual researchers to become equipped with knowledge, skills, and attitudes for taking responsibility, with a specific focus on the identification of ethical implications of SC research.

As the field of SC research has a plethora of ethical implications, this proposal for the responsibilization of SC researchers is not exhaustive and serves as an example of how such responsibilization could take place. However, the proposed blueprint for responsibilization can aid organizations and SC researchers in identifying other ethical implications and accompanying responsibilities of their research, considering how these responsibilities should be distributed, and recognizing what individual stakeholders need regarding governance frameworks, organizational support, and knowledge, attitudes, and skills to fulfill these responsibilities.

While it is worthwhile for every SC researcher to understand the ethical dimensions and implications of their work, it is questionable whether all SC researchers should be fully responsibilized to the point of dealing with the soft impacts of their research. Instead, researchers who are motivated to take an extra step should have the opportunity to become better equipped and help to ensure the ethical conduct and translation of SC research in general.

Lastly, although this chapter focused primarily on the SC researcher, other stakeholders, such as ethicists and (other) educators, play a crucial role in the responsibilization and responsible conduct of SC researchers. Ethicists can aid SC researchers by offering education about the ethical dimension and how research integrity could be fostered through virtue-based training. Moreover, ethicists and moral philosophers still have many challenges, as developments in SC research such as SCB-EM, chimeras, and complex forms of neural and cerebral organoids challenge the conception of moral status and desirability.

References

Alahmad, Ghiath, Sarah Aljohani, and Muath Fahmi Najjar. 2020. "Ethical Challenges Regarding the Use of Stem Cells: Interviews with Researchers from Saudi Arabia." *BMC Medical Ethics* 21: article no. 35. https://doi.org/10.1186/s12910-020-00482-6.

Andrews, P. W., D. Baker, N. Benvinisty, B. Miranda, K. Bruce, O. Brüstle, et al. 2015. "Points to Consider in the Development of Seed Stocks of Pluripotent Stem Cells for Clinical Applications: International Stem Cell Banking Initiative (ISCBI)." *Regenerative Medicine* 10 (2) (supplement): 1–44. https://doi.org/10.2217/rme.14.93.

Antes, Alison L., Stephen T. Murphy, Ethan P. Waples, Michael D. Mumford, Ryan P. Brown, Shane Connelly, and Lynn D. Devenport. 2009. "A Meta-analysis of Ethics Instruction Effectiveness in the Sciences." *Ethics & Behavior* 19 (5): 379–402. https://doi.org/10.1080/10508420903035380.

Assen, Lars S., Karin R. Jongsma, Rosario Isasi, Marianna A. Tryfonidou, and Annelien L. Bredenoord. 2021. "Recognizing the Ethical Implications of Stem Cell Research: A Call for Broadening the Scope." *Stem Cell Reports* 16 (7) (July 13): 1656–1661. https://doi.org/10.1016/j.stemcr.2021.05.021.

Assen, Lars S., Karin R. Jongsma, Rosario Isasi, Marianna A. Tryfonidou, and Annelien L. Bredenoord. 2022. "Roles and Responsibilities in Stem Cell Research: A Focus Group Study with Stem Cell Researchers and Patients." *Regenerative Medicine* 17 (7): 445–459. https://doi.org/10.2217/rme-2022-0019.

Bauer, Gerhard, Magdi Elsallab, and Mohamed Abou-El-Enein. 2018. "Concise Review: A Comprehensive Analysis of Reported Adverse Events in Patients Receiving Unproven Stem Cell-Based Interventions." *Stem Cells Translational Medicine* 7 (9) (September): 676–685. https://doi.org/10.1002/sctm.17-0282.

Boenink, Marianne. 2013. "The Multiple Practices of Doing 'Ethics in the Laboratory': A Mid-level Perspective." In *Ethics on the Laboratory Floor*, edited by Simone van der Burg and Tsjalling Swierstra, 57–78. Houndmills, UK: Palgrave Macmillan. https://doi.org/10.1057/9781137002938_4.

Boon, Wouter, Judith de Haan, Carien Duisterwinkel, Lauren Gould, Willem Janssen, Karin Jongsma, et al. 2022. "Meaningful Public Engagement in the Context of Open Science: Reflections from Early and Mid-career Academics." *Research for All* 6 (1). https://doi.org/10.14324/RFA.06.1.23.

Bouros, Demosthenes, and Geoff Laurent. 2013. "Regenerative Medicine and Stem Cells: Prometheus Revisited." *Respiration* 85 (1) (December): 1–2. https://doi.org/10.1159/000345622.

Bouter, Lex M. 2015. "Commentary: Perverse Incentives or Rotten Apples?" *Accountability in Research* 22 (3): 148–161. https://doi.org/10.1080/08989621.2014.950253.

Brown, Brian. 2021. "Responsibilization and Recovery: Shifting Responsibilities on the Journey through Mental Health Care to Social Engagement." *Social Theory & Health* 19 (1) (March): 92–109. https://doi.org/10.1057/s41285-019-00097-x.

Carter, Lucy, Aditi Mankad, and Elizabeth V. Hobman. 2023. "Is Public Engagement in Bioengineering and Synthetic Biology Improving Research Outcomes?" *OMICS: A Journal of Integrative Biology* 27 (2) (February): 47–50. https://doi.org/10.1089/omi.2022.0181.

Chan, Sarah. 2017. "Current and Emerging Global Themes in the Bioethics of Regenerative Medicine: The Tangled Web of Stem Cell Translation." *Regenerative Medicine* 12 (7): 839–851. https://doi.org/10.2217/rme-2017-0065.

Clarkeburn, Henriikka, J. Roger Downie, and Bob Matthew. 2002. "Impact of an Ethics Programme in a Life Sciences Curriculum." *Teaching in Higher Education* 7 (1): 65–79. https://doi.org/10.1080/13562510120100391.

Coeckelbergh, Mark. 2006. "Regulation or Responsibility? Autonomy, Moral Imagination, and Engineering." *Science, Technology, & Human Values* 31 (3) (May): 237–260. https://doi.org/10.1177/0162243905285839.

Collingridge, David. 1980. *The Social Control of Technology*. New York: St. Martin's.

Day, Michael. 2019. "Disgraced Tracheal Transplant Surgeon Is Handed 16 Month Prison Sentence in Italy." *BMJ* 367: article no. l6676. https://doi.org/10.1136/bmj.l6676.

de Wert, Guido, and Christine Mummery. 2003. "Human Embryonic Stem Cells: Research, Ethics and Policy." *Human Reproduction* 18 (4) (April): 672–682. https://doi.org/10.1093/humrep/deg143.

Dougherty, Carol. 2006. *Prometheus*. London: Routledge.

Ellison, Brooke. 2016. "Stem Cell Research and Social Justice: Aligning Scientific Progress with Social Need." *Current Stem Cell Reports* 2 (4): 328–335. https://doi.org/10.1007/s40778-016-0063-3.

Fabbri, Morris, Margaret Ginoza, Lars Assen, Karin Jongsma, and Rosario Isasi. 2023. "Modeling Policy Development: Examining National Governance of Stem Cell-Based Embryo Models." *Regenerative Medicine* 18 (2): 155–168. https://doi.org/10.2217/rme-2022-0136.

Fisher, Erik, Roop L. Mahajan, and Carl Mitcham. 2006. "Midstream Modulation of Technology: Governance from Within." *Bulletin of Science, Technology & Society* 26 (6) (December): 485–496. https://doi.org/10.1177/0270467606295402.

Gerrits, Elianne M., Lars S. Assen, Liesbeth Noordegraaf-Eelens, Annelien L. Bredenoord, and Marc H. W. van Mil. 2023. "Moral Imagination as an Instrument for Ethics Education for Biomedical Researchers." *International Journal of Ethics Education* 8 (2) (December): 275–289. https://doi.org/10.1007/s40889-023-00171-z.

Gianni, Robert. 2021. "Scientific and Democratic Relevance of RRI: Dimensions and Relations." In *Assessment of Responsible Innovation: Methods and Practices*, edited by Emad Yaghmaei and Ibo van de Poel, 11–41. Abingdon, UK: Routledge. https://doi.org/10.4324/9780429298998.

Goddiksen, Mads Paludan, and Mickey Gjerris. 2022. "Teaching Phronesis in a Research Integrity Course." *Facets* 7 (January): 139–152. https://doi.org/10.1139/facets-2021-0064.

Gopalan, Nishakanthi, Siti Nurani Mohamed Noor, and Mohd Salim Mohamed. 2021. "The Pro-medical Tourism Stance of Malaysia and How It Affects Stem Cell Tourism Industry." *Sage Open* 11 (2) (April). https://doi.org/10.1177/21582440211016837.

Grene, David. 1940. "Prometheus Bound." *Classical Philology* 35 (1) (January): 22–38. https://doi.org/10.1086/362316.

Grunwald, Armin. 2013. "Responsible Research and Development: Roles of Ethicists on the Laboratory Floor." In *Ethics on the Laboratory Floor*, edited by Simone van der Burg and Tsjalling Swierstra, 38–56. Houndmills, UK: Palgrave Macmillan. https://doi.org/10.1057/9781137002938_3.

Haven, Tamarinde, H. Roeline Pasman, Guy Widdershoven, Lex Bouter, and Joeri Tijdink. 2020. "Researchers' Perceptions of a Responsible Research Climate: A Multi Focus Group Study." *Science and Engineering Ethics* 26 (6): 3017–3036. https://doi.org/10.1007/s11948-020-00256-8.

Hong, Sungook. 2008. "The Hwang Scandal That 'Shook the World of Science.'" *East Asian Science, Technology and Society* 2 (1): 1–7. https://doi.org/10.1215/s12280-008-9041-x.

Hyun, Insoo. 2010. "The Bioethics of Stem Cell Research and Therapy." *Journal of Clinical Investigation* 120 (1): 71–75. https://doi.org/10.1172/JCI40435.

Hyun, Insoo. 2022. "Stem Cell Ethics and Policy: What's Old Is New Again." *Med* 3 (12) (December 9): 820–823. https://doi.org/10.1016/j.medj.2022.11.008.

Isasi, Rosario, Peter W. Andrews, Jay M. Baltz, Annelien L. Bredenoord, Paul Burton, Ing-Ming Chiu, et al. 2014. "Identifiability and Privacy in Pluripotent Stem Cell Research." *Cell Stem Cell* 14 (4) (April 3): 427–430. https://doi.org/10.1016/j.stem.2014.03.014.

Isasi, Rosario, Margaret Ginoza, Karin Jongsma, Lars Assen, and Morris Fabbri. 2022. "Mending the Gaps: Ethically Sensitive Cells and the Evolution of European Stem Cell Policy." *Regenerative Medicine* 17 (8): 581–595. https://doi.org/10.2217/rme-2022-0043.

Johnson, Mark. 1993. *Moral Imagination: Implications of Cognitive Science for Ethics*. Chicago: University of Chicago Press.

Jonas, Hans. 1979. *Das Prinzip Verantwortung: Versuch einer Ethik für die technologische Zivilisation*. 8th ed. Frankfurt a.M.: Suhrkamp.

Jongsma, Karin R., and Annelien L. Bredenoord. 2020. "Ethics Parallel Research: An Approach for (Early) Ethical Guidance of Biomedical Innovation." *BMC Medical Ethics* 21: article no. 81. https://doi.org/10.1186/s12910-020-00524-z.

Kamenova, Kalina, and Timothy Caulfield. 2015. "Stem Cell Hype: Media Portrayal of Therapy Translation." *Science Translational Medicine* 7 (278) (March 11): 1–5. https://doi.org/10.1126/scitranslmed.3010496.

King, Nancy M. P., and Jacob Perrin. 2014. "Ethical Issues in Stem Cell Research and Therapy." *Stem Cell Research & Therapy* 5: article no. 85. https://doi.org/10.1186/scrt474.

Knoppers, Bartha M., and Rosario Isasi. 2010. "Stem Cell Banking: Between Traceability and Identifiability." *Genome Medicine* 2: article no. 73. https://doi.org/10.1186/gm194.

Kramer, Bianca, and Jeroen Bosman. 2024. "Recognition and Rewards in Academia—Recent Trends in Assessment." In *Talent Management in Higher Education*, edited by Marian Thunnissen and Paul Boselie, 55–75. Leeds, UK: Emerald Publishing Limited. https://doi.org/10.1108/978-1-80262-685-820241004

Kuhlmann, Stefan, Peter Stegmaier, and Kornelia Konrad. 2019. "The Tentative Governance of Emerging Science and Technology—a Conceptual Introduction." *Research Policy* 48 (5) (June): 1091–1097. https://doi.org/10.1016/j.respol.2019.01.006.

Lindner, Ralf, Stefan Kuhlmann, Sally Randles, Bjørn Bedsted, Guido Gorgoni, Erich Griessler, Allison Loconto, and Niels Mejlgaard, eds. 2016. *Navigating towards Shared Responsibility in Research and Innovation: Approach, Process and Results of the Res-AGorA Project*. Karlsruhe: Fraunhofer Institute for Systems and Innovation Research ISI. http://pure.au.dk/portal/files/98634660/RES_AGorA_ebook.pdf.

Longstaff, Holly, Catherine A. Schuppli, Nina Preto, Darquise Lafrenière, and Michael McDonald. 2009. "Scientists' Perspectives on the Ethical Issues of Stem Cell Research." *Stem Cell Reviews and Reports* 5 (2) (June): 89–95. https://doi.org/10.1007/s12015-009-9068-y.

Lovell-Badge, Robin, Eric Anthony, Roger A. Barker, Tania Bubela, Ali H. Brivanlou, Melissa Carpenter, et al. 2021. "ISSCR Guidelines for Stem Cell Research and Clinical Translation: The 2021 Update." *Stem Cell Reports* 16 (6) (June 8): 1398–1408. https://doi.org/10.1016/j.stemcr.2021.05.012.

MacPherson, Amanda, and Jonathan Kimmelman. 2019. "Ethical Development of Stem-Cell-Based Interventions." *Nature Medicine* 25 (7) (July): 1037–1044. https://doi.org/10.1038/s41591-019-0511-6.

Master, Zubin, Kirstin R. W. Matthews, and Mohamed Abou-el-Enein. 2021. "Unproven Stem Cell Interventions: A Global Public Health Problem Requiring Global Deliberation." *Stem Cell Reports* 16 (6) (June 8): 1435–1445. https://doi.org/10.1016/j.stemcr.2021.05.004.

McCabe, Christopher, and Douglas Sipp. 2016. "Undertested and Overpriced: Japan Issues First Conditional Approval of Stem Cell Product." *Cell Stem Cell* 18 (4) (April 7): 436–437. https://doi.org/10.1016/j.stem.2016.03.006.

Mejlgaard, Niels, Lex M. Bouter, George Gaskell, Panagiotis Kavouras, Nick Allum, Anna-Kathrine Bendtsen, et al. 2020. "Research Integrity: Nine Ways to Move from Talk to Walk." *Nature* 586 (7829) (October 15): 358–360. https://doi.org/10.1038/d41586-020-02847-8.

Nejati, Mehran, and Azadeh Shafaei. 2018. "Leading by Example: The Influence of Ethical Supervision on Students' Prosocial Behavior." *Higher Education* 75 (1) (January): 75–89. https://doi.org/10.1007/s10734-017-0130-4.

Niemansburg, Sophie L., Tjidde H. Tempels, Wouter J. A. Dhert, Johannes J. M. van Delden, and Annelien L. Bredenoord. 2015. "Societal Impacts of Regenerative Medicine: Reflections on the Views of Orthopedic Professionals." *Regenerative Medicine* 10 (1): 17–24. https://doi.org/10.2217/rme.14.69.

Nollkaemper, Andre. 2018. "The Duality of Shared Responsibility." *Contemporary Politics* 24 (5): 524–544. https://doi.org/10.1080/13569775.2018.1452107.

Owen, Richard, Phil Macnaghten, and Jack Stilgoe. 2012. "Responsible Research and Innovation: From Science in Society to Science for Society, with Society." *Science and Public Policy* 39 (6) (December): 751–760. https://doi.org/10.1093/scipol/scs093.

Peels, Rik, Jeroen de Ridder, Tamarinde Haven, and Lex Bouter. 2019. "Value Pluralism in Research Integrity." *Research Integrity and Peer Review* 4: article no. 18. https://doi.org/10.1186/s41073-019-0076-4.

Pennock, Robert T. 2015. "Fostering a Culture of Scientific Integrity: Legalistic vs. Scientific Virtue-Based Approaches." *Professional Ethics Report* 28 (2) (Spring): 1–3. https://doi.org/10.1126/srhrl.acr8257.

Pennock, Robert T., and Michael O'Rourke. 2017. "Developing a Scientific Virtue-Based Approach to Science Ethics Training." *Science and Engineering Ethics* 23: 243–262. https://doi.org/10.1007/s11948-016-9757-2.

Politi, Vincenzo, and Alexei Grinbaum. 2020. "The Distribution of Ethical Labor in the Scientific Community." *Journal of Responsible Innovation* 7 (3): 263–279. https://doi.org/10.1080/23299460.2020.1724357.

Power, Carl, and John E. J. Rasko. 2008. "Whither Prometheus' Liver? Greek Myth and the Science of Regeneration." *Annals of Internal Medicine* 149 (6) (September 16): 421–426. https://doi.org/10.7326/0003-4819-149-6-200809160-00009.

PytlikZillig, Lisa M., and Alan J. Tomkins. 2011. "Public Engagement for Informing Science and Technology Policy: What Do We Know, What Do We Need to Know, and How Will We Get There?" *Review of Policy Research* 28 (2) (March): 197–217. https://doi.org/10.1111/j.1541-1338.2011.00489.x.

Rip, Arie, and Douglas K. R. Robinson. 2013. "Constructive Technology Assessment and the Methodology of Insertion." In *Early Engagement and New Technologies: Opening Up the Laboratory*, edited by Neelke Doorn, Daan Schuurbiers, Ibo van de Poel, and Michael E. Gorman, 37–53. Dordrecht: Springer. https://doi.org/10.1007/978-94-007-7844-3_3.

Robertson, John A. 2001. "Human Embryonic Stem Cell Research: Ethical and Legal Issues." *Nature Reviews Genetics* 2 (1) (January): 74–78. https://doi.org/10.1038/35047594.

Rose, Nikolas. 1993. "Government, Authority and Expertise in Advanced Liberalism." *Economy and Society* 22 (3): 283–299. https://doi.org/10.1080/03085149300000019.

Rose, Nikolas. 2013. "Personalized Medicine: Promises, Problems and Perils of a New Paradigm for Healthcare." *Procedia – Social and Behavioral Sciences* 77 (April 22): 341–352. https://doi.org/10.1016/j.sbspro.2013.03.092.

Sawai, Tsutomu, Hideya Sakaguchi, Elizabeth Thomas, Jun Takahashi, and Misao Fujita. 2019. "The Ethics of Cerebral Organoid Research: Being Conscious of Consciousness." *Stem Cell Reports* 13 (3) (September 10): 440–447. https://doi.org/10.1016/j.stemcr.2019.08.003.

Schneider, Michael D. 2004. "Prometheus Unbound." *Nature* 432 (7016) (November 25): 451–453. https://doi.org/10.1038/432451a.

Sipp, Douglas, and Margaret Sleeboom-Faulkner. 2019. "Downgrading of Regulation in Regenerative Medicine." *Science* 365 (6454) (August 16): 644–646. https://doi.org/10.1126/science.aax 6184.

Sleeboom-Faulkner, Margaret. 2019. "Regulatory Brokerage: Competitive Advantage and Regulation in the Field of Regenerative Medicine." *Social Studies of Science* 49 (3) (June): 355–380. https://doi.org/10.1177/0306312719850628.

Sugarman, Jeremy, Amander Clark, James Fishkin, Kazuto Kato, Kevin McCormack, Megan Munsie, Michael J. Peluso, Nancy René, and Susan L. Solomon. 2023. "Critical Considerations for Public Engagement in Stem Cell-Related Research." *Stem Cell Reports* 18 (2) (February 14): 420–426. https://doi.org/10.1016/j.stemcr.2023.01.002.

Swierstra, Tsjalling. 2015. "Identifying the Normative Challenges Posed by Technology's 'Soft' Impacts." *Etikk i praksis* 9 (1): 5–20. https://doi.org/10.5324/eip.v9i1.1838.

Swierstra, Tsjalling, and Jaap Jelsma. 2005. "Trapped in the Duality of Structure: An STS Approach to Engineering Ethics." In *Inside the Politics of Technology: Agency and Normativity in the Co-Production of Technology and Society*, edited by Hans Harbers, 199–227. Amsterdam: Amsterdam University Press. https://doi.org/10.1515/9789048503841-010.

Swierstra, Tsjalling, and Hedwig te Molder. 2012. "Risk and Soft Impacts." In *Handbook of Risk Theory: Epistemology, Decision Theory, Ethics, and Social Implications of Risk*, edited by Sabine Roeser, Rafaela Hillerbrand, Per Sandin, and Martin Peterson, 1049–1066. Dordrecht: Springer. https://doi.org/10.1007/978-94-007-1433-5_42.

Tijdink, Joeri K., Reinout Verbeke, and Yvo M. Smulders. 2014. "Publication Pressure and Scientific Misconduct in Medical Scientists." *Journal of Empirical Research on Human Research Ethics* 9 (5) (December): 64–71. https://doi.org/10.1177/1556264614552421.

Universiteiten van Nederland. 2019. *Room for Everyone's Talent: Towards a New Balance in the Recognition and Rewards of Academics*. https://recognitionrewards.nl/wp-content/uploads/2020/12/position-paper-room-for-everyones-talent.pdf.

van der Burg, Simone. 2009. "Taking the 'Soft Impacts' of Technology into Account: Broadening the Discourse in Research Practice." *Social Epistemology* 23 (3–4): 301–316. https://doi.org/10.1080/02691720903364191.

Waelbers, Katinka. 2009. "Technological Delegation: Responsibility for the Unintended." *Science and Engineering Ethics* 15 (1): 51–68. https://doi.org/10.1007/s11948-008-9098-x.

Walhout, Bart, Stefan Kuhlmann, Gonzalo Ordóñez-Matamoros, and Jakob Edler. 2016. "Res-AGorA Concepts and Approach." In *Navigating towards Shared Responsibility in Research and Innovation: Approach, Process and Results of the Res-AGorA Project*, edited by Ralf Lindner, Stefan Kuhlmann, Sally Randles, Bjørn Bedsted, Guido Gorgoni, Erich Griessler, Allison Loconto, and Niels Mejlgaard, 47–53. Karlsruhe, DE: Fraunhofer Institute for Systems and Innovation Research ISI. http://pure.au.dk/portal/files/98634660/RES_AGorA_ebook.pdf.

Watts, Logan L., Kelsey E. Medeiros, Tyler J. Mulhearn, Logan M. Steele, Shane Connelly, and Michael D. Mumford. 2017. "Are Ethics Training Programs Improving? A Meta-analytic Review of Past and Present Ethics Instruction in the Sciences." *Ethics & Behavior* 27 (5): 351–384. https://doi.org/10.1080/10508422.2016.1182025.

Wetenschappelijke Raad voor het Regeringsbeleid. 2017. *Weten is nog geen doen: Een realistisch perspectief op redzaamheid*. The Hague: Wetenschappelijke Raad voor het Regeringsbeleid.

Lars Assen is a postdoctoral researcher at the University of Twente in Enschede, the Netherlands. His interests lie at the intersection of technological developments in biomedicine and its philosophical and ethical implications. He obtained his PhD in bioethics, during which he conducted research on the responsibilities of stem cell researchers to anticipate and deal with the ethical implications of their work. To this end, Assen combines insights from philosophy of technology, bioethics, and science and technology studies.

Chapter 11
The ABCs of Enhancement: AI, Biohacking, and CRISPR Culture

Rina Bliss

Abstract Recently, research laboratories and biomedical startups promising significant medical enhancement to our minds and bodies have flooded the landscape of science and biotechnology, making what once seemed eugenic hyperbole a thriving market. This chapter explores the ethical, legal, and social implications of one corner of the market: medical brain enhancement technologies. Analyzing the emerging fields of neurotech enabled by artificial intelligence, biohacking of one's genes and genomes, and human gene editing research and development against the historical backdrop of biomedical research and development, I elucidate the potential dangers around how society conceptualizes race and ability, and how it addresses racism and bias. I argue that our present culture of innovation dovetails with extant inequalities in medicine and healthcare that stand to perpetuate and amplify racial inequality and bias in our algorithmic and social systems.

Keywords Artificial intelligence · Genetics · Genomics · CRISPR · Biohacking

11.1 Introduction

In February 2024, Elon Musk's artificial intelligence (AI) embedded brain-computer interface company Neuralink made headlines when the company reported successfully transplanting its AI brain implant "Telepathy" into Neuralink's first human subject (Madhok 2024). Brain-computer interfaces, also called brain-machine interfaces, are technologies that make an electrical link that transfers data between an individual's brain and some external device, such as a robotic medical prosthetic or a computer (Maiseli et al. 2023). The connection that Telepathy provided enabled the research subject's brain's electrical activity to control an external device's hardware and software without using neuromuscular energy (Carpenter 2024). Musk told the press that the patient, later revealed to be thirty-year-old quadriplegic Noland Arbaugh, was doing well and able to move a computer cursor with his thoughts

R. Bliss (✉)
Rutgers University, New Brunswick, NJ, USA
e-mail: catherine.bliss@rutgers.edu

M. C. Altman and D. Schwan (eds.), *Ethics and Medical Technology*, The International Library of Bioethics 113, https://doi.org/10.1007/978-3-031-94690-5_11

(Mann 2024). Musk simultaneously released a video calling for more quadriplegics to participate in Neuralink trials, asking them to help the company "redefine the boundaries of human capability" (Neuralink 2023). In promotional publicity and interviews, Musk made it clear that his goal with Neuralink's brain-enhancing technology was to develop medical brain enhancement technologies that any human on earth could use to expand their everyday abilities (Regalado 2023). Musk characterized Neuralink as a passage toward a permanent merging of human bodies and minds with AI to achieve a hyperintelligence beyond all measure (Niemeyer 2024).

While Neuralink's advances set off a media frenzy, further investigations revealed that Neuralink is just the tip of the iceberg in AI-based medical enhancements (Eisenstein 2024). Other brain-computer interface companies such as Cognixion, BrainGate, Synchron, and BlackRock Neurotech have also received Food and Drug Adminstration (FDA) clearance to implant AI computer chips into human brains to collect, analyze, and enhance brain activity in quadriplegics. The FDA has designated Neuralink's Telepathy, Cognixion's ONE, BrainGate's BrainGate2, Synchron's Stentrode, and BlackRock Neurotech's Neuralace "breakthrough therapies" in order to prioritize them for clinical testing and commercialization. What once seemed like science fiction is now a government-approved path to market, creating a world in which highly technologized medical enhancements are presumed to benefit society writ large.

This chapter explores some of the latest neural enhancement technologies emerging from AI neurotech, biohacking, and gene-editing science to determine their ethical, legal, and social implications. Analysis of company leaders' mission and vision statements will reveal how present-day marketing tropes for technologies sold as healthcare fixes for severely disabled patients are in fact promoting elective enhancements that correspond to historical visions of eugenics on a massive nonmedical scale. Looking closely at implications for racism and bias, I will show how founders and funders like Musk instill a new biomedicalized paradigm of health and human potential that, though absent of race talk, supports supremacist thinking and practice. Moreover, as leaders roll out enhancement technologies into a political economy of racialized science, enhancement technologies intersect with and intensify systematic racism and bias in medicine and the wider society. As AI enters the clinic via medical diagnostics, staff support, electronic medical records, and polygenic indexing, and as technologies reach beyond healthcare and medicine to educational systems and settings, species-altering medical enhancement technologies stand to entrench racial injustice while spreading a genetically deterministic concept of racial difference that masks deeply rooted social inequalities in science, medicine, education, and public health.

11.2 The Rise of "Next Human" Medicine

In 2003, Adele Clarke et al. (2003) wrote that American society was being overtaken by a culture of biomedical enhancement. Whereas medical research and development had once aimed to heal the sick, New Millennium technologies had metamorphosed to enhance the healthy. Clarke and colleagues called this shift *biomedicalization*: "the increasingly complex, multisited, multidirectional processes of medicalization that today are being both extended and reconstituted through emergent social forms and practices of a highly and increasingly technoscientific biomedicine" (162). Regardless of health status or the presence of an illness, members of society would increasingly be invited to medically transform their minds and bodies "from the inside out" in ways that would forever changing the limits of human ability and the nature of humanity.

True to this proclamation, a seismic shift in medical enhancement was underway. With the rise of social media and personalized genomics, people began availing themselves of personal genetic tests, off-label pharmaceuticals, and implant technology to hack their health the way one would hack a computer. In 2003, a cottage industry of transformative mobile health apps called "mHealth" entered the market, forevermore blurring the lines between authoritative medical practice and recreational health and wellness (Istepanian 2022). Two years later, nationally acclaimed inventor Ray Kurzweil released *The Singularity Is Near: When Humans Transcend Biology* (2005), a popular book on humanity's amalgamation with AI to become superhuman. At the core of many biohacking efforts of this era were visions to genetically and technologically enhance humans so that they could stave off or reverse aging and cognitive decline as well as enable humans to merge with computer systems to elevate cognitive and physical prowess (Gangadharbatla 2020). By the end of the first decade of the new millennium, companies were marketing personal genomic DNA tests to healthy consumers interested in managing their health without the oversight of medical experts (Hogarth and Saukko 2017). Biotech firms told the public that control over one's genes, mind, and body was a human right (Phillips 2024). Company leaders championed a new era of biomedical autonomy and democracy through self-determination of health using the latest in science and technology.

In 2012, geneticists working with DNA molecules called "CRISPR" (Clustered Regularly Interspaced Short Palindromic Repeats) found that they could manipulate genetic variants to cut and paste strands of DNA (Cribbs and Perera 2017). The following year, researchers applied CRISPR to human cells, reprogramming cells with sickle cell disease to be disease-free (Li et al. 2023). In 2018, the first gene-edited babies were born, twins born of IVF (in vitro fertilization) and engineered to be HIV resistant using genetic variants also known to be associated with cognitive function (Regalado 2018). Shortly after, as clinical trials for the world's first CRISPR-based pharmaceutical therapy got underway, a biotech firm edited the genomes of six people to enhance brain activity (Swain 2023). At a time when developers were engineering the world's first generative networks and transformers, bioengineering was fusing with public health efforts to forge beyond curing disease to a new frontier of medical enhancement (Mansuri 2024). Again, leaders celebrated what they viewed as gaining greater control over our personal destiny using the latest in science and technology.

Amid these developments, technology companies bringing medical brain enhancements to market articulated a vision of a New Human, a cyborg of machine learning and human intelligence able to supersede mental and physical limitations to become "super" or "trans"-human (Dunn and Brueck 2022). Founders and funders of AI-based brain-computer interface technology did not see their inventions as being limited to the disabled or diseased populations on whom they tested enhancements in clinical trials. Instead, company leaders envisioned medical brain enhancements as technologies for the masses of health-seeking humans who simply wanted to be the best they could be using the latest in science and technology.

Musk, for one, told reporters in 2021 that he had designed a stylish white chair to administer brain implant surgery, an outpatient surgery that he pictured consumers would undergo in a casual thirty-minute MedSpa session (Regalado 2021). He declared then that his motivation for engineering medical brain enhancements was to boost human intelligence by way of a "symbiosis with AI" so that machine intelligence would not outpace human intelligence. Less than one month into Telepathy's clinical trials, Musk pivoted from the company's original research questions of neurodegeneration and disease to direct his team of engineers to design an enhancement technology capacious enough to address mood disorders, learning disabilities, and other mental and emotional challenges (Shankland 2024). Musk has since maintained that this "fitbit for your skull" will eventually empower humans to have "superhuman cognition," affording them mind-reading capabilities via an integrated system of human-machine AI (Newton 2024).

BlackRock Neurotech's funder Christian Angermeyer has also touted the company's Neuralace implant—a brain-computer interface technology that dusts the brain with ultrasound-based smart chips—as a whole-brain solution to cognitive function, mental illness, and emotional well-being ("Brain Chips" 2021). Moreover, Angermeyer has articulated a "Next Human Agenda," what he describes as making all humans hyperintelligent and happy via neural implants (GQ Staff 2023). Through his private investment firm Apeiron (named after the Greek word for "infinite"), and his neurotech venture capital firm re.Mind, Angemeyer finances an array of gene therapies and neurotech that is claimed to be "enabling millions to find freedom, fulfillment, and happiness," not simply quadriplegics or other patients living with disabling disorders ("re.Mind Capital" 2024).

Similarly, BlackRock Neurotech's mainstay investor Peter Thiel (2019) envisions mass-marketed brain enhancements as the salve for any and all mental and emotional limitations (Shead 2021b). Thiel, who founded the Singularity Summit and has a Machine Intelligence Research Institute, wants medical brain enhancements armed with large language models to rewire people to feel content and optimistic throughout their daily lives, so that they can take on the power of AI to rule the world (Thiel 2019). Like Musk and Angermeyer, Thiel finances research and development to shape human ability in order to permanently alter the species, the end goal being to propagate a fitter, more powerful human being and human race (Olson 2024).

Investors like Thiel have their sights set on creating technologies that can enhance their minds and bodies irrespective of disease (Shead 2021a).

11.3 Deep Roots in Eugenics

As much as these technology developers proclaim a novel, “first ever seen” transformation of what human brains can do, their motivations and inspirations driving their rollout of contemporary medical enhancement culture are nothing new. The promise of a “next human” enhancement of the species by way of science and technology, and the comingling of medical and recreational activities to engender control over biological destinies, are eugenic cultural scripts and tactics that have been at the heart of research and development since the dawn of modern medicine (Bliss 2023).

Even the most venerated leading scientists of the early modern era articulated eugenic missions and visions for society. In the latter half of the nineteenth century, following his journey on the *HMS Beagle*, Charles Darwin (1859) characterized evolution as a process in which all members of a species could potentially mate with one another and pass on their genes. Darwin wrote that, because organisms that possessed traits well-suited to particular environments would be more likely to survive, there was not one set of traits that was superior to all others. Still, Darwin claimed that human brain development and intelligence had genetically advanced further in the environmental context of Europe (Bernasconi and Lott 2000). Though he opposed slavery, Darwin maintained that whites had superior intellectual capacity and therefore naturally ruled over people of color. As a result of his “scientific” conclusions, he called for the controlled breeding of European populations to improve the human species (Desmond and Moore 1992).

Darwin’s cousin Francis Galton popularized this notion by coining the term “eugenics.” In 1883, Galton wrote that eugenics was

> the science of improving stock, which is by no means confined to questions of judicious mating, but which, especially in the case of man, takes cognizance of all influences that tend in however remote a degree to give to the more suitable races or strains of blood a better chance of prevailing speedily over the less suitable than they otherwise would have had. (1883, 25)

Galton’s research spurred and heavily influenced many fledging fields, including genetics, statistics, anthropology, and psychology, where his goal of creating “a highly-gifted race of men” became the leading authoritative science (Galton 1869, 1). However, Galton’s largest reach was in inspiring politicians (e.g., Theodore Roosevelt and Winston Churchill), funding agencies (e.g., the Carnegie and Rockefeller Foundations), and laypeople (e.g., parents of the winners of Better Babies and Fitter Families contests) who adopted Galton’s twin strategies of encouraging those deemed superior to breed and preventing those deemed unfit (what scientists then called “feebleminded,” “moronic,” “idiotic,” or “imbecilic”) to breed (Bashford and Levine 2010). Moving into the twentieth century, those propounding a medicalized enhancement of the human species to improve the race could be found in doctors' offices, at county fairs, as well as in the highest offices of government.

Even without the existence of technologies that manipulate genomes or implant computers into the brain, throughout the twentieth century, scientists and medical experts created and marshalled the latest medical technologies to produce their version of the next human. All told, the US government forcibly sterilized approximately 65,000 American citizens leading up to World War II, and one-third of all Puerto Rican citizens in the postwar period (Lazar 2021). In other parts of the world, millions more were sterilized, interned, and exterminated in order to, as Musk would later put it in his campaign for hyperintelligence, "redefine the boundaries of human capability."[1] Even as race science and white supremacism were challenged in the final decades of the twentieth century, the notion that intelligence was genetically endowed and present in greater quantity in certain hereditary lineages continued to predominate.

11.4 Whither Eugenics?

At the turn of the twenty-first century, a science of genome-mapping took hold all over the world, starting with the Human Genome Project—an international collaboration involving over twenty nations, yet primarily funded and administered by the US government, that was dedicated to creating a picture of what all the DNA in one human being looked like. Initially, race was absent from scientific discussions over how to go about collecting, analyzing, and explaining human DNA. It seemed as though eugenics was dead in science and medicine, and that human genomics would be the first science to be able to divorce race from genetics.

Yet as the Human Genome Project got underway, geneticists on the project as well as those working in other labs began to ask whether they should be concerned about human variation and, even possibly, race (Bliss 2012). Many sought to distance themselves from a genetic science steeped in scientific racism and eugenics, and they believed that mapping a human genome would lead humanity to a greater understanding of the nature of race. Some additionally believed that genomic findings about human diversity would be an antidote to racist and eugenic beliefs. Scientists reflected on the Eurocentrism of past genetic research and development, and they determined to gain greater representation of racial minority groups so that genomics could be a science for the public good of all.

One genome project that emerged amid the first phase of the Human Genome Project to solve these puzzles and fight Eurocentrism was the Human Genome Diversity Project. The Human Genome Diversity Project set out to collect and compare DNA from populations across the globe to reveal the truth about humanity's diversity. Yet despite the project's intent to battle Eurocentrism, in the mid-1990s,

[1] While Musk is not focused on genetic transmission, he is envisioning enhancement as a permanent species-level transformation that would be passed on across generations.

as project scientists began amassing sample collections from inside and outside the United States got underway, several indigenous American groups protested against the Human Genome Diversity Project, claiming that genome projects were inescapably Eurocentric and eugenicist no matter what their leaders' intent happened to be (Reardon 2004). Though the Human Genome Diversity Project reached out to African American advocates who could consult the project on its policies around sampling and racial representation, to potentially revise its aims and objectives, and though project leaders simultaneously acknowledged and decried scientific racism, the project eventually lost public and governmental support, and project leaders abandoned their grandest aims of being the first explicitly antiracist genome project.

In 2003, a team of African American geneticists working at Howard University attempted a new kind of genome project that would make the question of race a central focus of its research. Calling the effort the African American Diversity Project, its leaders sought to once and for all divorce genetic science from scientific racism. That year, as the Human Genome Project came to a close, its chief scientists also determined to create a new global diversity mapping project that could tackle the question of race head on. The International HapMap Project aimed to collected DNA from people living on the African, American, Asian, and European continents. Though project leaders did not want to reinforce the notion of genetic variation by continental race, the DNA collections that they amassed and later distributed adhered to a continental racial schematic (Bliss 2012). In the early decades of the twenty-first century, with the rise of technologies and projects designed to map the whole genomes of individual organisms (what researchers call "whole-genome sequencing"), racial stratification of the latest advances in biomedical technology took new pervasive forms. Despite anti-eugenic and antiracist sentiments to the contrary, the substrate of biomedical innovation was decidedly racial, and genomic science inadvertently systematized racially structured DNA collections.

Today, biomedical and social scientific research databases (e.g., All of Us, UK Biobank, 23andMe) and cohort studies (e.g., Add Health, PAARTNERS, TEDS, ULADS) spanning research communities across the world often individually sample, cluster, database, data mine, distribute, and disseminate by race. They also harmonize their own individual standards into more widespread comprehensive algorithmic protocols where a genetic account of race is reinforced as individual databases combine existing algorithmic structures in an "invisible matching process" (Lampland and Star 2009, 6). Their protocols are structuring research and setting a field of possibilities for healthcare and education to know, treat, and administer the individual patients and students in their midst, and they are doing so in a way that maintains race at the core of scientific knowledge production. Far from an absence of race science, the latest in genomic technology has reified race and entrenched it in innovation.

11.5 Humankind 2.0

I share this racial backdrop of genomic science because, today, amid the rise of genome-wide sequencing and analysis, and the development of implantable chip technology, a new eugenic discourse of intellectual ability has emerged that has the potential to invigorate a tenacious form of eugenics despite our best attempts to prevent it. Researchers working toward intellectual enhancement and better learning outcomes have begun articulating a vision of manipulating social policy and educational enrichment in order to aid individuals to grow into the best version of themselves. Like their historical forebears in early modern genetics and medicine, these project leaders imagine designing medical technologies that can be applied to anyone, healthy or diseased, so that they can control their destiny while enriching society as a whole. Though the language of race has gradually fallen out of most articulations and claims in this arena, the specter of race and racism continue to haunt it.

One strand of medical enhancement culture trained on the brain concerns the proposal to use human gene-editing to edit out of existence genetic alleles associated with low intelligence or low educational attainment. In 2005, a team of researchers working in a laboratory specializing in genomic analyses of microcephaly, led by geneticist Bruce Lahn, wrote that genes responsible for large brain size were more common in Asian and European people than in African people (Evans et al. 2005). They went on to suggest that Asian and European brains were still evolving into larger brains with higher cognitive function (Richardson 2011). In 2013, geneticists at Beijing Genomics Institute (BGI) embarked upon a high intelligence genome project to sequence the whole genomes of people with high IQ test scores (test scores of 160 or above) to locate more evidence of genetic determinants of high intelligence (Yong 2013). UK-based behavior geneticist Robert Plomin, a staunch advocate of the genetic determinism of intelligence (Plomin 2019), donated 1,600 DNA samples to the project. Members of this research team working in China, the United Kingdom, and the United States suggested that researchers could eventually use gene editing technologies to enhance human cognition and possibly edit low intelligence out of existence (Richardson 2015).

In recent years, one member of BGI, Steven Hsu of the biotech firm Genomic Prediction, has suggested that parents use IVF and the form of genetic testing that many now refer to as "genomic prediction" to select and implant offspring with greater potential for high intelligence and educational attainment (Walters 2019). He also continues to maintain that, with CRISPR, we will one day be able to edit human brains to be hyperintelligent such that the gene pool of our species is permanently enhanced (Metzl 2019).

Another strand of this form of medical enhancement culture concerns the proposal to use genetic intelligence tests and learning chips to dictate educational regimes (Wilby 2014). This field has been referred to as "personalized" or "precision" education because it combines medical technology with genetically tailored curricula, but it can also be seen as a more social form of biohacking that manipulates social environments to boost the brain (Williamson 2018). Plomin, for example, in collaboration with Kathryn Asbury has articulated one version of genetically tailored education with his notion of the "Learning Chip," a computer chip that holds genetic assessments of a person's intelligence and neurobiology which can be used to predict their behavior and assign them to learning environments that are supposedly best suited to their innate ability and limitations (Asbury and Plomin 2013). Clinical psychologist Kathryn Paige Harden similarly advances the use of genetic educational attainment tests to determine individualized education plans so that schools and communities can hack genetically endowed weaknesses to become strengths (Harden 2021).

In these two strands of enhancement culture, as with AI-based applications like Telepathy, much of the language of race has fallen away. Many technology developers make no mention of race in their statements, communiques, and publications. And when they are asked about race, many claim that their research does not make assessments or predictions by race. Yet there are structural reasons why race remains central to these claims beyond overt adherences to race, as in the case of the Lahn laboratory's overt racial comments. For one, genetic tests and prediction software employ algorithms that utilize IQ scores, and IQ data is notoriously racially biased (Benjamin 2019). As nearly half a century of research has shown, IQ tests hold cultural and even racial biases in their structure and content (Holden and Tanenbaum 2023). Likewise, IQ scores reflect deep socioeconomic and intersectional inequalities in society that are driven in part by structural racism (Jencks and Phillips 1998). IQ scores attributed to people of color, especially African Americans, often inaccurately determine those individuals to be of lower intelligence than the mean—in other words, lower than the majority population of white, English-speaking test takers on whom averages are based (Wade 1980). Though IQ scores have been rising in all groups along with a rising standard of living worldwide, people of color, especially Black and Indigenous Americans, continue to be systemically discriminated against and are therefore disproportionately more likely to reside in and be schooled in underserved and under-resourced social environments that have a subpar standard of living (Dickens and Flynn 2006). Black, Indigenous, and other people of color (what some researchers currently refer to as "BIPOC") are still systematically discriminated against in all areas of life, and they suffer the most deeply entrenched intergenerational inequities (Cities and Pilgrim 2022).

People of color also face what researchers call "stereotype threat" when taking IQ tests (Inzlicht and Schmader 2012). Stereotype threat is the process by which test takers incur lower test results than they are due as a result of thinking with stereotypes as they sit for a test. When a person of color takes an IQ test, simply being confronted with the test can remind them of the stereotypes about the group that they are associated with—stereotypes that pervade society claiming that they are intellectually inferior and destined to fail (Steele and Aronson 1995). The resulting fear and anxiety that test takers of color feel can lead them to perform worse on tests. Studies revealing the diverse array of sources of stereotype threat, and its pervasive social nature, prove that even the most bias-conscious test makers and test administrators cannot prevent stereotype threat from biasing test scores (Aronson et al. 2013).

As a result of these structural and psychological pressures, a gap in IQ scores between white Americans and members of other racial groups continues to exist even as living standards have improved, social institutions like the education system have been desegregated, and social environments in some parts of the world have grown more equitable. IQ is thus a poor and unfair basis for predicting intelligence. Any medical or recreational technology that relies on IQ scores to assign values to a person's intelligence so that they can enhance their personal lives as well as the health of the species will only reinforce the extant racial biases in science and society.

11.6 A Backdoor to Eugenics

Embryo selection and gene-editing for intellectual enhancements, and social engineering to boost the health and ability of the brain, explicitly deal in racially stratified genetic data and racially biased IQ data. But even medical enhancement technologies like Telepathy that have no apparent connection to stratified or biased data stand to worsen our already grave racial inequities due to systemic algorithmic biases in AI training data. As sociologist and policy expert Alondra Nelson has written: "DNA is the ultimate big data. Genetic data is multivocal and contains information that can be used in varied facets of society regardless of its source or its original intent of use" (2016, 8). Due to convergences in AI and genomic data through data training mechanisms, any plan to overhaul humanity's abilities by fusing AI and brain activity will hold the power to exacerbate racial hierarchies already in existence, ushering in what sociologist Troy Duster (2004) calls a "backdoor to eugenics"—a revival of eugenic thinking in contemporary technological innovation.

The most direct doorway for eugenics to reenter our world via medical enhancement technology is through an AI brain-computer interface technology's interpretations and uses of highly racialized data and misinformation about human difference to train its large language models, as well as the biased algorithm's subsequent influence on user thought and action. As my research into polygenic indexing—the creation of a personal risk score to predict an individual's likelihood of having a particular trait or disease using DNA analysis—has shown, biomedical training data is racially biased through our newest innovations around genomic health (Bliss 2018). In recent years, as genomic researchers have data mined racially stratified public health databases such as that of the International HapMap Project and carceral databases such as FBI's CODIS in order to home in on alleles associated with specific behaviors (e.g., criminality and/or delinquency) and specific social outcomes (e.g., committing violent acts and/or being incarcerated), research findings have cast behavioral traits and diseases as racially disparate. Downstream of research, members of the criminal justice and education systems have then applied technologies in ways that further structural racism, such as assessing recidivism risks and determining sentencing based on a person's DNA. These practices have reinforced racial stratification within the larger corpora of data, making genetic factors of health and behavior (such as antisocial tendencies and academic success) appear to be innately stratified by race, when in fact it is the social collection, databasing, dissemination, and analysis by race, as well as the biased application of racially stratified technologies and deep racial injustices in society that drive disparities in behavioral traits, mental illnesses, and social outcomes.

The end result of having racially biased AI directing thought and action could be a fomentation of prejudice and a corruption of identity formation due to racisms being fed to users in their minds. Psychological analyses of cognitive processes around race and identity have shown that people learn to hold implicit racial biases from their earliest social interactions (Meltzoff and Gilliam 2024). In preschool and early elementary school, American children tend to show a preference for whiteness no matter what their racial background is, even when they have been told to think positively about their own in-group (Newheiser and Olson 2012). As youth learn the racial stereotypes of their society, they form biased thoughts that can lead to an internalized belief in superiority or inferiority (Qian et al. 2019). Misinformation about human difference abounds, so it has been impossible to avoid creating AI systems that echo the racism in our wider society (Buolamwini 2024). With AI developers reducing their efforts to stave off misinformation (Huang and O'Reagan 2024), adding algorithmic biases in AI systems to these processes will likely cement stereotypic and prejudiced thinking and action in users' minds, leading to prejudicial thought and treatment as well as bolstered beliefs in superiority and inferiority reaching to the core of a person's identity formation.

For youth, this could be particularly problematic in terms of identity development given the move that many educational systems are making to implement AI in the classroom. Currently, schools around the world are adopting AI technologies for the classroom that market themselves as an "all-in-one," "one stop shop" of academic and disciplinary systems (Rosenbaum 2024). Similar to the AI used in AI-based brain implants, companies with names like "MagicSchool" and "SchoolAI" employ large language models to make predictions about what an educator should know about and do with a particular student (Milano et al. 2023). However, like AI medical enhancement technology that is trained on racially biased biomedical corpora, the large language models used in educational AI are trained on racially biased educational and psychological corpora (Warr et al. 2023). These systems are embedded with the power to further reinforce standards and classifications that, as Martha Lampland and Susan Leigh Star write, "produce advantages for some groups and disadvantages for others" (2009, 6). As racially biased medical and educational statistics are rendered corpora for AI EdTech programs that generate personalized plans for their diverse students while assessing, surveilling, and directing the conduct of those students in real-time, AI brain-computer interface technologies synced with AI programs in the classroom could add another layer of racial data-streaming to already biased and prejudicial cognitive processes, including but not limited to how a student sees themselves and others and thinks about their own learning potential and their potential to succeed in an educational environment.

11.7 More Doorways to Eugenics

Another less direct but equally dangerous route to a racist form of eugenics in medical enhancement technology is via the digital divide that prevents the likelihood of AI-based brain implants reaching medically underserved populations. Due to the devastating legacy of racial segregation, people of color continue to face stark health disparities in access to medical technologies and therapies, especially high-cost innovations involving emerging research and development (Saeed and Masters 2021). There is nothing preventing mass-marketed brain enhancements like AI-based brain implants and gene-editing for cognitive advantage from passing by members of racial minority groups. If that were to happen, the world of medical enhancement could become populated by a distinct overclass and underclass. The overclass would possess medically enhanced brains with the capacity for superhuman thought as well as the inclination toward racially biased and prejudicially predictive thought. Far from redefining the boundaries of human capability across the human species, this would enhance those already in dominant positions, a biosocial engineering that would cause irreparable damage to society.

Already we see racial and socioeconomic divides emerging in several areas of medical research and development. In the realm of genomic databases, researchers have found that databases formed for recreational purposes, such as selling people direct-to-consumer DNA tests, predominantly hold DNA samples from individuals who identify as white or "of European descent," whereas databases formed for criminal justice purposes, such as cataloguing the DNA of criminals, predominantly hold DNA samples from individuals who identify as Black or "of African descent" (Chow-White and Duster 2011). In other words, people who are taking part in medical markets in which they can benefit from genomic information that they can use to improve their health and avoid disease are overwhelmingly white, while those who are coerced to enter their DNA into a system designed to penalize and incarcerate potential threats to society are overwhelmingly Black.

Similarly, in the realm of clinical trials and drug development, researchers have found that pharmaceutical companies view whites as potential patients and/or consumers (as Kaushik Sunder Rajan [2006] writes, "patients-in-waiting") while they see people of color as potential research subjects and/or drug testers ("subjects-in-waiting"). When recruiting for clinical trials, companies set their sights on what they see as non-European genetic populations. Meanwhile, when developing marketing campaigns and targeted ads, they set their sights on individuals that they believe to be members of the dominant white group. As a result, there is a racial disparity in whom pharmaceutical companies target for risky clinical trials versus those whom they target to receive cutting-edge pharmaceutical therapies.

In addition to these divides in medical research and development, researchers are witnessing the emergence of a divide in global markets in medical tourism for those seeking cutting-edge medical enhancements (Stoney et al. 2022). Individuals of high socioeconomic status have the ability to travel anywhere to avail themselves of innovative therapies, especially those that remain unapproved by governmental agencies in their own countries (i.e., stem cell therapies and gene-editing therapies). The first CRISPR brain enhancement, for example, was conducted by a US-based company on American citizens who had to travel to Mexico due to the various moratoria on CRISPR clinical trials designated by leading members of the American scientific community. Those seeking this medical brain enhancement had to be able to afford not only to travel but also to receive their postoperative care in offshore medical facilities. This inequitable pattern in medical enhancement markets suggests that those in a society who already hold disproportionate wealth will be able to access whatever medical brain-enhancement technologies emerge, while those who lack access to basic healthcare may never see the benefits of such technologies. Musk's white chair may be a harbinger of the racial divides that already plague medical research and development, but that will only be more devastating if paired with AI.

11.8 Conclusion

In *The Nature of Race: How Scientists Think and Teach about Human Difference* (2011), Ann Morning argued that the way we as a society conceptualize race and human difference matters greatly to the possibility for equality between racial groups, because societies focused on genetic origins tend to ignore the social origins of the problems in their midst. Analyzing different kinds of racial conceptualization from the postwar period to the early 2000s in the United States, Morning found that genetic conceptualizations of human difference have held sway in American society despite the nation's ideological shift toward a belief in fostering civil rights and racial equality. With a core concept of human difference as genetic, it has therefore been difficult to dislodge the pervasive notion that race is attributable to differences in DNA as opposed to one's position in a racist society. As DNA tests, DIY genomics, gene therapies, and medical enhancement technologies have proliferated in the postgenomic era, researchers and developers have continued to portray race as an essential property of one's genetic heritage (TallBear 2013). Even ancestry tests that companies claim can reveal a person's unique combination of admixed "Old World" or "premigration" genetic lineages have been shown to reinforce the idea of original genetic races (Bliss 2008). With genetically deterministic conceptualizations of race holding sway, it is no surprise that members of society looking to improve on the status quo look to hack the body with medical enhancement technologies like CRISPR and AI instead of hacking structural racism with sociological solutions aimed at racial wealth gaps, stereotypes, microaggressions, and the like.

Likewise, society has continued to conceptualize intellectual ability in terms of DNA, as if learning outcomes and educational attainment are caused by innate genetic factors and not the sociological factors perpetuating inequality, such as structural racism and bias (Bliss 2025). Genomic hunts for intelligence involving associations of gene variants spanning the genome (what researchers call "genome-wide association studies" or "GWAS") have snowballed alongside brain enhancement technology in recent years, as geneticists have applied the latest research algorithms to identify potential targets for the treatment of cognitive function and neurodegenerative illnesses. Though Americans no longer adhere to eugenic doctrines and policies that direct government officials, medical professionals, and members of the criminal justice system and military to conduct forcible sterilizations, internment, incarceration, or genocide on people with low IQ scores, markets in DNA IQ tests and apps have flourished. Yet, as with race, holding even a remotely genetically deterministic conceptualization of intelligence only perpetuates the belief that it is our biology that needs fixing (in this case, our brains and neurobiology), not our social system that is rife with educational inequality, unequal (and what for some is adversely toxic) living and working environments, unsafe neighborhoods, and the like. Together, these misdirected aims of medical enhancement lead us to a return to biological, gene-targeted innovations that mask pressing social factors.

Though there are many parallels between historical forms of eugenics and today's version of eugenics, current medical enhancement technologies could create irreversible harm in a way that goes beyond anything we have ever witnessed. The old eugenics of Darwin and Galton's time pivoted on an overt biological sorting by race and class and an imperative to breed and kill to conjure a superior new man. Thus, the eugenics of the past relied on inculcating eugenic beliefs and strategies into specific social actors and mobilizing those actors. Because the new eugenics is subtle, flying under the radar of most citizens as it reaches market, and because it is widely embraced as a healthcare boon by those in the know, it has the potential to do far more damage. The eugenics of the present may lead to drastic changes in our society undertaken with little government awareness or regulatory oversight or action. One company alone can enact changes that could affect all of humanity.

Medical brain enhancements are entering into a world of biased and inequitable social systems. This is why when companies advocate for technologies that can supposedly permanently and indelibly enhance human brains for the good of the species, we must attend to the racial implications of that message. With human differences in ancestry and intelligence being widely conceptualized as genetic, with genomic and pharmaceutical research and development further classifying and stratifying by race, and with inequitably accessible AI systems being trained on racially stratified, genetically deterministic data, our entire system of medical enhancement rests on systems of racial bias. The race-free language of "human" voiced in the "next human agenda," must instead be qualified as "members of the dominant group," and promises of medical enhancement for all must be read as a bait-and-switch for technologies that can enable those already in power to consolidate their power.

References

Aronson, Joshua, Diana Burgess, Sean M. Phelan, and Lindsay Juarez. 2013. "Unhealthy Interactions: The Role of Stereotype Threat in Health Disparities." *American Journal of Public Health* 103 (1) (January): 50–56. https://doi.org/10.2105/AJPH.2012.300828.

Asbury, Kathryn, and Robert Plomin. 2013. *G Is for Genes: The Impact of Genetics on Education and Achievement*. Chichester, UK: Wiley Blackwell.

Bashford, Alison, and Philippa Levine. 2010. *The Oxford Handbook of the History of Eugenics*. Oxford: Oxford University Press.

Benjamin, Ruha. 2019. *Race after Technology: Abolitionist Tools for the New Jim Code*. Cambridge: Polity.

Bernasconi, Robert, and Tommy Lee Lott. 2000. *The Idea of Race*. Indianapolis: Hackett.

Bliss, Catherine. 2008. "Mapping Race through Admixture." *International Journal of Technology, Knowledge & Society* 4 (4): 79–83. https://doi.org/10.18848/1832-3669/CGP/v04i04/55899.

Bliss, Catherine. 2012. *Race Decoded: The Genomic Fight for Social Justice*. Stanford: Stanford University Press.

Bliss, Catherine. 2018. *Social by Nature: The Promise and Peril of Sociogenomics*. Stanford: Stanford University Press.

Bliss, Rina. 2023. *Rethinking Intelligence: A Radical New Understanding of Our Human Potential*. New York: HarperCollins.

Bliss, Rina. 2025. *What's Real about Race? Untangling Science, Genetics, and Society*. New York: Norton.

"Brain Chips to Become 'More Common Than Pacemakers,' Says Investor, as Blackrock Neurotech Raises $10m." 2021. *Stack*. May 19. https://www.thestack.technology/blackrock-neurotech-brain-machine-interfaces-peter-thiel/.

Buolamwini, Joy. 2024. *Unmasking AI: My Mission to Protect What Is Human in a World of Machines*. New York: Random House.

Carpenter, Susan. 2024. "Musk Says Neuralink Device Implanted in Human Brain Successfully." *Spectrum News 1*. January 31. https://spectrumnews1.com/ca/southern-california/health-and-medicine/2024/01/30/msuk-s-neuralink-implants-device-in-human-brain-for-the-first-time.

Chow-White, Peter A., and Troy Duster. 2011. "Do Health and Forensic DNA Databases Increase Racial Disparities?" *PLoS Medicine* 8 (10) (October): e1001100. https://doi.org/10.1371/journal.pmed.1001100.

Cities, Living, and Aminah Pilgrim. 2022. *Systemic Racism 101: A Visual History of the Impact of Racism in America*. New York: Simon & Schuster.

Clarke, Adele E., Janet K. Shim, Laura Mamo, Jennifer Ruth Fosket, and Jennifer R. Fishman. 2003. "Biomedicalization: Technoscientific Transformations of Health, Illness, and U.S. Biomedicine." *American Sociological Review* 68 (2) (April): 161–194. https://doi.org/10.2307/1519765.

Cribbs, Adam P., and Sumeth M. W. Perera. 2017. "Science and Bioethics of CRISPR-Cas9 Gene Editing: An Analysis Towards Separating Facts and Fiction." *Yale Journal of Biology and Medicine* 90 (4) (December): 625–634. https://www.ncbi.nlm.nih.gov/pmc/articles/PMC5733851/.

Darwin, Charles. 1859. *On the Origin of Species by Means of Natural Selection; or the Preservation of Favoured Races in the Struggle for Life*. London: John Murray.

Desmond, Adrian, and James R. Moore. 1992. *Darwin*. New York: Penguin.

Dickens, William T., and James R. Flynn. 2006. "Black Americans Reduce the Racial IQ Gap: Evidence from Standardization Samples." *Psychological Science* 17 (10) (October): 913–920. https://doi.org/10.1111/j.1467-9280.2006.01802.x.

Dunn, Andrew, and Hilary Brueck. 2022. "Why Tech Billionaires Like Elon Musk, Bill Gates, and Jeff Bezos Are All Investing in Biotech Startups That Want to Link Your Computer Directly to Your Brain." *Business Insider*. December 21. https://www.businessinsider.com/elon-musk-bill-gates-jeff-bezos-invest-in-brain-implants-2022-12.

Duster, Troy. 2004. *Backdoor to Eugenics*. London: Routledge.

Eisenstein, Michael. 2024. "Seven Technologies to Watch in 2024." *Nature* 625 (7996) (January 22): 844–848. https://doi.org/10.1038/d41586-024-00173-x.

Evans, Patrick D., Sandra L. Gilbert, Nitzan Mekel-Bobrov, Eric J. Vallender, Jeffrey R. Anderson, Leila M. Vaez-Azizi, Sarah A. Tishkoff, Richard R. Hudson, and Bruce T. Lahn. 2005. "Microcephalin, a Gene Regulating Brain Size, Continues to Evolve Adaptively in Humans." *Science* 309 (5741) (September 9): 1717–1720. https://doi.org/10.1126/science.1113722.

Galton, Francis. 1869. *Hereditary Genius: An Inquiry into Its Laws and Consequences*. London: Macmillan.

Galton, Francis. 1883. *Inquiries into Human Faculty and Its Development*. New York: Macmillan.

Gangadharbatla, Harsha. 2020. "Biohacking: An Exploratory Study to Understand the Factors Influencing the Adoption of Embedded Technologies within the Human Body." *Heliyon* 6 (5) (May): e03931. https://doi.org/10.1016/j.heliyon.2020.e03931.

GQ Staff. 2023. "German Entrepreneur and Investor Christian Angermayer Is on a Mission to Find a Cure for Ageing." *GQ*. April 18. https://www.gqmiddleeast.com/gq-partnership/christian-angermayer-ageing.

Harden, Kathryn Paige. 2021. *The Genetic Lottery: Why DNA Matters for Social Equality*. Princeton, NJ: Princeton University Press.

Hogarth, Stuart, and Paula Saukko. 2017. "A Market in the Making: The Past, Present and Future of Direct-to-Consumer Genomics." *New Genetics and Society* 36 (3): 197–208. https://doi.org/10.1080/14636778.2017.1354692.

Holden, LaTasha R., and Gabriel J. Tanenbaum. 2023. "Modern Assessments of Intelligence Must Be Fair and Equitable." *Journal of Intelligence* 11 (6) (June): 126. https://doi.org/10.3390/jintelligence11060126.

Huang, Kalley, and Sylvia Varnham O'Reagan. 2024. "Meta Cuts Funding for Fact-Checking on WhatsApp as Elections Loom." *The Information*. https://www.theinformation.com/articles/meta-cuts-fact-checking-efforts-on-whatsapp-as-elections-loom.

Inzlicht, Michael, and Toni Schmader. 2012. *Stereotype Threat: Theory, Process, and Application*. New York: Oxford University Press.

Istepanian, Robert S. H. 2022. "Mobile Health (M-Health) in Retrospect: The Known Unknowns." *International Journal of Environmental Research and Public Health* 19 (7) (April 1): 3747. https://doi.org/10.3390/ijerph19073747.

Jencks, Christopher, and Meredith Phillips. 1998. *The Black-White Test Score Gap: Why It Persists and What Can Be Done*. Brookings. March 1. https://www.brookings.edu/articles/the-black-white-test-score-gap-why-it-persists-and-what-can-be-done/.

Kurzweil, Ray. 2005. *The Singularity Is Near: When Humans Transcend Biology*. New York: Viking.

Lampland, Martha, and Susan Leigh Star. 2009. *Standards and Their Stories: How Quantifying, Classifying, and Formalizing Practices Shape Everyday Life*. Ithaca, NY: Cornell University Press.

Lazar, Alexandra. 2021. "La Operación: Coerced Sterilization of Puerto Rican Women in the 20th Century and the Complexity of Free Choice." B.A. thesis, Union College. https://digitalworks.union.edu/theses/2427/.

Li, Tianxiang, Yanyan Yang, Hongzhao Qi, Weigang Cui, Lin Zhang, Xiuxiu Fu, Xiangqin He, Meixin Liu, Pei-feng Li, and Tao Yu. 2023. "CRISPR/Cas9 Therapeutics: Progress and Prospects." *Signal Transduction and Targeted Therapy* 8 (1) (January 16): 1–23. https://doi.org/10.1038/s41392-023-01309-7.

Madhok, Diksha. 2024. "Elon Musk Says the First Human Patient Has Received a Brain Implant from Neuralink." *CNN Business*. January 30. https://www.cnn.com/2024/01/30/business/elon-musk-brain-implant-neuralink-intl-hnk/index.html.

Maiseli, Baraka, Abdi T. Abdalla, Libe V. Massawe, Mercy Mbise, Khadija Mkocha, Nassor Ally Nassor, Moses Ismail, James Michael, and Samwel Kimambo. 2023. "Brain-Computer Interface: Trend, Challenges, and Threats." *Brain Informatics* 10: article no. 20. https://doi.org/10.1186/s40708-023-00199-3.

Mann, Jyoti. 2024. "Elon Musk Says Neuralink's First Patient Can Move a Computer Mouse 'by Just Thinking.'" *Business Insider*. February 20. https://www.businessinsider.com/neuralink-elon-musk-first-human-patient-control-mouse-with-mind-2024-2.

Mansuri, Misbaah. 2024. "Neuropriming and CRISPR Technologies Are Empowering 'Super Athletes.'" *Wired.* July 30. https://wired.me/technology/crispr-neuropriming-sports/.

Meltzoff, Andrew N., and Walter S. Gilliam. 2024. "Young Children & Implicit Racial Biases." *Daedalus* 153 (1) (Winter): 65–83. https://doi.org/10.1162/daed_a_02049.

Metzl, Jamie. 2019. *Hacking Darwin: Genetic Engineering and the Future of Humanity.* Naperville, IL: Sourcebooks.

Milano, Silvia, Joshua A. McGrane, and Sabina Leonelli. 2023. "Large Language Models Challenge the Future of Higher Education." *Nature Machine Intelligence* 5 (4) (April): 333–334. https://doi.org/10.1038/s42256-023-00644-2.

Morning, Ann. 2011. *The Nature of Race: How Scientists Think and Teach about Human Difference.* Berkeley: University of California Press.

Nelson, Alondra. 2016. *The Social Life of DNA: Race, Reparations, and Reconciliation after the Genome.* Boston: Beacon.

Neuralink. 2023. "PRIME Video Release." *X.* November 21. Accessed November 26, 2024. https://x.com/neuralink/status/1727135227565547810.

Newheiser, Anna-Kaisa, and Kristina R. Olson. 2012. "White and Black American Children's Implicit Intergroup Bias." *Journal of Experimental Social Psychology* 48 (1) (January): 264–270. https://doi.org/10.1016/j.jesp.2011.08.011.

Newton, Chrissy. 2024. "'The Future Is Going to Be Weird.' Elon Musk Predicts Brain Chips Will Eventually Replace Phones." *Debrief.* July 17. https://thedebrief.org/the-future-is-going-to-be-weird-elon-musk-predicts-brain-chips-will-eventually-replace-phones/.

Niemeyer, Kenneth. 2024. "Elon Musk Says Neuralink Could Help Humans Compete with AI: 'Let's Give People Superpowers.'" *Business Insider.* August 3. https://www.businessinsider.com/elon-musk-says-neuralink-help-humans-compete-with-ai-2024-8.

Olson, Parmy. 2024. "Peter Thiel's Doping Games and Tech's Quest for a Superhuman." *Deccan Herald.* July 12. https://www.deccanherald.com//opinion/peter-thiels-doping-games-and-techs-quest-for-a-superhuman-3104240.

Phillips, Zach. 2024. "The Impact of 23&Me's Marketing Strategies." McMillan & Phillips. Accessed November 26, 2024. https://mcmillanphillips.com/podcast/the-impact-of-23mes-marketing-strategies/.

Plomin, Robert. 2019. *Blueprint: How DNA Makes Us Who We Are.* Cambridge, MA: MIT Press.

Qian, Miao K., Gail D. Heyman, Paul C. Quinn, Genyue Fu, and Kang Lee. 2019. "Differential Developmental Courses of Implicit and Explicit Biases for Different Other-Race Classes." *Developmental Psychology* 55 (7) (July): 1440–1452. https://doi.org/10.1037/dev0000730.

Rajan, Kaushik Sunder. 2006. *Biocapital: The Constitution of Postgenomic Life.* Durham, NC: Duke University Press.

Reardon, Jenny. 2004. *Race to the Finish: Identity and Governance in an Age of Genomics.* Princeton, NJ: Princeton University Press.

re.Mind Capital. 2024. Accessed November 26, 2024. https://www.f6s.com/re.mind-capital.

Regalado, Antonio. 2018. "Chinese Scientists Are Creating CRISPR Babies." *MIT Technology Review.* November 25. https://www.technologyreview.com/2018/11/25/138962/exclusive-chinese-scientists-are-creating-crispr-babies/.

Regalado, Antonio. 2021. "Brain Implants Could Be the Next Computer Mouse." *MIT Technology Review.* October 27. https://www.technologyreview.com/2021/10/27/1036821/brain-computer-interface-implant-mouse/.

Regalado, Antonio. 2023. "Elon Musk Wants More Bandwidth between People and Machines. Do We Need It?" *MIT Technology Review.* September 29. https://www.technologyreview.com/2023/09/29/1080472/elon-musk-bandwidth-brains/.

Richardson, Sarah S. 2011. "Race and IQ in the Postgenomic Age: The Microcephaly Case." *BioSocieties* 6 (4) (December): 420–446. https://doi.org/10.1057/biosoc.2011.20.

Richardson, Sarah S. 2015. "The Trustworthiness Deficit in Postgenomic Research on Human Intelligence." *Hastings Center Report* 45 (S1) (September-October): S15–S20. https://doi.org/10.1002/hast.493.

Rosenbaum, Eric. 2024. "AI Is Getting Very Popular among Students and Teachers, Very Quickly." *CNBC*. June 11. https://www.cnbc.com/2024/06/11/ai-is-getting-very-popular-among-students-and-teachers-very-quickly.html.

Saeed, Sy Atezaz, and Ross MacRae Masters. 2021. "Disparities in Health Care and the Digital Divide." *Current Psychiatry Reports* 23 (9) (September): article no. 61. https://doi.org/10.1007/s11920-021-01274-4.

Shankland, Stephen. 2024. "Neuralink's Brain Chip Is Running in a Human. Your Skull Is Safe, for Now." *CNET*. March 22. https://www.cnet.com/health/medical/neuralinks-brain-chip-is-running-in-a-human-your-skull-is-safe-for-now/.

Shead, Sam. 2021a. "Elon Musk's Brain Computer Start-Up Raises $205 Million from Google Ventures and Others." *CNBC*. July 30. https://www.cnbc.com/2021/07/30/elon-musks-neuralink-backed-by-google-ventures-peter-thiel-sam-altman.html.

Shead, Sam. 2021b. "Peter Thiel Is Backing a Rival to Elon Musk's Brain Implant Company." *CNBC*. May 19. https://www.cnbc.com/2021/05/19/peter-thiel-is-backing-a-rival-to-elon-musks-neuralink-.html.

Steele, Claude M. and Joshua Aronson. 1995. "Stereotype Threat and the Intellectual Test Performance of African Americans." *Journal of Personality and Social Psychology* 69 (5) (November): 797–811. https://doi.org/10.1037//0022-3514.69.5.797.

Stoney, Rhett J., Phyllis E. Kozarsky, Allison T. Walker, and Joanna L. Gaines. 2022. "Population-Based Surveillance of Medical Tourism among U.S. Residents from 11 States and Territories: Findings from the Behavioral Risk Factor Surveillance System." *Infection Control & Hospital Epidemiology* 43 (7) (July): 870–875. https://doi.org/10.1017/ice.2021.245.

Swain, Frank. 2023. "Inside the Secretive Life-Extension Clinic." *Wired*. May 1. https://www.wired.com/story/bioviva-gene-therapies-liz-parrish-longevity/.

TallBear, Kim. 2013. *Native American DNA: Tribal Belonging and the False Promise of Genetic Science*. Minneapolis: University of Minnesota Press.

Thiel, Peter. 2019. "Peter Thiel on 'The Straussian Moment.'" By Peter Robinson. *Uncommon Knowledge*. September 5. https://www.youtube.com/watch?v=iRleB034EC8&list=PL-hIxnwiNB0XqnZL3a7E2PakQPR81ngJk&index=16.

Wade, Daniel L. 1980. "Racial Discrimination in IQ Testing – Larry P. v. Riles." *DePaul Law Review* 29 (4) (Summer): 1193–1214. https://via.library.depaul.edu/law-review/vol29/iss4/12/.

Walters, Pat, host. 2019. "Unnatural Selection." Radiolab (podcast). July 25. Accessed November 26, 2024. https://radiolab.org/podcast/g-unnatural-selection.

Warr, Melissa, Nicole Jakubczyk Oster, and Roger Isaac. 2023. "Implicit Bias in Large Language Models: Experimental Proof and Implications for Education." *Social Science Research Network*. November 6. https://doi.org/10.2139/ssrn.4625078.

Wilby, Peter. 2014. "Psychologist on a Mission to Give Every Child a Learning Chip." *Guardian*. February 18. https://www.theguardian.com/education/2014/feb/18/psychologist-robert-plomin-says-genes-crucial-education.

Williamson, Ben. 2018. "Scientists Seek Genetic Data to Personalize Education." Connected Learning Alliance. https://clalliance.org/blog/scientists-seek-genetic-data-to-personalize-education/.

Yong, Ed. 2013. "Chinese Project Probes the Genetics of Genius." *Nature* 497 (7449) (May 16): 297–299. https://doi.org/10.1038/497297a.

Rina Bliss is Associate Professor of Sociology at Rutgers University, USA. She is the author of *What's Real About Race? Untangling Science, Genetics, and Society* (2025), *Rethinking Intelligence: A Radical New Understanding of Our Human Potential* (2023), *Social by Nature: The Promise and Peril of Sociogenomics* (2018), and *Race Decoded: The Genomic Fight for Social Justice* (2012). Her work explores the personal and societal significance of emerging genetic sciences.

Chapter 12
Mental Augmentation, Human Rights, and the Future of Choice

Łukasz Szoszkiewicz and Stephen Damianos

Abstract This chapter emphasizes the role of international human rights law in guiding the integration of mental augmentation into clinical practice. Mental augmentation refers broadly to efforts aimed at improving human cognition and behavior through direct recording and manipulation of neural activity. Utilizing neurotechnologies, mental augmentation increasingly involves interventions aimed at enhancing cognitive and emotional functioning such as memory, attention, sensation, and problem-solving beyond innate capabilities. The chapter reviews relevant treaties, such as the Convention on Economic, Social, and Cultural Rights (ICESCR), the Convention on the Rights of Persons with Disabilities (CRPD), and the Convention on the Rights of the Child (CRC), which stress the importance of empowering individuals to meaningfully exercise their rights. The analysis grants special focus to the implications for persons in vulnerable situations, including persons with disabilities and children, whose evolving decision-making capacities require robust safeguards and ongoing interdisciplinary dialogue. The commentary calls for ethical, legal, and regulatory frameworks that ensure that mental augmentation technologies support decision-making while upholding human rights.

Keywords Mental augmentation · Neurotechnologies · Human rights · Children · Persons with disabilities

12.1 Introduction

Humanity has long concerned itself with progress, striving to maximize opportunity and achieve higher standards of living. This drive to advance the human condition has fueled monumental developments across time, including within medicine and

Ł. Szoszkiewicz
Adam Mickiewicz University, Poznań, Poland

S. Damianos (✉)
Neurorights Foundation, New York, NY, USA
e-mail: stephen.damianos@gmail.com

M. C. Altman and D. Schwan (eds.), *Ethics and Medical Technology*, The International Library of Bioethics 113, https://doi.org/10.1007/978-3-031-94690-5_12

healthcare. In the medical domain, advancements such as vaccines, anesthesia, and large-scale sanitation campaigns not only saved countless lives but reshaped the way humanity understands and manages health. This progress improved public health, increased global life expectancy, and altered the human experience by engineering greater control over health outcomes and the ability to flourish.

Across time, innovation has supported breakthroughs that were once inconceivable, transforming societies and individuals alike. Society is now on the brink of yet another profound shift, one that will revolutionize our understanding of the human experience. This new frontier is marked by the rise of neurotechnologies, which are devices that record or alter the activity of the nervous system, including the brain, the spinal cord, and the peripheral nerves. The medical community is hardly a stranger to this technology: electrical brain stimulation has been used in clinical settings since the early 1900s, with a vast array of applications related to brain imaging and neurostimulation (Selimbeyoglu and Parvizi 2010). However, neurotechnologies are rapidly expanding in terms of technical capacity and functionality, offering new ways of influencing brain functions.

Mental augmentation is a fast-emerging field that lacks formal boundaries and consensus regarding definitions and scope. For example, scholars use terms such as "cognitive enhancement," "neuroenhancement," "cognitive augmentation," and "brain augmentation" (at times interchangeably) to refer to a variety of interventions, both medical and non-medical. These can include pharmaceutical approaches (e.g., performance-enhancing drugs), technological methods (e.g., neurostimulation) and lifestyle practices (e.g., dieting and exercise) (Beck et al. 2024). For the purposes of this chapter, mental augmentation refers broadly to efforts aimed at improving human cognition and behavior through direct recording and manipulation of neural activity. Utilizing neurotechnologies, mental augmentation increasingly involves interventions aimed at enhancing cognitive and emotional functioning such as memory, attention, sensation, and problem-solving beyond innate capabilities. Examples include electroencephalogram (EEG) neurofeedback[1] (Iodice et al. 2022), speech neuroprotheses (Metzger et al. 2023; Card et al. 2024; Tankus et al. 2025), and cochlear implants (Arambula et al. 2022), among others.

As neurotechnologies continue to evolve, new challenges arise in ensuring that mental augmentation practices are grounded in robust ethical and legal frameworks. One such challenge involves decision-making, and the tensions between approaches prioritized by the medical community and international human rights law. This chapter explores these dynamics, analyzing how international human rights law can inform and guide the integration of mental augmentation technologies in healthcare settings.

[1] Neurofeedback is a noninvasive technique that monitors brain activity in real time and uses that information to help individuals learn to regulate their neural processes, thereby enhancing cognitive and emotional functioning.

12.2 The Relevance of International Human Rights Law to Medical Professionals

International human rights law is a body of legal norms and standards designed to protect the fundamental rights of every individual. It is primarily established through nine core international treaties adopted under the auspices of the United Nations (UN), such as the International Covenant on Economic, Social and Cultural Rights (ICESCR), the Convention on the Rights of the Child (CRC), and the Convention on the Rights of Persons with Disabilities (CRPD). These treaties are legally binding on states, which means that states must incorporate the standards set within each treaty into their domestic legal frameworks. Alongside these treaties, specialized UN Treaty Bodies[2] are tasked with monitoring state compliance, interpreting treaty provisions, and to a more limited extent, ensuring access to remedy through complaint mechanisms. The combined impact of these instruments exerts influence on domestic legal frameworks, including those governing healthcare.

All UN member states have ratified at least one treaty affirming the right to health,[3] which means that medical professionals operate within national systems increasingly shaped by international norms.[4] State obligations extend to the regulation of healthcare provision, access to medical treatments and innovations, as well as adequate training, facilities, and support for healthcare professionals (ESCR Committee 2000).[5] Their normative content is interpreted by the UN Treaty Bodies in the form of General Comments and General Recommendations. These documents are developed through a process that actively engages various stakeholders—including governments, NGOs, academic institutions, and individual researchers—whose written submissions help shape their final form. The process is highly informal and does not require specialized procedural knowledge, with submissions coming from representatives across all sectors, including healthcare professionals.

Governments are required to review and regularly reform their laws and policies to meet standards set out in the General Comments. UN Treaty Bodies monitor

[2] These bodies are composed of independent experts with recognized expertise in human rights, elected by states for fixed terms.

[3] For instance, Article 12 of the ICESCR (1966) recognizes "the right of everyone to the enjoyment of the highest attainable standard of physical and mental health." Article 25 of the Universal Declaration of Human Rights (1948) recognizes that "everyone has the right to a standard of living adequate for the health and well-being of himself and of his family, including food, clothing, housing and *medical care* and necessary social services, and the right to security in the event of unemployment, sickness, disability, widowhood, old age or other lack of livelihood in circumstances beyond his control" (emphasis added).

[4] Obligations related to the right to health are derived from the treaties such as the International Covenant on Economic, Social and Cultural Rights (Article 12); the Convention on the Rights of Persons with Disabilities (Article 25); and the Convention on the Rights of the Child (Article 24).

[5] For instance, during the drafting of the General Comments on the Rights of Children in the Digital Environment, the CRC Committee received 279 written submissions (available here: https://www.ohchr.org/en/documents/general-comments-and-recommendations/general-comment-no-25-2021-childrens-rights-relation).

compliance and issue recommendations that frequently address health-related issues, from access to medical treatment and adoption of public health strategies to patients' rights in clinical settings. For instance, the Committee on the Rights of Persons with Disabilities (CRPD Committee) takes an uncompromisingly negative stance on the substitute decision-making paradigm (2014, para. 3), which compels states to shift toward supported decision-making mechanisms for persons with disabilities, a move that has sparked significant debate within the medical community (Scholten and Gather 2018).

Importantly, non-governmental actors play an active role in this process by submitting so-called shadow reports that are reviewed by UN Treaty Bodies. This mechanism allows representatives of the medical community and patients, through their written submissions, to influence regulatory frameworks and public policies.[6] Additionally, the monitoring process serves as a forum for addressing complex and sometimes controversial legal solutions, such as the availability of termination of pregnancy (abortion) services or the permissibility of facilities that enable the anonymous abandonment of infants (see, for example, Sękowska-Kozłowska et al. 2024). This ensures that a broad range of perspectives is considered.

Medical professionals implement international human rights standards in day-to-day practice. By engaging with UN Treaty Bodies, they can help shape standards on complex health-related issues to ensure that policies and practices meet both medical standards and human rights norms. This engagement is increasingly important as new technologies such as mental augmentation expand within clinical settings. Human right standards are designed to be universal and future-proof, with general guidance that can be applied to a range of emerging scenarios. At the same time, harmonizing innovations with human rights frameworks often falls partly upon practitioners, especially as national and subnational regulations lag behind the pace of scientific progress. Clinicians may find themselves navigating uncharted territories, such as how to manage neural data or assess the appropriateness of mental augmentation in a given situation, when clear legal guidelines are still evolving. In these cases, international human rights law can provide guidance. The next sections will explore two groups in relation to whom the medical community will increasingly need guidance with regard to mental augmentation and patient autonomy: persons with disabilities and children.

[6] For instance, during consideration of the latest periodic report of Ireland (2024) by the UN Committee on Economic, Social and Cultural Rights, shadow reports were submitted by civil society actors such as Mental Health Reform, Disability Federation Ireland, and Independent Living Movement Ireland. In the context of the latest periodic review of Romania (2024), the report was submitted by the Association for Spina Bifida and Hydrocephalus in Romania (ARSBH). See ESCR Committee, Concluding Observations from 2024: Ireland (E/C.12/IRL/4) and Romania (E/C.12/ROU/6).

12.3 Equality before the Law for Persons with Disabilities

The Convention on the Rights of Persons with Disabilities (CRPD) reaffirms equality before the law as an absolute human right that cannot be limited under any circumstances.[7] The CRPD Committee's General Comment No. 1, which provides an authoritative interpretation of this right, emphasizes that every individual is entitled to legal capacity on an equal basis with others,[8] an entitlement that includes both legal standing and legal agency, regardless of cognitive abilities.[9] Still, in many countries, legal capacity depends upon assessments of "mental capacity," which refers to the ability of a person to make rational, informed, and voluntary decisions. In many jurisdictions, if mental capacity is considered to be impaired, a person's legal capacity is limited or entirely removed.

This limitation constitutes an unjustified violation of international human rights law and is a subject of constant criticism from the CRPD Committee in its General Comments and monitoring procedure.[10] As the Committee points out, "mental capacity is not, as is commonly presented, an objective, scientific and naturally occurring phenomenon" (CRPD Committee 2014, para. 14). Additionally, mental capacity is influenced by social and political factors, particularly those affecting the professions and practices that play a crucial role in evaluating mental capacity, such as evaluations conducted by clinical psychologists or psychiatrists, or legal determinations made by judges and lawyers. These assessments presume "to be able to accurately assess the inner-workings of the human mind" and—if a person does not reach certain thresholds—deny legal capacity (paras. 14–15). Still, numerous states maintain this practice and keep reservations to Article 12 of the CRPD.[11] This issue also raises controversies among medical professionals (Nilsson and Series 2018),

---

[7] "There are no permissible circumstances under international human rights law in which a person may be deprived of the right to recognition as a person before the law, or in which this right may be limited." See CRPD Committee (2014, para. 5).

[8] Article 12(2) of the CRPD: "States Parties shall recognize that persons with disabilities enjoy legal capacity on an equal basis with others in all aspects of life."

[9] The CRPD Committee has explicitly stated that "perceived or actual deficits in mental capacity must not be used as justification for denying legal capacity." See CRPD Committee (2014, para. 13).

[10] Under the core international human rights instruments (including the CRPD), state parties submit periodic reports to treaty bodies that review and recommend measures for effective implementation. See, for example: CRPD, *Concluding Observations: Benin*, CRPD/C/BEN/CO/1, 2024, para. 23; CRPD, *Concluding Observations: Bahrain*, CRPD/C/BHR/CO/1–2, 2024, para. 25; CRPD, *Concluding Observations: Zambia*, CRPD/C/ZMB/CO/1, 2024, para. 23.

[11] In international law, a reservation is a unilateral statement made by a state upon signing or ratifying a treaty to exclude or modify the legal effect of specific provisions for itself. Several countries declared reservations to Article 12 to permit substitute decision-making (Canada, Ireland, the Netherlands, Norway, Uzbekistan), limit legal agency (Egypt, Estonia), or limit legal capacity (Georgia, Kuwait, Poland, Singapore, Syria, Venezuela).

particularly regarding the permissibility of substitute decision-making for individuals with impaired decision-making capacities (Scholten and Gather 2018), as well as the use of coercive interventions.[12]

In this context, mental augmentation technologies, such speech-decoding brain–computer interfaces and AI-based communication aids, present both transformative opportunities and new ethical challenges. These innovations enable the restoration of speech-based communication (and, in the future, potentially via avatar-based facial gestures and synthesized voice modulation), representing a breakthrough for individuals with intact cognitive functions who experience significant impairments in speech production, as seen in conditions such as amyotrophic lateral sclerosis (ALS) or locked-in syndrome. The following section examines how these emerging neurotechnologies intersect with the right to equality before the law under the CRPD, addressing two core issues: the promise of best interpretation of will and preferences, and the implications of AI-based communication aids that depend on the processing of neural data.

12.3.1 Best Interpretation of Will and Preferences versus Best Interests

The CRPD abandoned the model of the "best interests" assessment to one that emphasizes the best interpretation of an individual's will and preferences.[13] Mental augmentation offers novel tools, such as advanced speech-decoding systems, that can capture and convey a person's authentic desires more accurately than conventional assessments. Invasive speech decoding neurotechnologies, which involve devices implanted directly in the brain, can currently interpret intended speech with remarkable precision, reaching an accuracy of 97.5% in some cases, allowing individuals with severe paralysis to communicate by decoding neural activity from the speech motor cortex (Card et al. 2024). Noninvasive approaches, such as wearable EEG-based headsets, are advancing rapidly and currently achieve around 48% accuracy, although they are unlikely to match the performance of their invasive counterparts in the foreseeable future (if ever).[14]

At the same time, the CRPD mandates a "best interpretation" approach, acknowledging that some uncertainty—stemming, for example, from technical limitations—will always remain. For instance, speech decoding neurotechnologies perform better on closed vocabularies (devices which are trained on a limited number of phrases),

[12] Some maintain that cases such as organic confusional states can justify coercive interventions, a claim supported by surveys of those who have experienced involuntary treatment. See Szmukler (2019).

[13] The "will and preferences" paradigm must replace the "best interests" paradigm to ensure that persons with disabilities enjoy the right to legal capacity on an equal basis with others. See CRPD Committee (2014, para. 21).

[14] Note that noninvasive speech decoding studies primarily involve persons without disabilities. See Sato et al. (2024).

which diminishes the freedom to express one's will and preferences compared to individuals who lack communication impediments. However, scientists are gradually expanding these vocabularies, currently reaching up to 125,000 words, compared to 170,000 words in the English language (Card et al. 2024). Further progress in this area will pave the way for more natural and fluent communication. Additionally, challenges remain regarding the speed of decoding both speech and gestures (such as when reconstructing a person's avatar) (Metzger et al. 2023), which affects interactions with the environment and will ultimately be evaluated under the "best interpretation of will and preferences" framework.

By translating neural signals into coherent communication, these technologies help ensure that decisions reflect the individual's own choices rather than substitute judgments. This ability to better interpret will and preferences aligns with the CRPD's approach and offers a pathway for its implementation in cases where communication barriers exist, for example, in individuals with ALS or locked-in syndrome, who maintain normal brain activity yet are unable to communicate effectively. The use of such neurotechnologies must therefore be integrated into supported decision-making frameworks that prioritize the individual's will and preferences over imposed interpretations. Standards for implementing such solutions and their minimum efficacy levels should be agreed upon by medical professionals and representatives of persons with disabilities. According to the international human rights framework, this process should be based on an ongoing dialogue between experts and affected individuals, and it must be grounded in the most advanced and up-to-date scientific knowledge (ESCR Committee 2020, para. 18).

12.3.2 Whose Interpretation of Will and Preferences?

Utilizing neurotechnologies to interpret will and preferences will require resolving the outcomes of human-machine interactions. Some elements, such as the legal acceptability of using speech-decoding neurotechnologies, will be determined by law, while the application in specific cases and the interpretation of the resulting data will likely be the responsibility of the medical personnel. The following section discusses two promising areas of research that are likely to capture the interest of both ethicists and policymakers: (1) the application of large language models, and (2) novel therapies involving early implantation.

One promising research avenue in speech decoding research is the use of industry-developed language models, with early results indicating their potential to improve decoding performance, particularly through their capacity to integrate conversational context into predictions (Silva et al. 2024). There are several approaches to integrating language models into speech decoding pipelines, with some yielding "drastically improved accuracy" (Sankaran et al. 2023) but at the expense of user agency (Maslen and Rainey 2021). Such solutions can enhance the flow of communication. However, from the perspective of assessing "will and preferences," they prompt consideration of the extent to which the language model influences the output. To maintain fluid communication, a person might prioritize response speed over accuracy, which could affect how their will and preferences are interpreted by external observers. Furthermore, proprietary language models may contain biases in their training data and face limitations due to technical constraints.

Solutions utilizing language models are already being tested by companies producing communication assistive devices, albeit in a different context. For instance, Australian neurotechnology company Synchron is collaborating with OpenAI to leverage large language models to make communication smoother and more natural (Rao 2024). However, this approach relies on the language model proposing responses that an individual can either accept or reject. These limitations should not detract from the significance of such solutions, given their high (but not flawless) effectiveness, despite challenges such as the black-box or proprietary nature of the most powerful models. This is particularly relevant in cases where there is a discrepancy between assessments of "best interests" and "best will and preferences," with the latter taking precedence according to Article 12 CRPD.

Rapid advances in speech decoding pave the way for new therapeutic interventions in individuals at the early stages of cognitive or communicative decline. For example, a recent study on a speech neuroprosthesis demonstrated that training with overt speech data (i.e., audio recordings or transcripts of speech) enables patients to silently control the device with high accuracy, overcoming the challenges associated with aligning imagined speech (Tankus et al. 2022). This finding is particularly significant for persons with conditions such as ALS, where early intervention may help preserve communication abilities critical for independent living, as underscored by Article 19 of CRPD.[15] An additional yet equally complex question is whether individuals should have the right to calibrate their speech prostheses using their own neural data, even when other high-quality training datasets become eventually available. This might necessitate the early implantation of the device, even if it is not yet considered medically necessary. Again, CRPD mandates respect of a person's will and preferences, making it essential to establish procedures that ensure this right is upheld.

Mental augmentation, when aligned with the principles of the CRPD, offers a promising pathway to empower individuals by reinforcing their legal capacity. Yet this promise comes with substantial ethical considerations. The need for a more CRPD-based interpretation of will and preferences, and the appropriate timing of novel therapeutic interventions, demands rigorous safeguards and an unwavering commitment to respecting the person's inherent rights. Only by embedding these technologies within robust ethical and legal frameworks can society ensure that mental augmentation fulfills its potential as an empowering tool—one that upholds equality before the law for all, regardless of cognitive or communicative challenges.

[15] Article 19 of CRPD states: "States Parties to this Convention recognize the equal right of all persons with disabilities to live in the community, with choices equal to others, and shall take effective and appropriate measures to facilitate full enjoyment by persons with disabilities of this right and their full inclusion and participation in the community."

12.4 Evolving Capacities and Best Interests of the Child

International human rights law, particularly the Convention on the Rights of the Child (CRC), mandates that the best interests of the child be a primary consideration in all actions concerning children (Article 3(1)). The Committee on the Rights of the Child (CRC Committee) has emphasized that this principle must guide decision-making across various settings, including healthcare (2013, para. 30). In practice, this means that any decision affecting a child's health should result from a careful best-interests assessment that weighs all relevant factors in the individual context (para. 83). For example, in medical decisions, high-quality treatment is not the sole factor; psychological and social factors (such as the child's comfort or family well-being) also inform assessment of the child's best interests. States should establish strict safeguards to determine a child's best interests, ensuring the child's own views are meaningfully considered and that decisions can be reviewed periodically (para. 93). Ultimately, if there is a conflict (for example, parents refusing a life-saving treatment that the child requires), authorities may intervene to uphold the child's best interests, as the state's duty to protect the child can override parental choices that put the child at risk.

The CRC Committee recognizes the evolving capacities of children, meaning that a child's ability to make informed decisions grows with age and experience (2016, para. 19). Decision-making frameworks thus differentiate between very young children and adolescents, and they should promote individual capacity assessments rather than rigid age thresholds. The CRC Committee underlines that a child's age and health status never justify ignoring their views: all children, regardless of age or capacity, should be supported to participate to the fullest extent in decision-making about them. In this context, the Committee emphasizes that the "voluntary and informed consent of the adolescent should be obtained whether or not the consent of a parent or guardian is required for any medical treatment or procedure" (para. 39). To this end, states should introduce minimum legal age limits, which may be different than the age of maturity (para. 39). Furthermore, any child below that minimum age who can demonstrate sufficient understanding should have the right to either provide or withhold consent (para. 39).

12.4.1 Opportunities for Children and Adolescents

Advancements in neuroscience intersect with human rights principles by offering new ways to assess, support, and enhance children's cognitive capacities. Mental augmentation falls within the realm of healthcare, an area in which adolescents are entitled to stronger decision-making safeguards. Moreover, progress in neuroscience—and the need to regulate clinical mental augmentation interventions within a medical framework—may lead policymakers, in cooperation with medial community, to establish neural measurement approaches and define thresholds, for instance, for determining eligibility for medical treatment or deeming it medically necessary. Adopting such metrics would offer an alternative to relying solely on strict age limits or an adult's subjective judgment of a child's decision-making capacity. This evolution and the possibility of more widespread mental augmentation brings both opportunities and risks, which we will explore further below.

Decision-making is a complex process of reasoning through which individuals select a preferred course of action based on the information and cognitive capabilities available to them. Mental augmentation may present new opportunities to support the decision-making capabilities of children, especially children with disabilities. Technologies that monitor and enhance cognitive activity offer novel tools for improving focus, attention, emotional regulation, memory, and other functions that are relevant to the neural mechanisms underlying decision-making (Kelly and O'Connell 2015). This may yield particular benefit to children and adolescents, whose brains are actively in formation. For instance, a meta-analysis of studies on transcranial electrical stimulation highlighted promising results for improving reading and mathematical skills, particularly for children with specific learning disabilities (Fathi Azar et al. 2024).

A range of interdisciplinary scholars evidence the implications of brain development and cognitive maturation on decision-making at different ages (for a nuanced summary, see Icenogle and Cauffman 2021). Children exhibit different cognitive capabilities than adolescents, who in turn exhibit different cognitive capabilities than adults, in part because the areas of the brain involved in reasoning, risk assessment, and emotional regulation continue to develop and mature over time (Mairon et al. 2023). This fact was also recognized by the CRC Committee (2019), which acknowledged that child development and neuroscience indicates that "maturity and the capacity for abstract reasoning is still evolving in children aged 12 to 13 years" (para. 22), "adolescent brains continue to mature even beyond the teenage years, affecting certain kinds of decision-making" (para. 22), and "brain development continues into the early twenties" (para. 32).

While there are scientific bases for asserting that children and adolescents generally have different (and in many cases, reduced) decision-making capabilities compared to adults (Albert and Steinberg 2011; Guyer et al. 2016; Jansson-Boyd and Bright 2024), these same bases can be used to discredit youth autonomy and choice. This raises concerns about epistemic injustice in medical settings (Baumtrog and Peach 2019; Greenblatt et al. 2024).

Children are often infantilized or perceived as incapable of understanding their own wants and needs, whereas adolescents are widely seen as having poor decision-making skills, with parents, teachers, doctors, policymakers, and the media highlighting teen pregnancy, susceptibility to peer pressure, underage drinking, drug use, social media addiction, and other risky behaviors as evidence of poor judgment (Casey et al. 2011; Blakemore 2018). Indeed, there is a prevailing sense in many settings that children and adolescents lack the experience and maturity necessary for complex moral reasoning, impulse control, future-oriented planning, and assessments of social acceptability, risk, and consequence.[16]

Children and adolescents may therefore experience disadvantages both in terms of their decision-making capabilities and the perceptions of their decision-making capabilities. Mental augmentation has the potential to support individual decision-making as well as assessments of decision-making competence, maturity, and who should make the final decision. In terms of decision-making processes, mental augmentation devices may be able to support youth by enhancing focus, memory, stress management, emotional regulation, and other cognitive functions. For example, neurofeedback has proven successful in reducing impulsive decision-making and increasing psychophysiological self-regulation under stress (Bluschke et al. 2016; Iodice et al. 2022; Balconi et al. 2023). Mental augmentation could likely help children and adolescents understand and control their emotional states by monitoring brain activity and providing feedback through interactive visual or auditory signals (e.g., in-app games designed to hone focus or manage stress). This could decrease stress, heighten emotional regulation, and support the optimization of cognitive resources throughout the decision-making process. In turn, this may foster a greater sense of autonomy and self-reliance, as well as perceptions that young people are competent decision-makers who can be trusted with more responsibility. These technologies can therefore contribute to the achievement of the highest attainable standard of health, as well as the right to development.

While mental augmentation has the potential to support all youth, it holds particular promise for children and adolescents living with disabilities. For example, attention deficit/hyperactivity disorder (ADHD) is associated with higher levels of risk-taking behavior (Pollak et al. 2019), with scholars noting that the impaired cognitive functioning associated with ADHD can exacerbate impulsive and risky decision-making in children and adolescents (Humphreys and Lee 2011; Dekkers et al. 2022; Rastikerdar et al. 2023). Autism is also correlated with impaired decision-making abilities in certain settings (and enhanced abilities in others), which can pose barriers to social inclusion, employment opportunity, and self-sufficiency (van der Plas et al. 2023; Fujino et al. 2024). In these cases and more, mental augmentation may provide additional support to decision-making processes. For example, clinical studies show that EEG neurofeedback can decrease impulsive decision-making among youth with ADHD (Bluschke et al. 2016) and increase cognitive functioning—including

[16] Note that risk-taking need not be negative, and that many young people are actively engaged in questions of future-making and morality. As others have noted, the dominant discourse around adolescent decision-making tends to focus on negative situations of danger and deviance, but there are many examples of prosocial risk-taking, courageous moral reasoning, and investment in the future (e.g., youth engagement in protest and social justice movements, climate justice, etc.). See Duell and Steinberg (2021) and Icenogle and Cauffman (2021).

decision-making and focus—in children with autism (Mercado et al. 2021; Saleem and Habib 2024).[17]

12.4.2 Challenges for Children and Adolescents

For youth with and without disabilities, mental augmentation holds the dual promise of improving cognitive functioning while also supporting assessments of individual capacity to make decisions about one's life. Still, the augmentation of child and adolescent brains raises ethical concerns that require careful thought and mitigation. Young brains exhibit particular plasticity because they are still actively developing. Childhood and adolescence are critical stages in human development, during which the foundations of identity, personality, and values are formed. The learning and stimuli experienced at these ages are accompanied by changes in the developing brain that endure into adulthood. This period of heightened plasticity makes children and adolescents especially sensitive to the influences around them, whether those influences come from caregivers, peers, media, or technology (Fandakova and Hartley 2020). There is a risk that mental augmentation will interfere with this process of identity formation, since childhood and adolescent years are crucial for the development of self-concept and social identity. At the same time, there are several risks associated with unresolved questions related to safety, side effects, and long-term effects, especially since children are severely underrepresented in clinical neurotechnology trials (UNICEF 2024). Moreover, research studies in cognitive neuroscience do not consistently report demographic information about their samples or examine how demographic variables influence outcomes (Dotson and Duarte 2020). This omission creates an even greater barrier to accessing the benefits of scientific progress, a benefit recognized as a human right in the Universal Declaration of Human Rights and affirmed in subsequent treaties.[18]

The extent to which mental augmentation could impact the emotional, cognitive, and identity-based development of children and adolescents is largely unknown. Also unknown is the extent to which mental augmentation will contribute to the monitoring, data profiling, and surveillance of young people. If neurotechnologies are integrated from early childhood into adolescence, enormous and longitudinal datasets of extremely sensitive data will amass over time. As noted in a recent UNICEF report, "neural data collected about children may give tremendous power to those holding, analysing or gaining access to the datasets, including the potential ability to track children's inner development and even mould them to specific ways of being.

[17] However, in a recent systematic review and meta-analysis of scientific evidence, neurofeedback was not found to be superior to stimulant medication, which calls for caution in overestimating its significance (Lee et al. 2023).

[18] Article 29 of the Universal Declaration of Human Rights (1948) reads as follows: "Everyone has the right freely to participate in the cultural life of the community, to enjoy the arts and to share in scientific advancement and its benefits."

These actors would range from states and police forces to marketing and insurance companies, and even potentially cybercriminals" (2024, 3).

For these reasons and more, there is urgent need for enhanced data security and privacy protections in the mental augmentation space. Given that mental augmentation directly affects the most intimate aspects of personality, it is essential that we develop enhanced privacy safeguards, for instance, similar to those afforded in the context of sexual and reproductive rights. Just as adolescents should, according to CRC (2016, para. 39), have the right to access confidential medical counseling without parental consent, mental augmentation interventions should be governed by robust protocols that protect individual privacy and autonomy, thereby upholding the integrity of personal identity.

12.5 Conclusion

The integration of international human rights law into medical practice is necessary to ensure that mental augmentation is administered in ways that respect and support decision-making. The legal frameworks established by core international treaties guide state obligations in regulating healthcare and safeguarding the rights of all individuals, with specific protections for certain groups, such as persons with disabilities and children. As healthcare professionals consider incorporating neurofeedback therapies and brain-computer interfaces, they will navigate complex ethical and legal questions that complicate the decision-making landscape. These technologies hold transformative potential to enhance cognitive function and support autonomy, yet without regulatory oversight and human rights guidance, they risk compromising individual rights and upholding traditional approaches that favor substitute decision-making.

Although not always medically necessary, the application of these mental augmentation technologies would support children and their capacity to make decisions. This raises tensions between balancing approaches and access based on medical necessity and those based on human rights frameworks. Eligibility or access on the sole basis of medical necessity should be rejected, and the medical community must work to accommodate the perspectives of international human rights law, especially when those perspectives provide new opportunities for supporting patient autonomy. Policymakers, medical professionals, and treaty body experts should engage in continuous interdisciplinary dialogue to develop legal standards for mental augmentation, ensuring that the future of choice is rooted in human rights.[19]

---

[19] The study was supported by a National Science Centre (Poland) grant: *Do we need the recognition of neurorights? The scope of State and business actors' human rights obligations in the area of neurotechnologies* (project no. 2023/49/B/HS5/02139).

References

Albert, Dustin, and Laurence Steinberg. 2011. "Judgment and Decision Making in Adolescence." *Journal of Research on Adolescence* 21 (1) (March): 211–224. https://doi.org/10.1111/j.1532-7795.2010.00724.x.

Arambula, Alexandra, Christoph Arnoldner, Athanasia Warnecke, and Hinrich Staecker. 2022. "The Augmented Cochlear Implant: A Convergence of Drugs and Cochlear Implantation for the Treatment of Hearing Loss." *Current Otorhinolaryngology Reports* 10 (4) (December): 349–356. https://doi.org/10.1007/s40136-022-00426-1.

Balconi, Michela, Laura Angioletti, and Davide Crivelli. 2023. "Neurofeedback as Neuroempowerment Technique for Affective Regulation and Interoceptive Awareness in Adolescence: Preliminary Considerations Applied to a Psychogenic Pseudosyncope Case." *Frontiers in Rehabilitation Sciences* 4: 1056972. https://doi.org/10.3389/fresc.2023.1056972.

Baumtrog, Michael D., and Harmony Peach. 2019. "They Can't Be Believed: Children, Intersectionality, and Epistemic Injustice." *Journal of Global Ethics* 15 (3): 213–232. https://doi.org/10.1080/17449626.2019.1695280.

Beck, Asad, Andreas Schönau, Kate MacDuffie, Ishan Dasgupta, Garrett Flynn, Dong Song, Sara Goering, and Eran Klein. 2024. "'In the Spectrum of People Who Are Healthy': Views of Individuals at Risk of Dementia on Using Neurotechnology for Cognitive Enhancement." *Neuroethics* 17 (2) (July): article no. 24. https://doi.org/10.1007/s12152-024-09557-2.

Blakemore, Sarah-Jayne. 2018. "Avoiding Social Risk in Adolescence." *Current Directions in Psychological Science* 27 (2) (April): 116–122. https://doi.org/10.1177/0963721417738144.

Bluschke, Annet, Felicia Broschwitz, Simon Kohl, Veit Roessner, and Christian Beste. 2016. "The Neuronal Mechanisms Underlying Improvement of Impulsivity in ADHD by Theta/Beta Neurofeedback." *Scientific Reports* 6: article no. 31178. https://doi.org/10.1038/srep31178.

Card, Nicholas S., Maitreyee Wairagkar, Carrina Iacobacci, Xianda Hou, Tyler Singer-Clark, Francis R. Willett, et al. 2024. "An Accurate and Rapidly Calibrating Speech Neuroprosthesis." *New England Journal of Medicine* 391 (7) (August 15): 609–618. https://doi.org/10.1056/NEJMoa2314132.

Casey, Bety J., Rebecca M. Jones, and Leah H. Somerville. 2011. "Braking and Accelerating of the Adolescent Brain." *Journal of Research on Adolescence* 21 (1) (March): 21–33. https://doi.org/10.1111/j.1532-7795.2010.00712.x.

CRC Committee. 2013. General Comment No. 14: The Right of the Child to Have His or Her Best Interests Taken as a Primary Consideration (Art. 3, Para. 1). https://www2.ohchr.org/english/bodies/crc/docs/gc/crc_c_gc_14_eng.pdf.

CRC Committee. 2016. General Comment No. 20: The Implementation of the Rights of the Child during Adolescence, CRC/C/GC/20. https://www.ohchr.org/en/documents/general-comments-and-recommendations/general-comment-no-20-2016-implementation-rights.

CRC Committee. 2019. General Comment No. 24: Children's Rights in the Child Justice System, CRC/C/GC/24. https://www.ohchr.org/en/documents/general-comments-and-recommendations/general-comment-no-24-2019-childrens-rights-child.

CRPD Committee. 2014. General Comment No. 1: Article 12: Equal Recognition Before the Law, CRPD/C/GC/1. https://www.ohchr.org/en/documents/general-comments-and-recommendations/general-comment-no-1-article-12-equal-recognition-1.

Dekkers, Tycho J., Erik de Water, and Anouk Scheres. 2022. "Impulsive and Risky Decision-Making in Adolescents with Attention-Deficit/Hyperactivity Disorder (ADHD): The Need for a Developmental Perspective." *Current Opinion in Psychology* 44 (April): 330–336. https://doi.org/10.1016/j.copsyc.2021.11.002.

Dotson, Vonetta M., and Audrey Duarte. 2020. "The Importance of Diversity in Cognitive Neuroscience." *Annals of the New York Academy of Sciences* 1464 (1) (March): 181–191. https://doi.org/10.1111/nyas.14268.

Duell, Natasha, and Laurence Steinberg. 2021. "Adolescents Take Positive Risks, Too." *Developmental Review* 62 (December): 100984. https://doi.org/10.1016/j.dr.2021.100984.

ESCR Committee. 2000. General Comment No. 14: The Right to the Highest Attainable Standard of Health, E/C.12/2000/4. https://www.ohchr.org/sites/default/files/Documents/Issues/Women/WRGS/Health/GC14.pdf.

ESCR Committee. 2020. General Comment No. 25 on Article 15: Science and Economic, Social and Cultural Rights, E/C.12/GC/25. https://docs.un.org/en/E/C.12/GC/25.

Elahe, Fathi Azar, Mahnaz Hejazi-Shirmard, and Hooshang Mirzaie. 2024. "Cognitive Enhancement Through Technology: A Review of Transcranial Electrical Stimulation (TES) Interventions in Children and Adolescents with Specific Learning Disabilities." *Child: Care, Health and Development* 50 (5) (September): e13318. https://doi.org/10.1111/cch.13318.

Fandakova, Yana, and Catherine A. Hartley. 2020. "Mechanisms of Learning and Plasticity in Childhood and Adolescence." *Developmental Cognitive Neuroscience* 42 (April): 100764. https://doi.org/10.1016/j.dcn.2020.100764.

Fujino, Junya, Shoko Okuzumi, and Shisei Tei. 2024. "Biological and Neurocognitive Aspects of Decision-Making in Adults with Autism Spectrum Disorder." In *Handbook of the Biology and Pathology of Mental Disorders*, edited by Colin R. Martin, Victor R. Preedy, Vinood B. Patel, and Rajkumar Rajendram, 1–16. Cham: Springer. https://doi.org/10.1007/978-3-031-32035-4_102-1.

Greenblatt, Andrea, Eunjung Lee, Rachelle Ashcroft, and Barbara Muskat. 2024. "Epistemic Justice and Injustice among Youth with Mental Health Concerns." *Children & Society* 38 (4) (July): 1039–1058. https://doi.org/10.1111/chso.12781.

Guyer, Amanda E., Jennifer S. Silk, and Eric E. Nelson. 2016. "The Neurobiology of the Emotional Adolescent: From the Inside Out." *Neuroscience & Biobehavioral Reviews* 70 (November): 74–85. https://doi.org/10.1016/j.neubiorev.2016.07.037.

Humphreys, Kathryn L., and Steve S. Lee. 2011. "Risk Taking and Sensitivity to Punishment in Children with ADHD, ODD, ADHD+ ODD, and Controls." *Journal of Psychopathology and Behavioral Assessment* 33 (3) (September): 299–307. https://doi.org/10.1007/s10862-011-9237-6.

Icenogle, Grace, and Elizabeth Cauffman. 2021. "Adolescent Decision Making: A Decade in Review." *Journal of Research on Adolescence* 31 (4) (December): 1006–1022. https://doi.org/10.1111/jora.12608.

Iodice, Pierpaolo, L. Cannito, A. Chaigneau, and R. Palumbo. 2022. "Learned Self-Regulation in Top-Level Managers through Neurobiofeedback Training Improves Decision Making under Stress." *Scientific Reports* 12: article no. 6127. https://doi.org/10.1038/s41598-022-10142-x.

Jansson-Boyd, Cathrine, and Peter Bright. 2024. *Consumer Neuroscience: Theory and Application.* Amsterdam: Elsevier.

Kelly, Simon P., and Redmond G. O'Connell. 2015. "The Neural Processes Underlying Perceptual Decision Making in Humans: Recent Progress and Future Directions." *Journal of Physiology-Paris* 109 (1–3) (February-June): 27–37. https://doi.org/10.1016/j.jphysparis.2014.08.003.

Lee, Clara S. C., Ting-ting Chen, Qingwen Gao, Chunzhuo Hua, Rui Song, and Xiu-ping Huang. 2023. "The Effects of Theta/Beta-Based Neurofeedback Training on Attention in Children with Attention Deficit Hyperactivity Disorder: A Systematic Review and Meta-analysis." *Child Psychiatry & Human Development* 54 (6) (December): 1577–1606. https://doi.org/10.1007/s10578-022-01361-4.

Mairon, Noam, Lior Abramson, Ariel Knafo-Noam, Anat Perry, and Mor Nahum. 2023. "The Relationship between Empathy and Executive Functions among Young Adolescents." *Developmental Psychology* 59 (11) (November): 2021–2036. https://doi.org/10.1037/dev0001639.

Maslen, Hannah, and Stephen Rainey. 2021. "Control and Ownership of Neuroprosthetic Speech." *Philosophy & Technology* 34 (3) (September): 425–445. https://doi.org/10.1007/s13347-019-00389-0.

Mercado, Jose, Lizbeth Escobedo, and Monica Tentori. 2021. "A BCI Video Game Using Neurofeedback Improves the Attention of Children with Autism." *Journal on Multimodal User Interfaces* 15 (3) (September): 273–281. https://doi.org/10.1007/s12193-020-00339-7.

Metzger, Sean L., Kaylo T. Littlejohn, Alexander B. Silva, David A. Moses, Margaret P. Seaton, Ran Wang, et al. 2023. "A High-Performance Neuroprosthesis for Speech Decoding and Avatar Control." *Nature* 620 (7976) (August 31): 1037–1046. https://doi.org/10.1038/s41586-023-06443-4.

Nilsson, Anna, and Lucy Series. 2018. "Article 12 CRPD: Equal Recognition before the Law." In *The UN Convention on the Rights of Persons with Disabilities: A Commentary*, edited by Ilias Bantekas, Michael Ashley Stein, and Dimitris Anastasiou, 339–382. Oxford: Oxford University Press. https://doi.org/10.1093/law/9780198810667.003.0013.

Pollak, Yehuda, Tycho J. Dekkers, Rachel Shoham, and Hilde M. Huizenga. 2019. "Risk-Taking Behavior in Attention Deficit/Hyperactivity Disorder (ADHD): A Review of Potential Underlying Mechanisms and of Interventions." *Current Psychiatry Reports* 21 (5) (May): article no. 33. https://doi.org/10.1007/s11920-019-1019-y.

Rao, Naveen. 2024. "GPT Has Entered the Chat: Inside Synchron's BCI-OpenAI Integration." *Forbes*. August 1. https://www.forbes.com/sites/naveenrao/2024/07/24/gpt-has-entered-the-chat-inside-synchrons-bci-openai-integration/.

Rastikerdar, Najmeh, Vahid Nejati, Negar Sammaknejad, and Jalil Fathabadi. 2023. "Developmental Trajectory of Hot and Cold Executive Functions in Children with and without Attention Deficit-Hyperactivity Disorder (ADHD)." *Research in Developmental Disabilities* 137 (June): 104514. https://doi.org/10.1016/j.ridd.2023.104514.

Saleem, Shemaila, and Syed Hamid Habib. 2024. "Neurofeedback Recuperates Cognitive Functions in Children with Autism Spectrum Disorders (ASD)." *Journal of Autism and Developmental Disorders* 54 (8) (August): 2891–2901. https://doi.org/10.1007/s10803-023-06037-z.

Sankaran, Narayan, David Moses, Winston Chiong, and Edward F. Chang. 2023. "Recommendations for Promoting User Agency in the Design of Speech Neuroprostheses." *Frontiers in Human Neuroscience* 17: 1298129. https://doi.org/10.3389/fnhum.2023.1298129.

Sato, Motoshige, Kenichi Tomeoka, Ilya Horiguchi, Kai Arulkumaran, Ryota Kanai, and Shuntaro Sasai. 2024. "Scaling Law in Neural Data: Non-invasive Speech Decoding with 175 Hours of EEG data." *arXiv*: 2407.07595. https://doi.org/10.48550/arXiv.2407.07595.

Scholten, Matthé, and Jakov Gather. 2018. "Adverse Consequences of Article 12 of the UN Convention on the Rights of Persons with Disabilities for Persons with Mental Disabilities and an Alternative Way Forward." *Journal of Medical Ethics* 44 (4) (April): 226–233. https://doi.org/10.1136/medethics-2017-104414.

Sękowska-Kozłowska, Katarzyna, Grażyna Baranowska, Joanna Grygiel-Zasada, and Łukasz Szoszkiewicz. 2024. "The Impact of the United Nations Human Rights Treaties on the Domestic Level in Poland." In *The Impact of the United Nations Human Rights Treaties on the Domestic Level: Twenty Years On*, 2nd ed., edited by Christof Heyns, Frans Jacobus Viljoen, and Rachel Murray, 823–898. Leiden: Brill.

Selimbeyoglu, Aslihan, and Josef Parvizi. 2010. "Electrical Stimulation of the Human Brain: Perceptual and Behavioral Phenomena Reported in the Old and New Literature." *Frontiers in Human Neuroscience* 4 (May): article no. 46. https://doi.org/10.3389/fnhum.2010.00046.

Silva, Alexander B., Kaylo T. Littlejohn, Jessie R. Liu, David A. Moses, and Edward F. Chang. 2024. "The Speech Neuroprosthesis." *Nature Reviews Neuroscience* 25 (7) (July): 473–492. https://doi.org/10.1038/s41583-024-00819-9.

Szmukler, George. 2019. "'Capacity,' 'Best Interests,' 'Will and Preferences' and the UN Convention on the Rights of Persons with Disabilities." *World Psychiatry* 18 (1) (February): 34–41. https://doi.org/10.1002/wps.20584.

Tankus, Ariel, Einat Stern, Guy Klein, Nufar Kaptzon, Lilac Nash, Tal Marziano, et al. 2022. "A Speech Neuroprosthesis in the Frontal Lobe and Hippocampus: Decoding High-Frequency Activity into Phonemes." *Neurosurgery* (96) (2) (February): 356–364. https://doi.org/10.1227/neu.0000000000003068.

UNICEF. 2024. "Neurotechnology and Children: Working Paper." June. https://www.unicef.org/innocenti/media/8956/file/UNICEF-Innocenti-Neurotechnology-and-Children-2024.pdf.

van der Plas, Elisa, David Mason, and Francesca Happé. 2023. "Decision-Making in Autism: A Narrative Review." *Autism* 27 (6) (August): 1532–1546. https://doi.org/10.1177/13623613221148010.

Łukasz Szoszkiewicz is Assistant Professor at the Faculty of Law and Administration and Cognitive Neuroscience Center at Adam Mickiewicz University in Poznan, Poland, and Director of European Affairs at the Neurorights Foundation. His research focuses on international human rights law—especially as it relates to emerging technologies such as artificial intelligence and neurotechnology—as well as child rights and the natural language processing of legal texts. His research experience includes collaboration with the EU Agency for Fundamental Rights in Vienna, the Global Campus of Human Rights, and a Fulbright-funded project at the Neurotechnology Center, Columbia University.

Stephen Damianos is the Executive Director of the Neurorights Foundation and an Adjunct Associate Researcher at Columbia University, USA. His research focuses on the intersection of technology and human rights, with focus on neurotechnologies as well as state violence enabled by digital bordering technologies. Damianos holds a PhD (DPhil) in International Development from the University of Oxford, where he studied as a Rhodes Scholar, an MPhil in Development Studies from the University of Cambridge, and a BA in Political Science from the University of Pennsylvania.

Part III
Data, Privacy, and Autonomy

Chapter 13
Bias and Disparities in the Electronic Health Record

Katharine Lawrence

Abstract Healthcare disparities, characterized by systematic differences in health outcomes among demographic groups, are often driven by bias, both explicit and implicit. Electronic Health Records (EHRs), integral to modern healthcare, pose unique bias and equity risks in healthcare delivery, which arise through EHR design, data entry, management practices, and clinical decision support tools. This chapter explores these risks and opportunities, identifying the "Four D's of a Bias-D EHR" system—design, data, documentation, and care delivery. It offers strategies to mitigate bias and emphasizes the importance of addressing these issues to promote health equity. Ensuring that EHR systems support fair, unbiased care is essential to improving outcomes across minoritized patient populations.

Keywords Health information technology · Electronic health record · Digital health equity · Bias · Health disparities

13.1 Introduction

Despite the strong professional, ethical, and moral responsibility of medical professionals to provide the best care to each of their patients (Hajar 2017), healthcare is not experienced equitably by all. Disparities in healthcare are pervasive, impacting patient outcomes and the quality of care provided across different populations (Braveman 2014; Lawrence 2022). Healthcare disparities refer to systematic differences in health outcomes between demographic groups, often driven by socioeconomic, racial, gender, or geographic factors rooted in unfair or avoidable differences (Weinstein et al. 2017). Bias, whether conscious or unconscious, plays a central role in perpetuating these inequities and is troublingly entrenched in medical school admissions, training, work environments, and interpersonal relations with both patients and colleagues (FitzGerald and Hurst 2017; Wheeler et al. 2019; Vela

K. Lawrence (✉)
New York University, New York, NY, USA
e-mail: katharine.lawrence@nyulangone.org

M. C. Altman and D. Schwan (eds.), *Ethics and Medical Technology*, The International Library of Bioethics 113, https://doi.org/10.1007/978-3-031-94690-5_13

et al. 2021). Conscious (explicit) bias involves a deliberate prejudice against an individual or group of people, while unconscious (implicit) bias refers to attitudes and beliefs about race, ethnicity, age, ability, gender, or other characteristics that operate outside conscious awareness and can influence healthcare professionals' decisions in negative ways (Sabin 2022).

The relatively recent "digital transformation" of healthcare into an electronically connected ecosystem of health-related data and information has brought new complexity to the issue of health disparities. In particular, the introduction of electronic health record (EHR) systems into US healthcare has resulted in an increasingly complex network of clinical documentation tools, medical decision-making support, patient data exchange and care connectivity, and health research. As defined by the Healthcare Information and Management Systems Society, an EHR is

> a longitudinal electronic record of patient health information generated by one or more encounters in any care delivery setting. Included in this information are patient demographics, progress notes, problems, medications, vital signs, past medical history, immunizations, laboratory data and radiology reports. … The EHR has the ability to generate a complete record of a clinical patient encounter—as well as supporting other care-related activities directly or indirectly via interface—including evidence-based decision support, quality management, and outcomes reporting. (quoted in Atherton 2011)

Broadly, EHR systems can help streamline care coordination, improve data accessibility, and enhance clinical decision-making (Menachemi and Collum 2011; Upadhyay and Hu 2022); however, EHRs also can also drive bias at technical, sociotechnical, and social levels, potentially jeopardizing the healthcare experience and outcomes of already minoritized patients.

This chapter argues that, rather than being an inherently neutral technology in a healthcare system, electronic health records can introduce or exacerbate critical biases in healthcare delivery that contribute to, and in some cases newly create, avoidable disparities for certain populations of patients. Specifically, the chapter outlines how unique biases emerge from the "Four D's of a Bias-D EHR"—design, data, documentation, and care delivery—and maintains that, as part of existing ethical imperatives to address inequities in both healthcare and emerging technologies, there is justification to resolve disparities driven by EHR-specific biases. Finally, the chapter offers ethically guided strategies to mitigate EHR biases. Addressing these issues is critical to improving health equity and ensuring that EHRs support, rather than hinder, fair and unbiased care.

13.2 Contexts of Bias in Electronic Health Records (EHRs) Systems

13.2.1 Systemic Bias in Healthcare

Biases in healthcare are deeply rooted in historical, social, and cultural contexts. The history of medical experimentation on minoritized populations within the United States is well-documented, including the infamous Tuskegee Syphilis Study (1932–1972), in which African American men with syphilis were deliberately left untreated after the discovery of penicillin in order to study the progression of the disease (Gamble 1997; Nuriddin et al. 2020; Paul et al. 2020). This and other events reflect a deeply embedded history of medicalized racism and structural violence within the healthcare system that has left a legacy of distrust and vulnerability among many communities (Jones 1997; Evans et al. 2020).

Bias in healthcare manifests in disparities in healthcare access and outcomes (Smedley et al. 2003; Riley 2012). Socioeconomic status significantly influences access to care, with poorer patients receiving less preventive care and experiencing worse outcomes. Racial minorities, particularly Black, Latino, and Indigenous populations, face barriers to healthcare rooted in both explicit and implicit bias (Krieger 2016). Gender bias is also a concern, with women (and particularly women of color) often dismissed or undertreated for their symptoms (Hay et al. 2019). Geographic disparities also exist, as patients in rural or underserved areas often lack access to high-quality care (Institute of Medicine 2008). These longstanding disparities, rooted in systemic bias, have implications for our modern healthcare technologies, including EHRs.

13.2.2 The "Four D's of a Bias-D EHR"

Bias within EHR systems arises from multiple points and can be categorized into four key domains: EHR Design and Development, Data Bias, Documentation Bias, and Care Delivery Bias. These "Four D's" collectively create an ecosystem where systemic biases in healthcare are reflected, perpetuated, and in some cases newly created, posing risks to equitable care delivery.

13.2.2.1 EHR Design and Development

The design and development phase of EHR systems is a critical introduction point for potential bias. In other fields—including software design, product design, and human-computer interaction—it has been well-documented that the design of a tool or technology can be inherently biased depending on for whom it is built and who is involved in creating it (Friedman et al. 1996; Ngalamou and Schmidbauer 2020). These biases are often invisible, stemming from assumptions designers make about user behavior or engineers make about user requirements, and they argue against the common belief that all technology is neutral (VanderLeest 2004; Price and Lloyd 2022). User- and human-centered design strategies (including the increasingly popular "Design Thinking" and "Agile" approaches) attempt to reduce potential biases by rigorously engaging with stakeholders and end-users in order to more effectively incorporate their needs and lived experiences into the design and deployment of new technologies or products (Beck et al. 2001; Altman et al. 2018). However, in practice these user-centered principles are inconsistently applied, and significant critiques of their real-world impacts—particularly regarding equity—have been raised (Pal 2023; Anderson et al. 2024). Diversity within the design teams responsible for building the EHR is also critical.

EHRs serve many needs, including medical documentation, billing and coding, and administrative organization. Often, however, the original design of the system is grounded in a single purpose (e.g., billing), with the structure, use, and outcomes of the system driven to prioritize that purpose (Rozier et al. 2022). As Michael Rozier, Kavita Patel, and Dori Cross explain, "The system itself indicates to its users what its highest value is; the users are thus habituated to adopt that value as their own" (2022, 137). In EHR systems, the choices made during the design phase, from how data is inputted to how information is displayed, can reflect the biases of the developers, whether intentional or not. For example, user interface (UI) and user experience (UX) decisions around how to display patient data can shape how clinicians interact with that data and choose to provide care based on it. A platform designer chooses which data fields are prominently displayed (e.g., a home screen) and how drop-down options are organized (e.g., "white" race showing first in a selection). A clinician may be impacted by these choices in their processes of ingesting, synthesizing, and making medical decisions based on the data "at hand."

Decisions around EHR accessibility can also impact minoritized individuals—both patients and clinicians. This includes font and color choices for those with limited vision, and speech-to-text and text-to-speech capabilities for the hearing impaired. Choices around languages supported (or not) in EHRs can impact accessibility but also create more nuanced biases—for example, in the use of gendered language (e.g., Spanish-language pronouns). It also includes choices about how to "platform" EHRs; whether they can be available on lap- versus desktops, web-based or mobile applications ("apps") can create barriers for users with structural barriers to accessing digital technology. For patients experiencing the "digital divide" (Sanders and Scanlon 2021), early design choices that support low-cost, universally available platforms such as web browsers or text messages can mean the difference between being able to access personal health data and being excluded from the ecosystem (although such design choices may introduce their own equity risks, particularly around data security and surveillance). Overall, the absence of thoughtful design features sensitive to both diverse clinician *and* patient end-users means that certain populations may not be served effectively by these systems.

13.2.2.2 EHR Data Bias

The computer science adage "garbage in, garbage out" applies strongly to EHR systems, where biased data inputs often lead to biased outputs and clinical decisions. EHR data bias most commonly arises from incomplete or missing data, variable data quality, and biased or skewed source data sets.

At baseline, the data available in EHRs often reflects only those patients who access healthcare, excluding a significant portion of the population due to historical and ongoing barriers that limit care access (Boyd et al. 2023). For patients who are able to access care, concerns around trust, security, and privacy may influence health or other disclosures to clinicians, resulting in incomplete medical records. This includes both omissions in conversations (e.g., recent substance use) and explicit requests not to document (e.g., immigration status). When patient-reported outcomes (PROs) are collected via patient portals, those without access to technology or with literacy challenges are excluded.

EHRs rely on clinical guidelines and coding systems such as ICD-10 codes to document patient conditions, but research indicates that certain conditions disproportionately affecting marginalized populations, such as chronic pain, may be undercoded, while others, such as noncompliance or substance use disorders, are overcoded (Hoffman et al. 2016; Geskey et al. 2023). This discrepancy in data entry practices can result in misdiagnosis and mistreatment, perpetuating healthcare disparities for vulnerable groups. Additionally, EHR systems frequently fail to prioritize the collection of social determinants of health (SDOH), which include critical factors such as socioeconomic status, housing, and education; many EHR systems do not routinely collect or organize SDOH data in a usable format, deprioritizing its role in clinical decision-making (Boyd et al. 2023). This lack of comprehensive data deprives clinicians of a full understanding of their patients' health.

More recently, scholars have raised alarm on the unique bias and equity risks of artificial intelligence and machine learning techniques applied to EHRs (Gianfrancesco et al. 2018). Many widely used health algorithms have been shown to reinforce health inequities, from heart-failure risk scores that inappropriately categorize Black patients as being in need of less care to algorithms that under-diagnose cancers in people of color (Owens and Walker 2020; Vyas et al. 2020). Much of the current medical evidence underlying AI models is generated from clinical trials with predominately white participants, which does not ensure that the conclusions drawn are safe and effective for all populations (Boyd et al. 2023). These models are then deployed into EHR clinical decision support (CDS) tools to suggest risk factors, diagnoses, treatments, and supportive services, even as the underlying logic of these tools limit applicability.

13.2.2.3 Documentation Bias

Documentation bias is one of the most direct ways bias manifests in EHR systems. Healthcare professionals, like the general population, harbor implicit biases that reflect societal stereotypes about race, gender, and ethnicity; such biases, inadvertently recorded in EHRs, contribute to perpetuating healthcare inequities (Perets et al. 2024). Studies show that physicians convey negative impressions in encounter notes by suggesting that patients are not being truthful, expressing disapproval of patients' decisions or behaviors, revealing racial or social class stereotypes of patients, displaying personal frustrations, and implying that patients are unreasonable (Park et al. 2021). Conversely, physicians portray patients positively by using compliments, showing approval, sharing feelings of respect toward patients, minimizing blame when patients are not adherent to treatments, and incorporating patient preferences into treatment plans (Perets et al. 2024). For example, Black patients are often documented as being less compliant or more likely to engage in risky behavior compared to their white counterparts, even when the circumstances are similar. In one study, psychiatrists and medical students were more likely to pair African American faces with words such as noncompliance (Londono Tobon et al. 2021). In another, researchers described how negative patient descriptors were more likely to be found in history and physical notes for Black and Latino patients (Sun et al. 2022).

The documentation process in EHRs also reflects biases in how diagnoses and care plans are recorded. A clinician's decision to diagnose a patient with a particular condition may be influenced by stereotypes or assumptions, which are then perpetuated when this data is used to inform future care decisions. Because EHRs store historical data, biased documentation can have a cumulative effect, influencing future interactions and treatment decisions. Use of negative terms in clinical notes may perpetuate prejudice from healthcare providers who read the notes prior to seeing a new patient and are biased against them as a result. A misdiagnosis or biased characterization in the medical record may follow a patient throughout their care journey, creating a cycle of poor or inequitable treatment. Finally, as patients increasingly access their medical records through patient portals, there is a risk that they will internalize negative language about themselves or lose trust or rapport with their providers.

13.2.2.4 Care Delivery Bias

One of the most direct consequences of bias in EHR systems is the increased likelihood of diagnostic errors. Research has shown that physicians often rely on heuristics—such as focusing on chest pain for heart attack diagnosis—when making clinical decisions; this can lead to the over-testing of low-risk patients while under-testing high-risk patients, particularly those from minority populations (Tertulien et al. 2022; Perets et al. 2024). Similarly, a clinician relying on an EHR algorithm that underrepresents certain populations or conditions may overlook critical risk factors that disproportionately affect their minority patients. In the case of heart disease, EHR-based clinical decision support tools may not accurately flag ischemic symptoms in women; because EHR algorithms are frequently based on data from male patients, women who present with "atypical" symptoms such as fatigue, nausea, and shortness of breath (rather than the more commonly recognized chest pain) are at risk of being underscored in back-end algorithms that then make clinical recommendations to practitioners (Adedinsewo et al. 2022). In each of these cases, complex screening and scoring processes are applied to EHR data in order to provide diagnostic and treatment recommendations. These systems are frequently opaque to clinician end-users, lack potentially relevant clinical or social contexts to refine their outputs, and may obscure or disrupt the traditional cognitive processes clinicians use to come to correct medical decisions.

Even in scenarios where direct medical errors do not occur, clinicians' differential interactions with EHRs have been shown to result in different treatment decisions. Chao Yan et al. (2023) found that health professionals were less likely to append a medical note, view relevant patient information in the problem list or flowsheets, complete a medication reconciliation, or scan a barcode for minoritized patients compared to white patients. The findings raise concerns about EHR engagement as a key factor associated with racial and ethnic care delivery disparities that may drive differences in health outcomes. Studies of patient portals (the patient-facing offering of many EHRs) show similar results, with minoritized patients being less likely to be offered access or interacted with by their clinicians through portal systems (Richwine et al. 2023).

The problem of biased EHRs in healthcare delivery is not confined to the direct clinical care setting. EHR data are also widely used by healthcare organizations, insurers, pharmaceutical companies, and researchers to make decisions with far-reaching implications. Hospitals may use predictive models built on biased historical data to make decisions about patient discharge or care management plans. These tools can then be commercialized or otherwise shared, spreading the bias to other healthcare settings (Rozier et al. 2022). Insurers often use EHR data for risk stratification, determining which patients are most likely to benefit from certain treatments or interventions. If the data are less complete or less accurate for minority patients, the decisions made based on this information will likewise be flawed, reinforcing disparities in access to care and resource allocation. Finally, EHRs are increasingly utilized in clinical research (Boyd et al. 2023). While the benefits of "big data" may include increased inclusiveness or representativeness over large populations, it is widely recognized that data collected for one purpose may not be suitable for another and that there are serious issues to be considered in the reuse of EHR data or research purposes (Verheij et al. 2018).

13.3 Impacts of Bias in Electronic Health Records (EHRs)

Beyond errors in medical diagnosis and treatment, biases in EHR design, data, and implementation pose significant equity risks for minoritized patients. A significant risk lies in the inequitable allocation of healthcare resources based on faulty data or logic from EHR data. When EHR algorithms are biased and either under- or overrepresent minoritized populations in diagnosis, demographics, or social determinants, they can contribute to inequities in how healthcare resources are distributed. For example, many health systems use EHR data to determine which patients are most at risk for readmission or complications, guiding decisions about resource allocation and follow-up care (Flaks-Manov et al. 2020). However, if the algorithm is trained on biased data, it may overlook patients from minority or low-income backgrounds, who are often at higher risk for adverse health outcomes but are underrepresented in the data. This can result in these patients receiving fewer resources, less follow-up care, and lower prioritization for necessary interventions. Conversely, minoritized patients who are disproportionately labeled as "non-adherent" to treatment recommendations may be actively disenrolled in supportive social programs or made ineligible for life-saving treatments (e.g., organ transplants).

The intersection of EHR systems and healthcare payment can also have implications for minoritized patients. In value-based care models where healthcare providers are reimbursed based on patient outcomes, biased EHR data can affect the evaluation of a provider's performance and subsequent reimbursement. Providers serving predominantly minority or low-income populations may appear to have worse outcomes due to the structural disadvantages their patients face, even if they are delivering high-quality care; this can lead to underfunding or penalization of providers who serve marginalized communities (Aggarwal et al. 2021; Johnston et al. 2021). Similarly, SDOH such as housing stability, food access, and transportation are critical factors contributing to a patient's overall health. If EHR systems do not routinely collect or integrate SDOH data, this can lead to an incomplete understanding of patient care needs and misallocation of medical or other resources to support them.

The risks of bias in EHR systems extend beyond clinical and patient outcomes to ethical and legal domains. For minority populations, the perception of bias in EHR systems can reinforce existing mistrust of the healthcare system; patients who do not trust their healthcare providers are less likely to adhere to treatment plans, show up for follow-up appointments, or share sensitive health information (LaVeist et al. 2000). This can lead to poorer health outcomes, particularly for chronic conditions such as diabetes and hypertension that require ongoing management and specialty referral. When EHR systems rely on biased algorithms to make care recommendations, it can undermine patient autonomy and the right of patients to participate in their own care decisions. The use of biased EHR systems can also expose clinicians and health systems to legal liability, particularly in cases where biased algorithms or documentation leads to incorrect diagnoses or other medical errors. If a minoritized patient is consistently misdiagnosed or undertreated due to biased data in the EHR, they may have grounds for legal action. If an algorithm systematically disadvantages certain populations, leading to disparities in care, healthcare institutions may face lawsuits for violating anti-discrimination laws. In each of these cases, EHRs that are misaligned to the needs of patients cause damage to the patient experience and health outcomes.

13.4 De-biasing the EHR: Opportunities and Future Directions

A number of ethical frameworks support the view that health disparities are anathema to medicine (both as a philosophy and an avocation) and should be addressed both as part of medical practice and larger social efforts. First, addressing health disparities aligns with core bioethical principles of beneficence, maleficence, and distributive justice; equitable care delivery is considered by many health practitioners to be central to their vocation and, simply put, disparities provide no benefit, cause significant harm, and violate equity. Cynthia Jones (2010) presents contractarian, Kantian, and utilitarian ethical justifications for viewing health disparities as a moral wrong: social-contract theory views health disparities as morally unjust because they violate individuals' basic liberties by imposing health inequalities unrelated to inherent biological differences; Kantian ethics argues that addressing health disparities is a moral duty, as respect for all persons requires eliminating preventable differences in health outcomes; and finally, from a utilitarian perspective, health disparities are ethically wrong and should be addressed because they harm a large group and undermine the goal of maximizing overall happiness. Stephen Bradley (2021) uses similar arguments to make the case for a population-level imperative to address health disparities; this includes a call for healthcare providers to engage in advocacy, policymaking, and other society-wide efforts to change health practices and promote health equity. There is also precedent for considering general ethics of emerging technologies, and to address inequities in these tools as they arise. James Moor argues that the rapid emergence of new technologies "should give us a sense of urgency in thinking about the ethical implications" of these technologies (2005, 111). Evie Kendal (2022), in a review of approaches for the ethics of emerging technologies, highlights the following: the Precautionary Principle, which outlines a precautionary approach to emerging technologies, particularly those involving potential harms (Hansson 2020); design ethics, particularly the concept of "value-sensitive design," which aims to identify and incorporate relevant human values during the research and development stages to ensure these values are "promoted and respected by the design" (Umbrello and van de Poel 2021, 283); the ethical technology assessment approach, which uses ethical concerns to guide decision-making and align technology with ethical standards (Palm and Hansson 2006); and finally some specific anticipatory approaches to emergent or future technology use-cases and concerns (Kendal 2022).

Pursuant to these arguments is the rationale to address inequities that may arise from applications of emerging technologies in healthcare, including the electronic health record. Fortunately, there are many opportunities to address bias and mitigate disparities in EHRs, guided by thoughtful applications of ethical principles in EHR design, deployment, and use. For example, Tim Jacquemard et al. propose a practical approach to identifying and addressing ethical issues that arise from electronic health records, acknowledging that "regard for ethical values during all stages of the technology's life-cycle from design, development, implementation through usage is paramount," given the tool's ubiquity and centrality to current medical practice

(2021, 2). They go on to identify specific content (including the purposes of the technology, its interested parties and stakeholders, and frames of reference such as regulation and codes of professional conduct) and contexts (such as data collection, data access, and digitally enabled care) that are relevant to an EHR, and suggest several critical questions at each point that should be considered when designing, building, and using the tool in practice. Relevant questions related to this work might include: Who are the stakeholders involved in the design and implementation of this tool? Who influences requirements engineering, design specification, implementation, and operational decisions about the uses and functionalities of the system or its data? What data are being included, and why? Who are the primary end-users? How will this tool be used? Who can benefit from or be harmed by the system?

Thinking through the "Four D's of a Bias-D EHR," the following examples illustrate potential solutions at each stage (Table 13.1). At baseline, it is critical to incorporate diverse patient populations into the design, development, and deployment of both EHR platforms and the data, algorithms, and other complex systems that underpin them. Equity-centered design approaches (e.g., inclusive design, liberatory design) can facilitate the more thoughtful and sustained inclusion of minoritized voices in this process (Pal 2023). These should be complemented by internal diversity, equity, and inclusion efforts that aim to build representative design and technical teams responsible for building the EHR itself. Standardized data collection practices that include comprehensive inclusions of race, ethnicity, gender, and SDOH data as well as patient-generated health information can provide a more complete picture of patient health and potentially reduce equity gaps in care delivery. Data, system, and software transparency and accountability are also essential, with regular audits and explainable models helping health system end-users identify and correct biases. Technical improvements in EHR design and data can be augmented by training clinicians to address implicit bias and reduce documentation bias in their own practices (Vela et al. 2022). Thoughtful ethnographic and other qualitative research can also be employed to evaluate EHRs "in the wild" to better understand how the translation of the tool into real-world settings exposes, exacerbates, mitigates, or newly creates biased practices from healthcare providers and other users.

While a significant source of potential bias in EHRs, advances in machine learning and AI can also offer opportunities to combat health inequities. Algorithms can be designed to identify patterns of incompleteness, skew, or other bias within EHR datasets, revealing data disparities that may not be immediately apparent to clinicians or researchers (Green et al. 2024). AI-based feedback and other training programs can help guide clinicians by flagging biased habits or patterns in their medical decision-making, documentation, or other aspects of their practice (Turner et al. 2024). And the more systematic inclusion of SDOH data into advanced decision support can provide a more comprehensive picture of patients' health risks and social needs (Guevara et al. 2024). These advances can allow the healthcare system to move toward true precision medicine that is sensitive to individual, community, and structural factors that drive health outcomes (Vyas et al. 2020). Lastly, collaboration among policymakers, institutions, and technologists is vital for promoting equity and addressing digital disparities in healthcare.

Table 13.1 Considerations and opportunities to mitigate bias in EHR design, data, documentation, and care delivery

1. *EHR Design and Technical Development Bias:* Diverse patient populations should be incorporated into the design and deployment stages of EHR platforms to ensure those systems reflect the needs of varied communities. Equity-centered design approaches, (e.g. inclusive and liberatory design) facilitate the inclusion of minoritized voices, while internal diversity, equity, and inclusion efforts ensure that representative teams are involved in creating the EHR infrastructure. *Questions to ask:* Are diverse and minoritized groups adequately represented in the design and testing phases of the EHR platform? What measures are in place to ensure that development teams reflect the diversity of the populations their platform serves? How can we prioritize minoritized perspectives? How are potential unintended equity consequences being anticipated?
2. *Data Bias:* Standardized data collection practices that include comprehensive information on race, ethnicity, gender, and social determinants of health (SDOH) can help create a more complete picture of patient health, improving personalized care and minimizing gaps in care delivery. Regular audits and the use of explainable, transparent models can further assist healthcare providers in recognizing and mitigating data bias within EHR systems. *Questions to ask:* Are data collection practices standardized in a way that accurately captures the diversity of race, ethnicity, gender, and SDOH data? Is there transparency around data sources, collection methodologies, and how data is used within decision-making tools? How frequently are data quality and inclusiveness assessed to prevent biased or incomplete data? What mechanisms are in place for identifying and mitigating biases in data algorithms?
3. *Documentation Bias*: Clinician training programs focused on implicit bias can help address documentation bias by promoting equity-aware documentation practices. AI tools could provide feedback that flags potentially biased patterns in clinicians' documentation, enabling them to adjust and improve their practices over time. *Questions to ask:* How are we training clinicians to recognize and counteract their own potential biases in documentation practices? How are we capturing and reviewing documentation outputs? What role can patients have in making and/or reviewing their own documentation?
4. *Care Delivery Bias*: Engage clinicians in health equity and/or social justice aimed at addressing health disparities. Collaboration among policymakers, institutions, and technologists is essential to establish standards that address digital disparities and promote equity within healthcare delivery. *Questions to ask:* How do we assess causation between EHR features/functionalities and individual medical decision-making? How do we assess causation between EHR features/functionalities and health outcomes, both individual and population?

The future of equitable EHR systems will require collaboration among clinical providers, health administrators, engineers and technologists, policymakers, and patients. Current EHR systems should be systematically evaluated and, where needed, dismantled and rebuilt to remove inequitable components; newly developed EHRs should commit to equity as a core technical, business, and social mission. When deployed, healthcare providers can monitor these systems to ensure they align with patient care needs, while health administrators and larger health system leaders can more broadly monitor their EHR product choices and vendor relationships. Technologists, engineers, and designers building EHRs can commit to equity-centered design and development processes, and engage with health systems in post go-live monitoring and mitigation of emergent biases. Policymakers must play a key role in establishing local and federal guidance to support and enforce an equitable digital health ecosystem. Finally, patient input is crucial in shaping systems that are accessible, user-friendly, and sustainable for diverse needs.

13.5 Conclusions

Bias within electronic health record systems is a reflection of broader systemic inequities in society. The four key areas where bias manifests in EHRs—design, data, documentation, and care delivery—create systemic inequities, particularly for minoritized populations, that can perpetuate diagnostic errors, unequal resource allocation, and discriminatory healthcare practices. There is both ethical and moral justification for addressing both general health inequities and inequities that arise from emerging technology, and, as such, a reasonable imperative to also address health disparities that result from EHRs. There are also clear, ethically guided opportunities to de-bias EHRs: more inclusive design and development processes, standardized data collection that fills existing data gaps and captures important contextualizing data such as social determinants of health, embedding transparency and accountability into the algorithms and AI that increasingly underpin EHR logic, and monitoring and mitigating biases as they emerge during real-world EHR use. Ultimately, creating equitable EHRs requires a collaborative effort involving clinicians, technologists, policymakers, and patients to build systems that support unbiased, patient-centered, and equitable care.

References

Adedinsewo, Demilade A., Amy W. Pollak, Sabrina D. Phillips, Taryn L. Smith, Anna Svatikova, Sharonne N. Hayes, et al. 2022. "Cardiovascular Disease Screening in Women: Leveraging Artificial Intelligence and Digital Tools." *Circulation Research* 130 (4) (February 18): 673–690. https://doi.org/10.1161/CIRCRESAHA.121.319876.

Aggarwal, Rahul, J. Gmerice Hammond, Karen E. Joynt Maddox, Robert W. Yeh, and Rishi K. Wadhera. 2021. "Association between the Proportion of Black Patients Cared for at Hospitals and Financial Penalties under Value-Based Payment Programs." *JAMA: Journal of the American Medical Association* 325 (12) (March 23/30): 1219–1221. https://doi.org/10.1001/jama.2021.0026.

Altman, Myra, Terry T. K. Huang, and Jessica Y. Breland. 2018. "Design Thinking in Health Care." *Preventing Chronic Disease* 15 (September 27): article no. 180128. https://doi.org/10.5888/pcd15.180128.

Anderson, Hannah L. Kakara, Xandro Xu, April Edwell, Laura Lockwood, Pricilla Cabral, and Anna Weiss, et al. 2024. "How Might We Build an Equitable Future? Design Justice, a Counternarrative to Dominant Approaches in Medical Education." *Teaching and Learning in Medicine*: 1–9. https://doi.org/10.1080/10401334.2024.2404008.

Atherton, Jim. 2011. "Development of the Electronic Health Record." *Virtual Mentor* 13 (3): 186–189. https://doi.org/10.1001/virtualmentor.2011.13.3.mhst1-1103.

Beck, Kent, Mike Beedle, Arie van Bennekum, Alistair Cockburn, Ward Cunningham, Martin Fowler, et al. 2001. "Manifesto for Agile Software Development." https://agilemanifesto.org/.

Boyd, Andrew D., Rosa Gonzalez-Guarda, Katharine Lawrence, Crystal L. Patil, Miriam O. Ezenwa, Emily C. O'Brien, et al. 2023. "Equity and Bias in Electronic Health Records Data." *Contemporary Clinical Trials* 130 (July): article no. 107238. https://doi.org/10.1016/j.cct.2023.107238.

Bradley, Stephen H. 2021. "The Ethics and Politics of Addressing Health Inequalities." *Clinical Medicine* 21 (2) (March): 147–149. https://doi.org/10.7861/clinmed.2020-0945.

Braveman, Paula. 2014. "What Are Health Disparities and Health Equity? We Need to Be Clear." *Public Health Reports* 129 (1), supplement 2 (January–February): 5–8. https://doi.org/10.1177/00333549141291S203.

Evans, Michele K., Lisa Rosenbaum, Debra Malina, Stephen Morrissey, and Eric J. Rubin. 2020. "Diagnosing and Treating Systemic Racism." *New England Journal of Medicine* 383 (3) (July 16): 274–276. https://doi.org/10.1056/NEJMe2021693.

FitzGerald, Chloë, and Samia Hurst. 2017. "Implicit Bias in Healthcare Professionals: A Systematic Review." *BMC Medical Ethics* 18: article no. 19. https://doi.org/10.1186/s12910-017-0179-8.

Flaks-Manov, Natalie, Einav Srulovici, Rina Yahalom, Henia Perry-Mezre, Ran Balicer, and Efrat Shadmi. 2020. "Preventing Hospital Readmissions: Healthcare Providers' Perspectives on 'Impactibility' beyond EHR 30-Day Readmission Risk Prediction." *Journal of General Internal Medicine* 35 (5) (May): 1484–1489. https://doi.org/10.1007/s11606-020-05739-9.

Friedman, Batya, Eric Brok, Susan King Roth, and John Thomas. 1996. "Minimizing Bias in Computer Systems." *ACM SIGCHI Bulletin* 28 (1) (January): 48–51. https://doi.org/10.1145/249170.249184.

Gamble, Vanessa Northington. 1997. "Under the Shadow of Tuskegee: African Americans and Health Care." *American Journal of Public Health* 87 (11) (November): 1773–1778. https://doi.org/10.2105/ajph.87.11.1773.

Geskey, Joseph M., Jodi Kodish-Wachs, Heather Blonsky, Samuel F. Hohman, and Steve Meurer. 2023. "National Documentation and Coding Practices of Noncompliance: The Importance of Social Determinants of Health and the Stigma of African-American Bias." *American Journal of Medical Quality* 38 (2) (March–April): 87–92. https://doi.org/10.1097/JMQ.0000000000000112.

Gianfrancesco, Milena A., Suzanne Tamang, Jinoos Yazdany, and Gabriela Schmajuk. 2018. "Potential Biases in Machine Learning Algorithms Using Electronic Health Record Data." *JAMA Internal Medicine* 178 (11) (November): 1544–1547. https://doi.org/10.1001/jamainternmed.2018.3763.

Green, B. Lee, Anastasia Murphy, and Edmondo Robinson. 2024. "Accelerating Health Disparities Research with Artificial Intelligence." *Frontiers in Digital Health* 6: article no. 1330160. https://doi.org/10.3389/fdgth.2024.1330160.

Guevara, Marco, Shan Chen, Spencer Thomas, Tafadzwa L. Chaunzwa, Idalid Franco, Benjamin H. Kann, et al. 2024. "Large Language Models to Identify Social Determinants of Health in Electronic Health Records." *NPJ Digital Medicine* 7: article no. 6. https://doi.org/10.1038/s41746-023-00970-0.

Hajar, Rachel. 2017. "The Physician's Oath: Historical Perspectives." *Heart Views* 18 (4) (October–December): 154–159. https://doi.org/10.4103/heartviews.heartviews_131_17.

Hansson, Sven Ove. 2020. "How Extreme Is the Precautionary Principle?" *NanoEthics* 14 (3): 245–257. https://doi.org/10.1007/s11569-020-00373-5.

Hay, Katherine, Lotus McDougal, Valerie Percival, Sarah Henry, Jeni Klugman, Haja Wurie, et al. 2019. "Disrupting Gender Norms in Health Systems: Making the Case for Change." *Lancet* 393 (10190) (June 22): 2535–2549. https://doi.org/10.1016/S0140-6736(19)30648-8.

Hoffman, Kelly M., Sophie Trawalter, Jordan R. Axt, and M. Norman Oliver. 2016. "Racial Bias in Pain Assessment and Treatment Recommendations, and False Beliefs about Biological Differences between Blacks and Whites." *Proceedings of the National Academy of the Sciences* 113 (16) (April 4): 4296–4301. https://doi.org/10.1073/pnas.1516047113.

Institute of Medicine (U.S.) Roundtable on Health Disparities. 2008. *Challenges and Successes in Reducing Health Disparities: Workshop Summary*. Washington, DC: National Academies. https://www.ncbi.nlm.nih.gov/books/NBK215371/.

Jacquemard, Tim, Colin P. Doherty, and Mary B. Fitzsimons. 2021. "The Anatomy of Electronic Patient Record Ethics: A Framework to Guide Design, Development, Implementation, and Use." *BMC Medical Ethics* 22: article no. 9. https://doi.org/10.1186/s12910-021-00574-x.

Johnston, Kenton J., David J. Meyers, Gmerice Hammond, and Karen E. Joynt Maddox. 2021. "Association of Clinician Minority Patient Caseload with Performance in the 2019 Medicare Merit-Based Incentive Payment System." *JAMA: Journal of the American Medical Association* 325 (12) (March 23/30): 1221–1223. https://doi.org/10.1001/jama.2021.0031.

Jones, Cynthia M. 2010. "The Moral Problem of Health Disparities." *American Journal of Public Health* 100 (S1) (April): S47–S51. https://doi.org/10.2105/AJPH.2009.171181.

Jones, James M. 1997. *Prejudice and Racism*. 2nd ed. New York: McGraw-Hill.

Kendal, Evie. 2022. "Ethical, Legal and Social Implications of Emerging Technology (ELSIET) Symposium." *Journal of Bioethical Inquiry* 19 (3) (September): 363–370. https://doi.org/10.1007/s11673-022-10197-5.

Krieger, Nancy. 2016. "Does Racism Harm Health? Did Child Abuse Exist before 1962? On Explicit Questions, Critical Science, and Current Controversies: An Ecosocial Perspective." *American Journal of Public Health* 93 (2) (February): 194–199. https://doi.org/10.2105/ajph.93.2.194.

LaVeist, T. A., Kim J. Nickerson, and Janice V. Bowie. 2000. "Attitudes about Racism, Medical Mistrust, and Satisfaction with Care among African American and White Cardiac Patients." *Medical Care Research and Review* 57 (1), supplement (November): 146–161. https://doi.org/10.1177/1077558700057001S07.

Lawrence, Katharine. 2022. "Digital Health Equity." In *Digital Health*, edited by Simon Lin Linwood, 121–130. Brisbane: Exon.

Londono Tobon, Amalia, José M. Flores, Jerome H. Taylor, Isaac Johnson, Angeli Landeros-Weisenberger, Okoduwa Aboiralor, Victor J. Avila-Quintero, and Michael H. Bloch. 2021. "Racial Implicit Associations in Psychiatric Diagnosis, Treatment, and Compliance Expectations." *Academic Psychiatry* 45 (1) (February): 23–33. https://doi.org/10.1007/s40596-020-01370-2.

Menachemi, Nir, and Taleah H Collum. 2011. "Benefits and Drawbacks of Electronic Health Record Systems." *Risk Management and Healthcare Policy* 4: 47–55. https://doi.org/10.2147/RMHP.S12985.

Moor, James H. 2005. "Why We Need Better Ethics for Emerging Technologies." *Ethics and Information Technology* 7: 111–119. https://doi.org/10.1007/s10676-006-0008-0.

Ngalamou, Lucien, and Harmony L. Schmidbauer. 2020. "Combating and Perpetuating Bias: The Relationship between Bias and Computer Science." *International Journal of Information Privacy, Security and Integrity* 4 (4): 296–313. https://doi.org/10.1504/IJIPSI.2020.115523.

Nuriddin, Ayah, Graham Mooney, and Alexandre I. R. White. 2020. "Reckoning with Histories of Medical Racism and Violence in the USA." *Lancet* 396 (10256) (October 3): 949–951. https://doi.org/10.1016/S0140-6736(20)32032-8.

Owens, Kellie, and Alexis Walker. 2020. "Those Designing Healthcare Algorithms Must Become Actively Anti-racist." *Nature Medicine* 26 (9) (September): 1327–1328. https://doi.org/10.1038/s41591-020-1020-3.

Pal, Arpita. 2023. "Liberatory Design Thinking for Equity-Centered Instructional Design: A Systems Thinking Analysis." *Journal of Applied Instructional Design* 12 (2) (August). https://doi.org/10.59668/722.13026.

Palm, Elin, and Sven Ove Hansson. 2006. "The Case for Ethical Technology Assessment (eTA)." *Technological Forecasting and Social Change* 73 (5) (June): 543–558. https://doi.org/10.1016/j.techfore.2005.06.002.

Park, Jenny, Somnath Saha, Brant Chee, Janiece Taylor, and Mary Catherine Beach. 2021. "Physician Use of Stigmatizing Language in Patient Medical Records." *JAMA Network Open* 4 (7) (July 14): e2117052. https://doi.org/10.1001/jamanetworkopen.2021.17052.

Paul, Dereck W. Jr., Kelly R. Knight, Andre Campbell, and Louise Aronson. 2020. "Beyond a Moment—Reckoning with Our History and Embracing Antiracism in Medicine." *New England Journal of Medicine* 383 (15) (October 8): 1404–1406. https://doi.org/10.1056/NEJMp2021812.

Perets, Oriel, Emanuela Stagno, Eyal Ben Yehuda, Megan McNichol, Leo Anthony Celi, Nadav Rappoport, and Matilda Dorotic. 2024. "Inherent Bias in Electronic Health Records: A Scoping Review of Sources of Bias." *medRxiv* [Preprint] (April 12). https://doi.org/10.1101/2024.04.09.24305594.

Price, Rebecca Anne, and Peter Lloyd. 2022. "Asking Effective Questions: Awareness of Bias in Designerly Thinking." In *Handbook of Engineering Systems Design*, edited by Anja Maier, Josef Oehmen, and Pieter E. Vermaas, 789–804. Cham: Springer. https://doi.org/10.1007/978-3-030-46054-9_24-4.

Richwine, Chelsea, Christian Johnson, and Vaishali Patel. 2023. "Disparities in Patient Portal Access and the Role of Providers in Encouraging Access and Use." *Journal of the American Medical Informatics Association* 30 (2) (February): 308–317. https://doi.org/10.1093/jamia/ocac227.

Riley, Wayne J. 2012. "Health Disparities: Gaps in Access, Quality and Affordability of Medical Care." *Transactions of the American Clinical and Climatological Association* 123: 167–174.

Rozier, Michael D., Kavita K. Patel, and Dori A. Cross. 2022. "Electronic Health Records as Biased Tools or Tools Against Bias: A Conceptual Model." *Milbank Quarterly* 100 (1) (March): 134–150. https://doi.org/10.1111/1468-0009.12545.

Sabin, Janice A. 2022. "Tackling Implicit Bias in Health Care." *New England Journal of Medicine* 387 (2) (July 14): 105–107. https://doi.org/10.1056/NEJMp2201180.

Sanders, Cynthia K., and Edward Scanlon. 2021. "The Digital Divide Is a Human Rights Issue: Advancing Social Inclusion through Social Work Advocacy." *Journal of Human Rights and Social Work* 6 (2) (June): 130–143. https://doi.org/10.1007/s41134-020-00147-9.

Smedley, Brian D., Adrienne Y. Stith, and Alan R. Nelson, eds. 2003. *Unequal Treatment: Confronting Racial and Ethnic Disparities in Health Care.* Institute of Medicine (US), Committee on Understanding and Eliminating Racial and Ethnic Disparities in Health Care. Washington, DC: National Academies. https://www.ncbi.nlm.nih.gov/books/NBK220358/.

Sun, Michael, Tomasz Oliwa, Monica E. Peek, and Elizabeth L. Tung. 2022. "Negative Patient Descriptors: Documenting Racial Bias in the Electronic Health Record." *Health Affairs* 41 (2) (February): 203–211. https://doi.org/10.1377/hlthaff.2021.01423.

Tertulien, Tarryn, Stephen T. Broughton, Gretchen Swabe, Utibe R. Essien, and Jared W. Magnani. 2022. "Association of Race and Ethnicity on the Management of Acute Non-ST-Segment Elevation Myocardial Infarction." *Journal of the American Heart Association* 11 (12) (June 21): e025758. https://doi.org/10.1161/JAHA.121.025758.

Turner, Laurah, Daniel A. Hashimoto, Shubha Vasisht, and Verity Schaye. 2024. "Demystifying AI: Current State and Future Role in Medical Education Assessment." *Academic Medicine* 99 (4S) (April): S42–S47. https://doi.org/10.1097/ACM.0000000000005598.

Umbrello, Steven, and Ibo van de Poel. 2021. "Mapping Value Sensitive Design onto AI for Social Good Principles." *AI and Ethics* 1 (3) (August): 283–296. https://doi.org/10.1007/s43681-021-00038-3.

Upadhyay, Soumya, and Han-fen Hu. 2022. "A Qualitative Analysis of the Impact of Electronic Health Records (EHR) on Healthcare Quality and Safety: Clinicians' Lived Experiences." *Health Services Insights* 15. https://doi.org/10.1177/11786329211070722.

VanderLeest, Steven H. 2004. "The Built-in Bias of Technology." Paper presented at the American Society for Engineering Education Annual Conference & Exposition, Salt Lake City, UT, June.

Vela, Monica B., Marshall H. Chin, and Monica E. Peek. 2021. "Keeping Our Promise—Supporting Trainees from Groups That Are Underrepresented in Medicine." *New England Journal of Medicine* 385 (6) (August 5): 487–489. https://doi.org/10.1056/NEJMp2105270.

Vela, Monica B., Amarachi I. Erondu, Nichole A. Smith, Monica E. Peek, James N. Woodruff, and Marshall H. Chin. 2022. "Eliminating Explicit and Implicit Biases in Health Care: Evidence and Research Needs." *Annual Review of Public Health* 43: 477–501. https://doi.org/10.1146/annurev-publhealth-052620-103528.

Verheij, Robert A., Vasa Curcin, Brendan C. Delaney, and Mark M. McGilchrist. 2018. "Possible Sources of Bias in Primary Care Electronic Health Record Data Use and Reuse." *Journal of Medical Internet Research* 20 (5) (May 29): e185. https://doi.org/10.2196/jmir.9134.

Vyas, Darshali A., Leo G. Eisenstein, and David S. Jones. 2020. "Hidden in Plain Sight—Reconsidering the Use of Race Correction in Clinical Algorithms." *New England Journal of Medicine* 383 (9) (August 27): 874–882. https://doi.org/10.1056/NEJMms2004740.

Weinstein, James N., Amy Geller, Yamrot Negussie, and Alina Baciu, eds. 2017. *Communities in Action: Pathways to Health Equity*. Washington, DC: National Academies. https://www.ncbi.nlm.nih.gov/books/NBK425848/.

Wheeler, Margaret, Shalila de Bourmont, Kimani Paul-Emile, Alanna Pfeffinger, Ashley McMullen, Jeff M. Critchfield, and Alicia Fernandez. 2019. "Physician and Trainee Experiences with Patient Bias." *JAMA Internal Medicine* 179 (12) (October 28): 1678–1685. https://doi.org/10.1001/jamainternmed.2019.4122.

Yan, Chao, Xinmeng Zhang, Yuyang Yang, Kaidi Kang, Martin C. Were, Peter Embí, et al. 2023. "Differences in Health Professionals' Engagement with Electronic Health Records Based on Inpatient Race and Ethnicity." *JAMA Network Open* 6 (10) (October 9): e2336383. https://doi.org/10.1001/jamanetworkopen.2023.36383.

Katharine Lawrence is a primary care physician, an Assistant Professor in the Department of Population Health at the NYU Grossman School of Medicine, and Clinical Innovations Lead at the Medical Center Information Technology (MCIT) FuturePractice at NYU Langone Health, New York, USA. She completed both her residency in internal medicine and a postdoctoral fellowship in healthcare delivery science at the NYU Grossman School of Medicine. Her research leverages digital innovations in healthcare—including telemedicine, remote patient monitoring, and generative AI for care delivery—to enhance patient-provider relationships, improve provider workflows and resilience, and promote digital health equity.

Chapter 14
Medical Data Privacy and Security in the AI Age

Sharona Hoffman

Abstract This chapter examines challenges to medical data privacy and security in the age of artificial intelligence (AI). It analyzes how AI intensifies concerns about health record privacy and security and evaluates key elements of federal legal oversight, including the HIPAA Privacy and Security Rules, the Americans with Disabilities Act (ADA), and the Genetic Information Nondiscrimination Act. The chapter identifies significant gaps in the current regulatory system, such as HIPAA's limited definition of covered entities, numerous exceptions allowing disclosure without consent, and lack of a private right of action. To address these shortcomings, the chapter proposes several reforms: expanding HIPAA's definition of covered entities, revising the ADA to prohibit discrimination based on AI-derived health predictions, mandating disclosure of AI use in decision-making, and potentially adding a private right of action for HIPAA breaches. These changes would go far to align US law with advancing AI capabilities and enhance Americans' medical data privacy.

Keywords Medical privacy · Data security · Health information disclosure · HIPAA Privacy Rule · Disability discrimination

14.1 Introduction

In May 2017, Google commenced a business relationship with the University of Chicago Medical Center (UCMC) by which UCMC would share its patients' electronic health records (EHRs) with Google. Google sought to use the EHR data to develop patented software that would employ machine learning to analyze the records, identify individuals' health conditions, and predict future medical problems. In June 2019, a former UCMC patient filed a class action in federal court against UCMC and Google. The complaint in *Dinerstein v. Google* (484 F. Supp. 3d 561 [N.D. Ill. 2020]) alleged that although the EHRs were largely de-identified, they improperly included date stamps for services as well as physicians' notes, which

S. Hoffman (✉)
Case Western Reserve University School of Law, Cleveland, OH, USA
e-mail: sharona.hoffman@case.edu

M. C. Altman and D. Schwan (eds.), *Ethics and Medical Technology*, The International Library of Bioethics 113, https://doi.org/10.1007/978-3-031-94690-5_14

could enable data re-identification. The plaintiff sought damages under various state statutory, tort, and contract theories. The court ultimately dismissed the case in part because the plaintiff failed to prove that the defendants' conduct caused him harm that justified money damages. But the *Dinerstein* claims highlight the tension that can exist between patient privacy and technological advancement, especially in the realm of artificial intelligence (AI) (Cassidy 2021, 3).

The allegations in *Dinerstein* grew out of a contractual relationship, but most privacy concerns arise in other ways. Data breaches and privacy violations are alarmingly common. Between October 2009 and December 2022, there were 5,150 large data breaches that exposed 382,262,109 healthcare records. Most commonly, contemporary breaches involve hacking (Murray-Watson 2024). Improper accessing and disclosure of personally identifiable health information can lead to a variety of harms, including loss of privacy, identity theft, and medical care disruption. In addition, data breach victims may experience financial losses, termination of employment, and even criminal prosecution if identity theft causes them to be wrongfully accused of misconduct (Perakslis et al. 2023, 529).

Privacy concerns have intensified as AI becomes prevalent in the medical arena. Some AI systems help diagnose, treat, or monitor patients. AI can also be used to assess the likelihood of patients' future health problems and to complete various administrative and office management tasks for healthcare providers. Insurers may develop AI to help review claims or complete other administrative tasks (Price et al. 2022, 123–124, 138–139).

As indicated in the *Dinerstein* case, AI algorithms that are used for all these purposes often need to be trained on vast amounts of data, and these data are gathered from healthcare providers, the Internet, or other sources (Marks and Haupt 2023; Minssen et al. 2023, 315). The flow of medical data to and from AI vendors makes health data more vulnerable to privacy breaches than ever before. Likewise, clinicians' use of tools such as ChatGPT, through which they disclose medical data to AI vendors, creates worrisome vulnerabilities.

A variety of federal and state laws address health information privacy and security, the most well-known of which is the HIPAA Privacy Rule. As used in this chapter, "data privacy" refers to the protection of data when they are collected, used, and shared (SNIA 2024). "Data security" is a more specific term that refers to mechanisms to protect "digital information from unauthorized access, corruption, destruction, modification, theft, or disclosure" (Taylor 2023).

American privacy provisions have always had significant gaps. These have been exacerbated, however, by the dual phenomena of AI development and increasingly sophisticated cyber-attacks.

This chapter will begin by describing the data privacy landscape. It will analyze why AI has intensified worries about health records' privacy and security. Next, the chapter will discuss three key elements of federal legal oversight: the HIPAA regulations, the Americans with Disabilities Act, and the Genetic Information Nondiscrimination Act. The chapter will also assess the troubling gaps that are embedded in the American regulatory system, and it will formulate recommendations for enhancing medical data protection.

14.2 Medical Data Privacy Threats

Individuals' medical data can be of great interest to a variety of parties. These parties include (1) employers who are seeking healthy employees; (2) lenders who hope their borrowers will be able to pay off loans; (3) advertisers and marketers who wish to tailor their ads to the needs of their recipients; (4) life, disability, and long-term care insurers that seek low-risk policy holders; and (5) hackers and other wrongdoers who perpetrate blackmail, fraud, and identity theft (Hoffman and Podgurski 2007, 334–335). Thus, medical information is valuable for anyone with an economic stake in people's health or with malicious intent to commit certain crimes.

Medical data security threats have been steadily growing in the last decade. In 2022, on average, 1.94 healthcare data breaches involving 500 or more health records (considered large breaches) were reported *every day*. By comparison, as recently as 2018, the number was one such breach per day. Between 2009 and 2023, a total of 5,789 large data breaches were reported to the US Department of Health and Human Services (HHS) Office of Civil Rights. 551 of these occurred in 2023 (Murray-Watson 2024). According to another source, over 112 million US patients had their data impermissibly exposed in 2023, a figure that is more than double the 2022 total of 48.6 million patients (Hales 2024).

To illustrate, one of the largest breaches in 2023 impacted 8,861,076 individuals, including patients and their parents, guardians, or guarantors. Managed Care of North America, a dental benefits administrator, had its systems infected with malicious code that enabled the attackers to access a wealth of personal information. This included "names, addresses, telephone numbers, email addresses, birth dates, Social Security numbers, driver's license numbers, government-issued ID numbers, health insurance information, Medicare/Medicaid ID numbers, group plan names and numbers, and information related to the dental and orthodontic care provided" (McKeon 2023). Some of the stolen data were leaked onto the dark web, and some data were held hostage for ransom.

14.2.1 The Dark Web

The dark web consists of hidden sites that are accessible only by means of special software and are not indexed by search engines such as Google, thus enabling website operators and users to avoid being identified or traced (Kumar and Rosenbach 2019). Many reported incidents have involved posting medical information on the dark web. In addition to the Managed Care of North America case, there were incidents at Miami's Leon Medical Centers, Texas' Nocona General Hospital (Collier 2021), and several Ontario hospitals (Wilhelm 2023). The material that was posted included personally identifying information, such as names, addresses, and birth dates, along with patients' diagnoses or procedures. Some hackers sell data on the dark web to individuals who then obtain medical care under a false identity so that the identity theft victims are billed for the services ("Hackers Are Stealing" 2019). Perpetrators can use false identities to commit other crimes as well. In some instances, hackers release a portion of the illegally obtained records onto the dark web in order to extort money from hacked organizations with the threat of releasing more files (Collier 2021).

14.2.2 Ransomware Attacks

A particularly threatening type of attack is ransomware, in which malware is used to encrypt files and prevent victims from accessing them and from using their devices. The perpetrators then demand a ransom in exchange for a decryption key (Cohen et al. 2017, 587). Attackers may post accessed data on the dark web if victims do not pay the ransom demanded.

For example, the infamous 2017 Wannacry ransomware attack was a coordinated, global attack allegedly launched by North Korea. In England alone, it infected at least eighty-one of the 236 National Health System hospitals along with 603 primary care and 595 other medical practices, causing over 19,000 appointments to be canceled (Riggi 2024). According to a study of US incidents, between January 2016 and October 2023, there were 539 ransomware attacks on 10,000 different healthcare facilities, and they affected over fifty-two million patient records (Olsen 2023).

14.2.3 Data Breach Harms and Litigation

Data breaches in the healthcare industry have led to a considerable amount of litigation and claims of compensable harm. A prominent example is the *Dinerstein* case discussed at the opening of this chapter (though the defendant ultimately prevailed). In other cases, plaintiffs asserted that data breaches caused them to experience more frequent suspicious calls, emails, and text messages; declines in their credit scores; fraudulent credit card charges; false unemployment benefits claims; fraudulent utility accounts established in their names; fraudulent bank or credit card accounts established in their names; posting of personal information on the dark web; and other harms. Plaintiffs sought damages based on numerous legal theories, including negligence, breach of contract, breach of implied contract, unjust enrichment, breach of implied covenant of good faith and fair dealing, breach of fiduciary duty, invasion of privacy, and violations of state statutes.[1] The reported cases generally involve

[1] See *Clemens v. ExecuPharm Inc.*, 48 F.4th 146 (3d Cir. 2022); *Resnick v. AvMed Inc.*, 693 F.3d 1317 (11th Cir. 2012); *In re Arthur J. Gallagher*, Data Breach Litig., 631 F. Supp. 3d 573 (N.D. Ill. 2022); *Graham v. Universal Health Serv., Inc.* 539 F. Supp. 3d 481 (E.D. Pa. 2021); *Opris v. Sincera Reprod. Med.*, 2022 WL 1639417 (E.D. Pa. May 24, 2022); *In re Blackbaud, Inc.*, Customer Data Breach Litig., 2021 WL 2718439 (D.S.C. July 1, 2021); *In re Am. Med. Collection Agency, Inc.*, Customer Data Sec. Breach Litig., 2021 WL 5937742 (D.N.J. Dec. 16, 2021); *In re Am. Med.*

motions to dismiss that are denied or partially denied by the courts, and several of the cases are known to have settled.[2]

14.3 Data Privacy and AI

AI's emergence in the field of healthcare has deepened concerns about privacy. Chatbots such as ChatGPT have generated particular anxiety because many people, including both patients and clinicians, now use them to seek medical information and advice. Chatbots are a form of large language models (LLMs), and LLMs are a type of generative AI system that creates "human-like language responses to a wide range of user questions and prompts" (Duffourc and Gerke 2023, 313). In response to queries, chatbots often prompt users to provide additional information for purposes of receiving better answers (Marks and Haupt 2023, 309). Clinicians may also use chatbots to efficiently produce medical notes, insurance documents, and other administrative material (Kanter and Packel 2023, 311).

If chatbots are not integrated into a healthcare organization, they likely are not subject to medical privacy laws (see Sects. 14.4.1 and 14.5.1). Thus, when individuals enter personal information for purposes of medical queries, they inadvertently provide chatbot developers (e.g., OpenAI) information that the companies could use for their own commercial purposes, such as selling it to marketers or data brokers (Marks and Haupt 2023). In addition, chatbots can be subject to software glitches, such as one in March 2023 that allowed ChatGPT users to see information about other users' chat histories and credit card details (Thorbecke 2023).

Another privacy challenge is that LLMs must be trained on massive data sets in order to function properly. Often, data sets are scraped from the Internet and other sources. These data may include personal information, and patients have no opportunity to object to their data's use for AI training purposes (Minssen et al. 2023, 315). In other instances, developers such as Google make special arrangements with healthcare entities to obtain patient records. These records are often purportedly de-identified to protect patient privacy, but AI may have the technological ability to re-identify "anonymized" data (Marks and Haupt 2023). One example of Google's AI pursuits was described in the *Dinerstein v. Google* case above. In another instance, Google undertook "Project Nightingale" in 2018, partnering with the largest US nonprofit health system, Ascension, to gain access to over fifty million patients' medical records in twenty-one states (Marks 2019).

Collection Agency, Inc., Customer Data Sec. Breach Litig., 2023 WL 6216542 (D.N.J. Sept. 21, 2023).

[2] See Saikali (2013) (reporting the outcome of *Resnick v. AvMed Inc.*); "Sincera Reproductive Medicine Data Breach" (2023) (reporting the outcome of the *Opris* case); "Blackbaud to Pay $49.5 Million" (2023) (reporting the outcome of the *In re Blackbaud, Inc.* case); Office of Attorney General, Commonwealth of Pennsylvania (2011) (announcing the outcome of the government's case against Am. Med. Collection Agency, Inc.).

AI can diminish medical privacy in another way as well. A *New York Times* writer who learned that researchers discovered his email by using the LLM GPT-3.5 Turbo warns of the "potential for ChatGPT, and generative A.I. tools like it, to reveal much more sensitive personal information with just a bit of tweaking" (White 2023). Indeed, AI can be used to derive health information about individuals from data that are not themselves health-related (Price 2021, 928–929). For example, purchasing records can indicate whether individuals go to a gym, eat nutritious food, smoke, refill their prescriptions, or are pregnant. Algorithms can infer a great deal about peoples' health status from their credit card purchasing records, grocery loyalty cards, earnings, demographics, and social media posts (Hoffman 2019, 132–134).

14.4 The Privacy and Anti-Discrimination Law Landscape

Numerous federal and state laws address medical privacy and security. The federal government's most comprehensive health privacy protection initiative consists of the Health Insurance Portability and Accountability Act (HIPAA) Privacy Rule and the HIPAA Security Rule (45 C.F.R. Part 160, 45 C.F.R. Part 164, Subpart A, E). This section discusses the key provisions of the HIPAA regulations.

American law also establishes a variety of anti-discrimination mandates that render certain data uses unlawful. Section 14.4.2 addresses two relevant federal laws: the Americans with Disabilities Act and the Genetic Information Nondiscrimination Act.

14.4.1 The HIPAA Privacy and Security Rules

In the Health Insurance Portability and Accountability Act of 1996, Congress required the Secretary of Health and Human Services to issue privacy regulations to govern individually identifiable health information if Congress did not itself pass privacy legislation within three years (US Department of Health and Human Services 2022a). The HIPAA Privacy Rule and the Security Rule took effect in 2003 and 2005, respectively. They were amended by the Health Information Technology for Economic and Clinical Health (HITECH) Act of 2009 (42 U.S.C.A. §§ 1320d to 1320d-9).

The HIPAA Privacy Rule protects health information that is individually identifiable and transmitted or maintained in electronic or other forms (45 C.F.R. § 160.103). It establishes standards for the disclosure of protected health information (PHI), allowing patients to retain a degree of control over their medical records. The Privacy Rule mandates that, with some exceptions that are discussed in Sect. 14.5.2, covered entities must obtain patients' authorization before disclosing their medical data to third parties such as employers and marketers (45 C.F.R. §§ 164.508-.510).

Another important HIPAA provision is the minimum necessary standard. Under this provision, parties lawfully requesting, using, or disclosing PHI must make reasonable efforts to limit the PHI to the minimum that is necessary to accomplish the task in question unless an exception applies (45 C.F.R. §§ 164.502[b], 164.514[d]).

The HIPAA Privacy Rule further requires that covered entities give patients notices of their privacy practices (45 C.F.R. § 164.520[a]) and allow patients to view their medical records, request that they be corrected, or ask for restrictions on their use (45 C.F.R. §§ 164.520, 164.522). Patients are also entitled to an accounting of PHI disclosures that were made in the last six years, with some exceptions (45 C.F.R. § 164.528). Furthermore, covered entities that experience breaches of unsecured data, such as incidents of hacking, must notify individuals whose data was exposed, HHS, and in cases of large breaches, the media (45 C.F.R. §§ 164.400-.408).[3]

The HIPAA Security Rule is less well-known but no less important. It delineates administrative, physical, and technical safeguards to protect the confidentiality, integrity, and availability of electronic health information (EHI) (45 C.F.R. §§ 164.302-.318). Administrative safeguards consist of security management processes, workforce security, information access management, security awareness and training, security incident procedures, and contingency plans (45 C.F.R. § 164.308). Of particular importance is the requirement that covered entities conduct risk assessments to identify their security vulnerabilities and determine how best to manage them. Physical safeguards include facility access controls, workstation security, and device and media controls (45 C.F.R. § 164.310). Technical safeguards are procedures to control EHI access (e.g., encryption), to audit EHI processing activities, to prevent improper modification or elimination of EHI, and to obtain authentication from anyone seeking EHI access (45 C.F.R. § 164.312). The regulations emphasize that the Security Rule is meant to be flexible and scalable, allowing covered entities to make judgments with respect to some of the requirements and to implement measures that are appropriate for their size, organizational structure, and risks (45 C.F.R. § 164.306[b]; American Medical Association 2024). HHS provides extensive Security Rule guidance material for covered entities (US Department of Health and Human Services 2023b).

The HIPAA Privacy and Security Rules provide important but limited privacy safeguards to American patients. They will be critiqued in Sect. 14.5.

14.4.2 Federal Anti-Discrimination Laws

Prohibiting unauthorized parties from accessing health information and implementing measures to prevent privacy violations is vital. But it is equally important

[3] The media must be notified if a breach involves "more than 500 residents of a State or jurisdiction" (45 C.F.R. § 164.406[a]). Unsecured protected health information means information "that is not rendered unusable, unreadable, or indecipherable to unauthorized persons through the use of a technology or methodology specified by the [HHS] Secretary," such as encryption (45 C.F.R. § 164.402).

to address the potential use of private medical information that any party possesses. Beyond the risk of hacking and other data breaches, a multitude of parties can lawfully acquire health information—for example, through preemployment examinations. Anyone with a financial stake in the health status of individuals, including employers, financial institutions, marketers, and others, might be tempted to use people's medical data to their own advantage and to the detriment of data subjects (Hoffman 2017, 778). Consequently, American law establishes a variety of anti-discrimination mandates to govern data utilization.

A prominent example is the Americans with Disabilities Act of 1990 (ADA). The ADA prohibits covered persons and entities from engaging in disability-based discrimination. Disability is defined as (1) a physical or mental impairment that substantially limits a major life activity, (2) a record of such an impairment, or (3) being regarded as having such an impairment (42 U.S.C.A. § 12102). Title I of the law applies to employers; Title II governs state and local government activities; and Title III regulates "public accommodations and services provided by private entities," such as banks, insurance offices, private educational institutions, and retailers (42 U.S.C.A. §§ 12101-89).

The ADA prohibits subjecting qualified individuals to adverse decisions and denying them services or opportunities because of their disabilities. To enjoy ADA protection, individuals with disabilities must be *qualified* for the opportunity or service in question. In the employment context, for example, this means that the person must be able to perform the essential job functions with or without a reasonable accommodation (42 U.S.C.A. § 12111[8]).

The ADA includes both non-discrimination and reasonable accommodation mandates. Covered entities must modify practices, policies, and procedures to accommodate individuals with disabilities so long as doing so is not unreasonably burdensome for the entity (42 U.S.C.A. § 12182[b][2][A]). To illustrate, physicians' offices should provide sign language interpreters to deaf patients but may not be required to make significant architectural modifications if doing so is structurally impossible or prohibitively expensive (ADA National Network 2020).

The Genetic Information Nondiscrimination Act (GINA) prohibits employers and health insurers from seeking genetic information and from discriminating against individuals based on genetic information (29 U.S.C.A. § 1182; 42 U.S.C.A. § 2000ff-1[a]). Consequently, employers and health insurers cannot make adverse decisions regarding individuals because of concern that genetic abnormalities may cause them to develop diseases in the future (29 U.S.C.A. § 1182[a]-[b]; 42 U.S.C.A. § 2000ff-1[a]).

14.5 Critique of the HIPAA Privacy and Security Rules

The HIPAA regulations are the most detailed and comprehensive medical privacy regulations in the United States, and therefore they merit careful analysis. While the HIPAA Rules provide important protections to the American public, those protections are characterized by several gaps. This section will focus on four primary limitations: (1) the definition of "covered entity," (2) the numerous Privacy Rule exceptions, (3) the definition of "protected health information," and (4) the absence of a private right of action (Hoffman 2016b, 275–279).

14.5.1 The Definition of "Covered Entities"

The HIPAA Privacy and Security Rules govern only a segment of parties that handle private health information. "Covered entities" are defined as including health plans, healthcare clearinghouses, healthcare providers who transmit health information electronically for purposes of HIPAA-relevant transactions, and their business associates (45 C.F.R. §§ 160.102-.103; 42 U.S.C.A. § 17934). Consequently, employers, marketers, website operators, and numerous other parties are left out even though they may handle vast amounts of health information (Hoffman and Podgurski 2007, 363–364).

Employers, for example, gain medical information by conducting medical inquiries and examinations to determine if individuals are qualified for particular jobs, as permitted by the ADA (42 U.S.C.A. § 12112[d]). They also can obtain records for purposes of workers' compensation claims, wellness programs, reasonable accommodation requests, or Family Medical Leave Act requests (Hoffman 2010, 409–410). The ADA has a brief provision mandating that medical data be "treated as confidential" and be kept in medical files that are separate from other employee records, but it provides no details as to how to achieve confidentiality. It also provides no guidance as to data security (42 U.S.C.A. § 12112[d][3][B]).

Patients themselves often willingly disclose data to noncovered entities, such as Fitbit vendors or website operators (Rutherford 2023, 354–358). To illustrate, WebMD's Symptom Checker asks users to provide details about their age, sex, zip code, email, and symptoms in order to identify their potential health conditions and suggest treatments. An additional example is mental health apps that connect users with licensed therapists, facilitate communication between therapists and patients, or even simulate therapy through AI tools such as automated chatbots (Park and West 2023). Individuals also divulge data about their own health through social media, blog posts, and other sources that are easily accessible to third parties who may have ill intent.

Purchasing information can likewise reveal a great deal about buyers. Retailers retain records of people's purchases of over-the-counter drugs, food, vitamins, home tests, and medical equipment. In one infamous case, Target discerned that a teen was pregnant and began sending her relevant marketing material, thereby alerting her father to her secret (Hill 2012). In the post-*Roe* era, the ability to extrapolate information about pregnancy may be particularly worrisome because it could lead to criminal prosecution of clinicians who provide reproductive care.

Even medical device manufacturers can obtain personal information about patients. Robots used for robotic surgery, for instance, collect detailed patient information before and during surgeries, which is then available to the companies that create the robots (Tschider 2021, 144–145; Rutherford 2023).

An entire industry of data brokers, which number in the thousands by some estimates, has emerged. Their business is to "buy, aggregate, disclose, and sell billions of data elements" and to build profiles of American citizens using proprietary algorithms (Electronic Privacy Information Center 2024; Weinberger 2023). Although their work consists of health data trafficking, data brokers are not covered entities.

Entities that are not covered by HIPAA remain free of its regulatory obligations. It is particularly worrisome that no matter how much health information they possess, they are not required to implement the HIPAA Security Rule's data security safeguards. In addition, noncovered entities are not bound by HIPAA's use and disclosure provisions. This leaves many of them at liberty to do as they please with individuals' most sensitive information, including employing it for AI development or marketing, without the data subjects' knowledge. This is not merely a hypothetical concern. As just one example, the Federal Trade Commission (FTC) filed a complaint against the mental health app BetterHelp for divulging users' IP addresses, emails, and intake questionnaire data to Meta, Snapchat, Criteo, and Pinterest, which sought the information for advertising purposes (In the Matter of BetterHelp 2023; Park and West 2023). The case alleged violations of Section 5 of the Federal Trade Commission Act, which prohibits "unfair or deceptive acts or practices in or affecting commerce." It settled for $7.8 million (15 U.S.C.A. § 45(a), (n); Nahara et al. 2023).

14.5.2 Permitted Disclosures without Consent

While the HIPAA Privacy Rule purports to furnish patients with control over their PHI, in truth, it features numerous exceptions that allow covered entities to disclose PHI without patients' knowledge or authorization. First, no consent is necessary when covered entities share patients' medical information for purposes of treatment, payment, and healthcare operations (45 C.F.R. § 164.506). Consequently, clinicians can consult colleagues, submit billing information to insurers, or handle data for any administrative reason without patients' knowledge. According to one estimate, up to 150 individuals, including doctors, nurses, medical technicians, and billing clerks, see a patient's records during a typical hospitalization (Foreman 2006).

Furthermore, covered entities need not obtain patient authorization for disclosures that are necessary for: (1) compliance with legal requirements; (2) public health activities; (3) handling cases of victim abuse, neglect, or domestic violence; (4) health oversight activities; (5) judicial and administrative proceedings; (6) law enforcement; (7) cadaveric organ, eye, or tissue donation; (8) medical research (with certain privacy safeguards in place); (9) averting a serious threat to health or safety; (10) specialized government functions, such as national security and intelligence activities; and (11) workers' compensation (45 C.F.R. §§ 164.502, 164.512).

The HIPAA exceptions are generally reasonable and logical. However, the HIPAA Privacy Rule is arguably less about patient consent than it is simply about notifying patients of how their data may be lawfully shared. Indeed, Americans often have little awareness of who is viewing their medical information and for what purposes it is being used.

14.5.3 "Protected Health Information" Definition and Data De-identification

It is also important to understand that the HIPAA Privacy and Security Rules protect a limited scope of data. The regulations define protected health information (PHI) as "individually identifiable health information" that is electronically or otherwise transmitted or maintained (45 C.F.R. § 160.103). Great volumes of information, however, are stored in de-identified form in databases used for research, quality assessment, public health initiatives, and AI development (Hoffman and Podgurski 2013). Properly de-identified data are entirely exempt from coverage by the HIPAA Privacy and Security Rules (45 C.F.R. § 46.116; Rothstein 2010, 4). Therefore, no patient authorization is needed for their use, and the HIPAA Security Rule standards do not apply to their storage.

The HIPAA Privacy Rule provides instructions regarding de-identification, and HHS has published detailed guidance about it (US Department of Health and Human Services 2022b). Health information can be deemed de-identified if: (1) a qualified expert determines that there is only a "very small" possibility that the data can be re-identified, and (2) the expert documents the analysis (45 C.F.R. § 164.514[b][1]).

In the alternative, covered entities can remove eighteen listed items to meet HIPAA de-identification standards (45 C.F.R. § 164.514[b][2][i]). These include names, geographic data, social security numbers, telephone numbers, email addresses, photographic images, and more.[4]

It is important to recognize, however, that even the most meticulous de-identification efforts cannot yield a guarantee that records will not be re-identified. As two prominent scholars explain, "the substantial increase in available personal information and advances in computing mean that individuals can often be identified in deidentified data by triangulating data sources" (Cohen and Mello 2019, 1141). For example, geolocation and other smartphone data could potentially be matched with

---

[4] In addition, information will not be considered de-identified if an entity has "actual knowledge that the information could be used alone or in combination with other information to identify an individual who is a subject of the information" (45 C.F.R. § 164.514[b][2][ii]). Note, however, that the HIPAA Privacy Rule relaxes the de-identification requirements for three purposes: research, public health, and healthcare operations. It allows covered entities to disclose "limited data sets" for these three uses without patient consent if data recipients sign data use agreements containing specified restrictions and privacy protections. Limited data sets remove most of the above-listed elements, but they retain dates and geographic locales, though not patients' exact addresses (45 C.F.R. § 164.514[e][1]-[4]).

de-identified EHRs that contain date stamps and physician notes (as in the *Dinerstein* case) to ascertain patients' identities. In fact, AI itself can be used to enable re-identification. To illustrate, in one study, researchers employed deep learning techniques to derive identities from chest x-rays (Price 2021, 926–929; Packhäuser et al. 2022).

One commentator points out that while AI raises privacy concerns, it could also be employed to enhance privacy protections and achieve more thorough de-identification (Price 2021). This is a promising path for future privacy and security endeavors.

14.5.4 No Private Cause of Action

The HIPAA Privacy and Security Rules do not offer data breach victims a private cause of action. Consequently, HIPAA enforcement is left entirely to the HHS Office for Civil Rights (OCR) and state attorneys general offices (45 C.F.R. § 160.306; 42 U.S.C.A. § 1320d-5[d]).

HIPAA authorizes the government to punish violators with harsh fines and imprisonment (42 U.S.C. §§ 1320d-5-d-6). On its website, OCR indicates that between 2003 and 2023 it received over 345,000 HIPAA complaints, and it initiated 1,179 compliance reviews on its own (US Department of Health and Human Services 2023a). OCR investigated and resolved 30,514 of these cases by offering technical assistance and requiring corrective action. In addition, OCR reached settlements or imposed civil money penalties in 138 cases, collecting a total of $137,018,772. OCR, however, found no HIPAA violation with respect to the vast majority of complaints it received.

State attorneys general have usually imposed penalties in only a handful of cases each year. However, 2023 was a particularly productive year for them, with fifteen cases listed as yielding penalties (Adler 2023).

In order to pursue personal remedies, aggrieved individuals must file state tort actions (Winn 2002). But prevailing in such cases can be challenging. First, data breach victims must show that they suffered actual harm, which often is not obvious (Citron and Solove 2022, 793). Second, breach of confidentiality lawsuits require that the plaintiff and defendant have a relationship of confidentiality, such as a doctor-patient relationship. If the wrongdoer is an insurer, clearinghouse, or business associate, that direct relationship will not exist (Oates 2007, 745).

Vigorous enforcement by federal and state agencies depends on resources and staffing, and private litigation depends on the ability to prove all elements of the relevant cause of action. Consequently, some covered entities may not be adequately incentivized to achieve full HIPAA compliance. They may calculate that regulatory violations are unlikely to be detected and severely punished and thus may not invest adequately in data security.

14.6 Predictive Data and Disability Discrimination Laws

The privacy laws are not the only statutes that exhibit shortcomings in the face of contemporary AI capabilities. Disability discrimination laws are also lacking. AI can be used to predict individuals' future health problems. Researchers have employed AI to analyze EHRs and other patient data to forecast liver disease, heart disease, Alzheimer's disease, cancers, and other conditions (Ghaffar Nia et al. 2023). It is possible that third parties such as employers will obtain these predictions through data brokers or other sources and exploit them for discriminatory purposes.

Recall that the ADA prohibits disability discrimination. But it is important to recognize that the law does not address discrimination based on predictions of future health problems unless they are based on detected genetic abnormalities and are covered by GINA. Rather, the ADA prohibits discrimination based on current disabilities, past disabilities, or being wrongly regarded as currently having a disability (42 U.S.C. § 12102[1]). It does not reach healthy individuals who are subjected to discrimination because they are suspected of being at risk of future health problems. Consequently, under the ADA, employers, lenders, educational institutions, or others are free to reject applicants or deprive individuals of opportunities because of anticipated medical conditions. Indeed, it may be difficult to resist the temptation of harnessing such data to avoid business risks and costs.

AI also raises concerns about algorithmic bias and discrimination. I have written about this topic elsewhere (Hoffman and Podgurski 2020), and it is covered in Chap. 3 of this book.

14.7 Aligning the Law with Technology

The federal privacy and disability discrimination laws discussed in this chapter were enacted several decades ago. In light of advancing technological and AI capabilities, they now feature significant statutory gaps. This section offers several strategies for addressing these shortcomings.

14.7.1 Expanding HIPAA's Definition of Covered Entity

Thanks to AI, a great deal of information can generate inferences about an individual's health status. Data sources are no longer limited to healthcare providers, insurers, billing companies, or their direct business associates (45 C.F.R. §§ 160.102-.103; 42 U.S.C.A. § 17934). Consequently, the definition of "covered entity" should be expanded to provide more comprehensive protection to the American public (Hoffman 2016a, 73–75; Hoffman 2019, 156–159).

A Texas statute features a broad definition of "covered entity" that could serve as a model for the HIPAA Privacy Rule. The law covers any person who,

> for commercial, financial, or professional gain, monetary fees, or dues, or on a cooperative, nonprofit, or pro bono basis, engages, in whole or in part, and with real or constructive knowledge, in the practice of assembling, collecting, analyzing, using, evaluating, storing, or transmitting protected health information. The term includes a business associate, health care payer, governmental unit, information or computer management entity, school, health researcher, health care facility, clinic, health care provider, or person who maintains an Internet site. (Tex. Health & Safety Code Ann. § 181.001[b][2][A]).

Protected health information should likewise be defined broadly to consist of "individually identifiable health information about an individual, including demographic information, which relates to the individual's past, present, or future physical or mental health condition, provision of health care, or payment for the provision of health care" (25 Tex. Admin. Code § 1.501). Unlike HIPAA's definition, this definition captures all health information, regardless of its source, and is not limited to data created or received by certain parties.[5]

These changes would have important benefits for data subjects. The "covered entity" definition would explicitly extend to website operators, which have raised significant privacy concerns. It is not, however, overly broad and would not, for instance, cover casual discussions among friends that relate to someone's health problems.

New covered entities would not be permitted to disclose PHI to third parties such as data brokers without patients' consent. When they lawfully disclose data, they would have to comply with the minimum necessary standard (45 C.F.R. § 164.502[b]). Upon request, they would need to provide patients with an accounting of PHI disclosures. Of particular importance would be the need to comply with the requirements of the HIPAA Security Rule for purposes of storing and processing PHI responsibly (Hoffman 2019; see Sect. 14.4.1).

In 2023, the FTC began pursuing health privacy enforcement actions against companies not covered by HIPAA for improper use and disclosure of health information. But such FTC actions are few in number, and the agency may only act when it deems an entity's conduct to be "unfair or deceptive" (15 U.S.C.A. § 45[a], [n]; Daniel and Kwon 2024). FTC enforcement, therefore, is not adequate to deter most health privacy violations and protect Americans who may be affected by them.

The proposed change may also benefit covered entities. Currently, some states have broad privacy laws that extend well beyond HIPAA (Huddleston and Salihu 2023). Other states have privacy laws that vary in scope. The state laws create a patchwork that can be confusing and burdensome for regulated entities, especially if they operate in multiple locations. The proposed broad definition of covered entities

---

[5] Currently, "health information" is defined more narrowly as information that "(1) Is created or received by a health care provider, health plan, public health authority, employer, life insurer, school or university, or health care clearinghouse; and (2) Relates to the past, present, or future physical or mental health or condition of an individual; the provision of health care to an individual; or the past, present, or future payment for the provision of health care to an individual" (45 C.F.R. § 160.103).

would create a uniform, national standard for determining which entities are covered by privacy regulations.

14.7.2 Revising the ADA

Predictive information about individuals' future health problems is becoming increasingly available. Consequently, the ADA and equivalent state laws should be amended to prohibit discrimination based on speculation that individuals who are now healthy will develop disabilities in the future.

A simple ADA modification could achieve this change. The ADA currently defines disability as including "being regarded as having such an impairment [i.e. a disability]" (42 U.S.C.A. § 12102[1][C]). This language could be amended to add "or are perceived as likely to develop such an impairment in the future" (Hoffman 2019, 158).

The proposed revision would not require employers or others to provide any additional reasonable accommodations. Individuals who are subjected to discrimination because of disease predictions would be healthy at present and therefore not require accommodations. Moreover, the ADA states explicitly that individuals who are covered solely based on being regarded as disabled (rather than being actually disabled) are not entitled to accommodations (42 U.S.C.A. § 12201[h]).

Proving discrimination is always challenging because it requires delving into the defendant's thought process and intent. Proving that a party regarded a healthy person as disabled or as likely to become disabled may be even more challenging. But, failing to recognize their vulnerability to an ADA challenge, some defendants might themselves inadvertently admit that they believe an individual is likely to develop an illness. In other cases, an affected individual may learn that defendants obtained predictive information shortly before taking adverse action. Employers, for example, are permitted to request workers' medical records to determine if they are qualified for particular job duties (42 U.S.C.A § 12,112(d)[3]-[4]). Medical records may contain risk assessments concerning potential future illnesses or could undergo AI analysis that derives health predictions from available data. Furthermore, the AI disclosure rule proposed in Sect. 14.7.3 would alert individuals to AI use and thus make it easier for them to prove that they were subjected to discrimination because of predictive analysis.

It makes little sense to prohibit discrimination based on predictive genetic information in GINA but to allow discrimination based on disease predictions that are rooted in other types of data and AI analysis. The proposed change, therefore, would align the ADA with GINA and promote uniformity among the anti-discrimination laws.

When Congress passed the ADA in 1990, it did not anticipate the widespread use of AI in medicine. Now, however, the law must be modified to account for new technologies and extend adequate protection to contemporary Americans.

14.7.3 Disclosing AI Use

Individuals will not be able to discern that they have been harmed by AI if they are unaware that it was utilized. Consequently, it is important that the law require disclosure of AI use in settings that might harm individuals (Hoffman 2017, 791–792).

A New York City law called "Automated Employment Decision Tools" provides a useful model as a disclosure mandate (N.Y.C. Admin. Code § 20–870 et seq.). This law requires New York City employers that use automated decision tools to screen candidates to disclose the tool's use to applicants who reside in New York City "no less than ten business days before such use and [to] allow a candidate to request an alternative selection process or accommodation." The disclosure must include the "job qualifications and characteristics" that the tool will assess. In addition, information about the type of data collected for the AI, its source, and the employer's data retention policy must be available on the employer's website or sent to candidates and employees upon written request within thirty days of the request.[6]

There is no reason that these prudent requirements should be limited to employers in New York City. For purposes of employment, the ADA should be amended to add a federal AI use disclosure mandate. With respect to medical data specifically, the statutory provision that governs medical examinations and inquiries could be revised to require employers to inform applicants and workers of any AI use intended to gather health information (42 U.S.C.A. § 12112[d]; Hoffman 2017, 791–792).

As noted in Sect. 14.2 above, numerous entities, such as lenders, insurers, educational institutions, and others have much to gain from health information about individuals. AI can enable actors to derive health data from countless sources other than medical records, and thus it exacerbates concerns about health privacy. Consequently, Congress would be wise to consider passing a federal law that requires any party that uses AI for purposes of making decisions about individuals to disclose AI use in a manner similar to that detailed in the New York City law.

14.7.4 Other Improvements

Right of action. State common law provides potential litigation vehicles for data breach victims, and both the federal and state governments are empowered to pursue enforcement actions. HHS and state attorneys general offices should ensure that HIPAA Privacy and Security Rule enforcement is a priority. Furthermore, to ensure that all HIPAA-covered entities are fully accountable for privacy violations, Congress could amend HIPAA's penalty provision (42 U.S.C.A. § 1320d-5) to add a private

[6] The New York City law also prohibits employers from using automated decision tools to screen candidates unless the tool has been subjected to an independent bias audit no more than a year before it is used, and the audit results are published on the employer's website. The audit is designed to ensure that the tool does not raise disparate impact discrimination concerns.

right of action. So long as successful plaintiffs must prove specific harm, this change will not open the floodgates of litigation or dramatically increase costs for covered entities.

Data Security Guidance and AI Utilization. Technology is evolving at a dizzying speed in ways that both benefit healthcare consumers and enable cyber attackers to detect and exploit security vulnerabilities more easily. Consequently, security regulations that are too rigid and specific are likely to become quickly outdated. Regulators must balance the dual goals of providing covered entities with adequate security guidance and ensuring that regulations are supple enough to remain useful in the long run. To support covered entities, HHS should continue to develop guidance documents that respond to emerging security threats. In addition, while AI can raise privacy concerns, it can also meaningfully enhance data security. Experts should harness AI capabilities to help de-identify data and promote greater protections for data subjects (Price 2021).

14.8 Conclusion

The HIPAA Privacy and Security Rules made important contributions to medical privacy in the early twenty-first century. Nevertheless, the work of ensuring comprehensive legal privacy protections in the United States is far from complete. This chapter has highlighted some of the existing regulatory shortcomings and called for reforms to help usher American law into the AI era.

References

ADA National Network. 2020. "Healthcare and the Americans with Disabilities Act." https://adata.org/factsheet/health-care-and-ada.

Adler, Steve. 2023. "HIPAA Enforcement by State Attorneys General." *HIPAA Journal*. September 1. https://www.hipaajournal.com/hipaa-enforcement-by-state-attorneys-general/.

American Medical Association. 2024. "HIPAA Security Rule and Risk Analysis." Accessed August 17, 2024. https://www.ama-assn.org/practice-management/hipaa/hipaa-security-rule-risk-analysis.

"Blackbaud to Pay $49.5 Million in Data Breach Settlement." 2023. Hunton Andrews Kurth. October 12. https://www.huntonprivacyblog.com/2023/10/12/blackbaud-to-pay-49-5-million-in-data-breach-settlement/.

Cassidy, Julia A. 2021. "Insights from the Google Health Data Lawsuit and the Competing Interests of Data, Technology, and Privacy." *Journal of Health and Life Sciences Law* 15 (1) (March): 2–10.

Citron, Danielle Keats, and Daniel J. Solove. 2022. "Privacy Harms." *Boston University Law Review* 102 (3) (April): 793–863. https://doi.org/10.2139/ssrn.3782222.

Cohen, I. Glenn, Sharona Hoffman, and Eli Y. Adashi. 2017. "Your Money or Your Patient's Life? Ransomware and Electronic Health Records." *Annals of Internal Medicine* 167 (8) (October 17): 587–588. https://doi.org/10.7326/M17-1312.

Cohen, I. Glenn, and Michelle M. Mello. 2019. "Big Data, Big Tech, and Protecting Patient Privacy." *JAMA: Journal of the American Medical Association* 322 (12) (August 9): 1141–1142. https://doi.org/10.1001/jama.2019.11365.

Collier, Kevin. 2021. "Hackers Post Detailed Patient Medical Records from Two Hospitals to the Dark Web." *NBC News*. February 5. https://www.nbcnews.com/tech/security/hackers-post-detailed-patient-medical-records-two-hospitals-dark-web-n1256887.

Daniel, Jodi, and Allison Kwon. 2024. "Recent Policy Changes in Health Data Privacy: Federal and State Policy Makers Scrutinize Non-HIPAA Health Data Use." *Westlaw Journal Health Law* 31 (11) (February 12): 3. https://today.westlaw.com/Document/I906f69ccbeb611ee8921fbef1a541940/View/FullText.html.

Duffourc, Mindy, and Sara Gerke. 2023. "Generative AI in Health Care and Liability Risks for Physicians and Safety Concerns for Patients." *JAMA: Journal of the American Medical Association* 330 (4) (July 6): 313–314. https://doi.org/10.1001/jama.2023.9630.

Electronic Privacy Information Center. 2024. "Data Brokers." Accessed August 17, 2024. https://epic.org/issues/consumer-privacy/data-brokers/.

Foreman, Judy. 2006. "At Risk of Exposure." *Los Angeles Times*. June 26. http://articles.latimes.com/2006/jun/26/health/he-privacy26.

Ghaffar Nia, Nafiseh, Erkan Kaplanoglu, and Ahad Nasab. 2023. "Evaluation of Artificial Intelligence Techniques in Disease Diagnosis and Prediction." *Discover Artificial Intelligence* 3: article no. 5. https://doi.org/10.1007/s44163-023-00049-5.

"Hackers Are Stealing Millions of Medical Records—and Selling Them on the Dark Web." 2019. *CBS News*. February 14. https://www.cbsnews.com/news/hackers-steal-medical-records-sell-them-on-dark-web/.

Hales, Maggie. 2024. "Trends from the Ten Largest Healthcare Data Breaches of 2023." *HIPAA E-Tool*. January 2. https://thehipaaetool.com/trends-from-the-ten-largest-healthcare-data-breaches-of-2023/.

Hill, Kashmir. 2012. "How Target Figured Out a Teen Girl Was Pregnant Before Her Father Did." *Forbes*. February 16. https://www.forbes.com/sites/kashmirhill/2012/02/16/how-target-figured-out-a-teen-girl-was-pregnant-before-her-father-did/.

Hoffman, Sharona. 2010. "Employing E-Health: The Impact of Electronic Health Records on the Workplace." *Kansas Journal of Law and Public Policy* 19 (3) (Spring): 409–432. https://core.ac.uk/download/pdf/214106457.pdf.

Hoffman, Sharona. 2016a. *Electronic Health Records and Medical Big Data: Law and Policy*. New York: Cambridge University Press.

Hoffman, Sharona. 2016b. "Medical Privacy and Security." In *The Oxford Handbook of U.S. Health Law*, edited by I. Glenn Cohen, Allison K. Hoffman, and William M. Sage, 267–290. New York: Oxford University Press. https://doi.org/10.1093/oxfordhb/9780199366521.013.13.

Hoffman, Sharona. 2017. "Big Data and the Americans with Disabilities Act." *Hastings Law Journal* 68 (4) (May): 777–794. https://repository.uclawsf.edu/hastings_law_journal/vol68/iss4/2.

Hoffman, Sharona. 2019. "What Genetic Testing Teaches about Predictive Health Analytics Regulation." *North Carolina Law Review* 98 (1): 123–163. https://scholarship.law.unc.edu/nclr/vol98/iss1/5.

Hoffman, Sharona, and Andy Podgurski. 2007. "In Sickness, Health and Cyberspace: Protecting the Security of Electronic Private Health Information." *Boston College Law Review* 48 (2) (March): 331–386. https://scholarlycommons.law.case.edu/faculty_publications/141.

Hoffman, Sharona, and Andy Podgurski. 2013. "The Use and Misuse of Biomedical Data: Is Bigger Really Better?" *American Journal of Law & Medicine* 39 (4) (December): 497–538. https://doi.org/10.1177/009885881303900401.

Hoffman, Sharona, and Andy Podgurski. 2020. "Artificial Intelligence and Discrimination in Health Care." *Yale Journal of Health Policy, Law and Ethics* 19 (3): 1–49. http://hdl.handle.net/20.500.13051/5964.

Huddleston, Jennifer, and Gent Salihu. 2023. "The Patchwork Strikes Back: State Data Privacy Laws after the 2022–2023 Legislative Session." CATO Institute. July 6. https://www.cato.org/blog/patchwork-strikes-back-state-data-privacy-laws-after-2022-2023-legislative-session-0.

In the Matter of BetterHelp, Inc. 2023. Complaint Before the Federal Trade Commission. Docket No. C-4796. https://www.ftc.gov/system/files/ftc_gov/pdf/2023169betterhelpcomplaintfinal.pdf.

Kanter, Genevieve P., and Eric A. Packel. 2023. "Health Care Privacy Risks of AI Chatbots." *JAMA: Journal of the American Medical Association* 330 (4) (July 6): 311–312. https://doi.org/10.1001/jama.2023.9618.

Kumar, Aditi, and Eric Rosenbach. 2019. "The Truth about the Dark Web." *International Monetary Fund*. September. https://www.imf.org/en/Publications/fandd/issues/2019/09/the-truth-about-the-dark-web-kumar.

Marks, Mason. 2019. "The Right Question to Ask about Google's Project Nightingale." *Slate*. November 20. https://slate.com/technology/2019/11/google-ascension-project-nightingale-emergent-medical-data.html.

Marks, Mason, and Claudia E. Haupt. 2023. "AI Chatbots, Health Privacy, and Challenges to HIPAA Compliance." *JAMA: Journal of the American Medical Association* 330 (4) (July 6): 309–310. https://doi.org/10.1001/jama.2023.9458.

McKeon, Jill, ed. 2023. "Biggest Healthcare Data Breaches Reported This Year, So Far." *Health IT Security*. June 26. https://healthitsecurity.com/features/biggest-healthcare-data-breaches-reported-this-year-so-far.

Minssen, Timo, Effy Vayena, and I. Glenn Cohen. 2023. "The Challenges for Regulating Medical Use of ChatGPT and Other Large Language Models." *JAMA: Journal of the American Medical Association* 330 (4) (July 6): 315–316. https://doi.org/10.1001/jama.2023.9651.

Murray-Watson, Rebecca. 2024. "Healthcare Data Breach Statistics." *HIPAA Journal*. Accessed January 18, 2025. https://www.hipaajournal.com/healthcare-data-breach-statistics/.

Nahara, Kirk J., Ali A. Jessani, Arianna Evers, and Samuel Kane. 2023. "FTC Continues Enforcement Focus on the Use and Disclosure of Health Information for Advertising." WilmerHale. March 7. https://www.wilmerhale.com/en/insights/client-alerts/20230307-ftc-continues-enforcement-focus-on-the-use-and-disclosure-of-health-information-for-advertising.

Oates, Daniel J. 2007. "HIPAA Hypocrisy and the Case for Enforcing Federal Privacy Standards under State Law." *Seattle University Law Review* 30 (3) (Spring): 745–776. https://digitalcommons.law.seattleu.edu/sulr/vol30/iss3/5/.

Office of Attorney General, Commonwealth of Pennsylvania. 2021. "AG Shapiro Announces Multistate Settlement with American Medical Collection Agency over 2019 Data Breach." March 11. https://www.attorneygeneral.gov/taking-action/ag-shapiro-announces-multistate-settlement-with-american-medical-collection-agency-over-2019-data-breach/.

Olsen, Emily. 2023. "Ransomware Attacks on Healthcare Facilities Cost $77.5B in Downtime, Report Finds." *Healthcare Dive*. October 27. https://www.healthcaredive.com/news/healthcare-ransomware-costs-comparitech-77-billion/698044/.

Packhäuser, Kai, Sebastian Gündel, Nicolas Münster, Christopher Syben, Vincent Christlein, and Andreas Maier. 2022. "Deep Learning-Based Patient Re-identification is Able to Exploit the Biometric Nature of Medical Chest X-ray Data." *Scientific Reports* 12: article no. 14851. https://doi.org/10.1038/s41598-022-19045-3.

Park, Eugene, and Darrell M. West. 2023. "Why Mental Health Apps Need to Take Privacy More Seriously." *Brookings*, November 30. https://www.brookings.edu/articles/why-mental-health-apps-need-to-take-privacy-more-seriously/.

Perakslis, Eric D., Megan L. Ranney, and Jennifer C. Goldsack. 2023. "Characterizing Cyber Harms from Digital Health." *Nature Medicine* 29 (3) (March): 528–531. https://doi.org/10.1038/s41591-022-02167-6.

Price, W. Nicholson II. 2021. "Problematic Interactions between AI and Health Privacy." *Utah Law Review* 2021 (4): 925–936. https://doi.org/10.26054/0d-th4e-sgvq.

Price, W. Nicholson II, Rachel E. Sachs, and Rebecca S. Eisenberg. 2022. "New Innovation Models in Medical AI." *Washington University Law Review* 99 (4): 1121–1174. https://openscholarship.wustl.edu/law_scholarship/293.

Riggi, John. 2024. "Ransomware Attacks on Hospitals Have Changed." *American Hospital Association Center for Health Innovation.* Accessed August 17, 2024. https://www.aha.org/center/cybersecurity-and-risk-advisory-services/ransomware-attacks-hospitals-have-changed.

Rothstein, Mark A. 2010. "Is Deidentification Sufficient to Protect Health Privacy in Research?" *American Journal of Bioethics* 10 (9) (September): 3–11. https://doi.org/10.1080/15265161.2010.494215.

Rutherford, Erin. 2023. "The Health Care Industry Is Ready for a Revolution: Its Privacy Laws Are Not." *Minnesota Journal of Law, Science and Technology* 24 (2): 345–374. https://scholarship.law.umn.edu/mjlst/vol24/iss2/6.

Saikali, Al. 2013. "$3,000,000 Settlement Reached in Data Breach Lawsuit." *Privacy & Data Security Law Journal.* October 22. https://www.datasecuritylawjournal.com/2013/10/22/3000000-settlement-reached-in-data-breach-lawsuit/.

"Sincera Reproductive Medicine Data Breach $1.2M Class Action Settlement." 2023. *Top Class Actions.* June 6. https://topclassactions.com/lawsuit-settlements/closed-settlements/sincera-reproductive-medicine-data-breach-1-2m-class-action-settlement/.

SNIA (Storage Networking Industry Association). 2024. "What Is Data Privacy?" Accessed August 17, 2024. https://www.snia.org/education/what-is-data-privacy.

Taylor, Sebastian. 2023. "Data Security." Corporate Finance Institute. October 23. https://corporatefinanceinstitute.com/resources/data-science/data-security/.

Thorbecke, Catherine. 2023. "Don't Tell Anything to a Chatbot You Want to Keep Private." *CNN.* April 6. https://www.cnn.com/2023/04/06/tech/chatgpt-ai-privacy-concerns/index.html.

Tschider, Charlotte A. 2021. "AI's Legitimate Interest: Towards a Public Benefit Privacy Model." *Houston Journal of Health Law and Policy* 21 (1): 125–184. https://houstonhealthlaw.scholasticahq.com/article/31666-ai-s-legitimate-interest-towards-a-public-benefit-privacy-model.

US Department of Health and Human Services. 2022a. "Summary of the HIPAA Privacy Rule." October 19. https://www.hhs.gov/hipaa/for-professionals/privacy/laws-regulations/index.html.

US Department of Health and Human Services. 2022b. "Guidance Regarding Methods for De-identification of Protected Health Information in Accordance with the Health Insurance Portability and Accountability Act (HIPAA) Privacy Rule." October 25. https://www.hhs.gov/hipaa/for-professionals/privacy/special-topics/de-identification/index.html.

US Department of Health and Human Services. 2023a. "Enforcement Highlights." December 15. https://www.hhs.gov/hipaa/for-professionals/compliance-enforcement/data/enforcement-highlights/index.html.

US Department of Health and Human Services. 2023b. "Security Rule Guidance Material." October 18. https://www.hhs.gov/hipaa/for-professionals/security/guidance/index.html.

Weinberger, Evan. 2023. "Data Brokers Eyed by CFPB for Selling Sensitive Info for Ads, AI." *Bloomberg Law.* August 15. https://news.bloomberglaw.com/banking-law/data-brokers-eyed-by-cfpb-for-selling-sensitive-info-for-ads-ai.

White, Jeremy. 2023. "How Strangers Got My Email Address from ChatGPT's Model." *New York Times.* December 22. https://www.nytimes.com/interactive/2023/12/22/technology/openai-chatgpt-privacy-exploit.html.

Wilhelm, Trevor. 2023. "Fourth Data Dump of Stolen Hospital Data Hits the Dark Web." *Windsor Star.* November 8. https://windsorstar.com/news/local-news/fourth-data-dump-of-stolen-hospital-data-hits-the-dark-web.

Winn, Peter A. 2002. "Confidentiality in Cyberspace: The HIPAA Privacy Rules and the Common Law." *Rutgers Law Journal* 33 (3) (Spring): 617–682.

Sharona Hoffman is the Edgar A. Hahn Professor of Law, Professor of Bioethics, and Co-Director of the Law-Medicine Center at Case Western Reserve University, USA. She has written over seventy journal articles and book chapters on health law and civil rights topics as well as two books. Much of her recent scholarship focuses on health information technology, aging, and public health. During sabbatical semesters, Dr. Hoffman worked with the Centers for Disease Control and Prevention and the National Institutes of Health. She has lectured nationally and internationally and frequently appears in the media. For more information see her website: http://sharonahoffman.com/.

Chapter 15
Surveillance Capitalism and the Right to Medical Privacy

Lauren Nuckols

Abstract This chapter examines medical privacy issues presented by surveillance capitalism outside the legally confidential clinical context. Working with family resemblance accounts of privacy, I argue that for-profit medical data commodification practices, including data collection, aggregation, predictive modeling, and sale, undermine informational and decisional medical privacy without sufficient justification. Although some privacy infringements may be justifiable with voluntary informed consent, for medical research or to prevent significant and likely harm to public health, for-profit data commodification practices do not usually serve the public interest, and meaningful voluntary informed consent usually is not obtained. These privacy infringements expose people to a number of harms, including chilling effects, emotional distress, intrusive targeted advertising, manipulation, decisional interference, and in some cases, legal repercussions, particularly in the wake of the *Dobbs* decision. I conclude by calling for improved legal and technical privacy protections, transparent privacy policies, and the minimization of unnecessary medical data collection.

Keywords Medical privacy · Surveillance · Big data

15.1 Introduction

Digital technologies have enabled the collection and commodification of medical data at an unprecedented scale. Personal medical data are created, collected, and inferred through search histories, web browsing activity, messages, apps, social media activity, purchase histories, surveys, sensors, and other sources (Terry 2013; Glenn and Monteith 2014). Location data are collected from smartphones, allowing for precise location tracking that can include visits to specific medical providers and services (Michael and Clarke 2013; Glenn and Monteith 2014). Newer vehicles from all major car manufacturers collect a stunning range of sensitive personal data,

L. Nuckols (✉)
Central Washington University, Ellensburg, WA, USA
e-mail: lauren.nuckols@cwu.edu

M. C. Altman and D. Schwan (eds.), *Ethics and Medical Technology*, The International Library of Bioethics 113, https://doi.org/10.1007/978-3-031-94690-5_15

including medical and genetic information (Caltrider et al. 2023). Once collected, personal health data are aggregated, analyzed, and shared or sold to data brokers, governments, law enforcement, researchers, public health agencies, and other parties (Glenn and Monteith 2014; Tanner 2017; Véliz 2019). While medical information collected by physicians' offices, hospitals, laboratories, pharmacies, insurance companies, and intermediaries is protected by confidentiality laws such as the Health Insurance Portability and Accountability Act of 1996 (HIPAA), it is also often shared or sold to other entities in de-identified form (Tanner 2017).

Shoshana Zuboff (2019) coined the term *surveillance capitalism* to refer to the economic system based on the commodification of personal data. Surveillance capitalism "unilaterally claims human experience as free raw material for translation into behavioral data" (8). The purpose of this chapter is to examine medical privacy issues in the context of contemporary surveillance capitalism. I argue that the for-profit, commercial trade in medical data undermines medical privacy in both informational and decisional forms without sufficient ethical justification. Although privacy violations are sometimes warranted for medical research and public health protection, most for-profit, commercial data practices violate medical privacy with few guardrails, minimal public benefit, and negative consequences for public health and safety. In my view, medical privacy is not dead, but we are rapidly losing it to unelected, unaccountable corporate and governmental entities.

Assuming a family resemblance model, I draw on Daniel Solove's (2008) and Anita Allen's (2011, 2021) taxonomies to examine the two forms of medical privacy that are most significantly undermined by surveillance capitalism: informational and decisional privacy. I then turn to the question of consent. The presence of consent can render privacy losses and violations acceptable, but the consent obtained under most privacy policies is neither fully voluntary nor fully informed. Finally, I acknowledge the limitations of privacy, as public health and safety protections sometimes require access to medical data. Some privacy losses are justifiable for meaningful and likely public benefit so long as checks and balances are enacted to prevent abuses. To that end, I apply Andrew Ferguson's (2021) "tyrant test" as a framework to help mitigate abuses.

15.2 The Meaning of Privacy

Privacy is a controversial and contested concept, and debates about its meaning and moral significance are ongoing. The earliest known philosophical treatment of privacy is Aristotle's distinction between public and private (domestic, familial) spheres of life, between the *polis* and *oikos* (1998, 1253b). One of the most influential definitions of privacy is attributed to Samuel D. Warren and Louis Brandeis (1890), who, under the influence of Thomas Cooley (1888), define privacy as the "right of the individual to be let alone" (Warren and Brandeis 1890, 33).

In general, the contemporary literature on privacy rights can be divided into two broad categories: what Carissa Véliz (2024) calls "access theories" and "control theories." Access theories view privacy as a matter of remaining unaccessed, including informational, physical, and sensorial access. Control theories distinguish information from the means of obtaining it, framing privacy as a matter of control over information and access. According to this view, privacy violations occur when consent to access is infringed or undermined (75). Combining the advantages of both access-based and control-based accounts, Véliz offers a "hybrid account of privacy" that encompasses both control and access (75).[1]

Although this is a helpful categorization of the literature, and the hybrid account has its advantages, the search for a singular, essential definition of privacy is overly reductive. It disregards well-established and useful meanings of privacy and leaves us unable to articulate the full range of privacy issues and losses. As an alternative, some theorists take a "cluster" or "family resemblance" approach,[2] discerning multiple meanings or forms of privacy (such as informational, sensorial, and decisional privacy) rather than seeking one essential definition (DeCew 1997; Solove 2008; Allen 2011, 2021; Beauchamp and Childress 2013). In this chapter, I assume such a model. Although family resemblance approaches are controversial and imperfect, they best capture the variety of meanings and practical implications of privacy as people use the concept (see Wittgenstein's "meaning as use").[3] As Judith DeCew argues, privacy is a "cluster concept covering multiple privacy interests," including control over access, information, and personal decision-making (1997, 73). Attempting to locate the essential nature of privacy fails to capture its complex, irreducible meanings and excludes significant privacy interests.

Working with a pragmatic, Wittgensteinian framework, Solove argues that privacy includes four broad categories, each of which is broken down into subcategories. These broader categories include *information collection*, *information processing*, *information dissemination*, and *invasion* (Solove 2008, 10–11). In Solove's analysis, attempts to locate one core essence of privacy have largely failed because the accounts are too narrow, too broad, or too vague, and because they have overlooked the plurality of meanings (12–38). His taxonomy provides a useful framework for

[1] Here Véliz distinguishes between privacy and the right to privacy. Privacy is a state in which "personal information or sensorial space … remain[s] unaccessed" but not necessarily inaccessible (2024, 76). The right to privacy, by contrast, is a matter of control, including the right to control actual and hypothetical access, as well as control over the means by which access is obtained.

[2] According to Wittgenstein, many concepts have a plurality of meanings that are related in a "family resemblance" of distinct but related terms (1958, §§ 66–67). Rather than one underlying core foundational essence, words in a family share commonalities, similarities, and complex relationships (§§ 66–70).

[3] Wittgenstein defends a theory of "meaning as use" in his *Philosophical Investigations* (1958, § 43). In Wittgenstein's view, the meaning of a word or concept resides in its use (or uses). Wittgenstein writes: "For a *large* class of cases—though not for all—in which we employ the word 'meaning' it can be defined thus: the meaning of a word is its use in the language" (§ 43). From this perspective, understanding the meaning of a word requires examining the meanings that it actually assumes as humans use it in context and practice.

understanding complex privacy issues, such as data aggregation and decisional interference, that cannot be adequately addressed by reducing privacy to informational or sensorial access. Moreover, by taking a Deweyan, problem-oriented approach, Solove is well-positioned to identify contemporary privacy infringements and gaps in existing protections.

Allen (2021) offers another cluster account, discerning five forms of medical privacy: informational, physical (or locational), associational, proprietary, and decisional privacy. Informational privacy is a state in which personal information remains unaccessed by unauthorized parties (pt. 1). Physical privacy refers to a state of physical or sensory inaccessibility; patients have "expectations that they will not be needlessly touched, crowded, gawked at or secretly filmed, recorded or imaged" (pt. 2). Associational privacy refers to social (in)accessibility and "selective intimacy": "People commonly want to reserve sharing the joys of medical experience with friends and family, no less than the agonies" (pt. 3). Proprietary privacy refers to proprietary interest in the body, genetic information, tissue samples, frozen embryos, and, in the context of identity theft, personal information (pt. 4). Finally, decisional privacy refers to autonomous decision-making on personal issues such as medical, sexual, and reproductive decisions (pt. 5). Allen's cluster account has the advantage of identifying complex forms of privacy that cannot be fully captured by a simple sum of narrow concepts. For example, associational privacy is not just "a combination of informational and sensorial access" (Véliz 2019, 2), though it does include those components. It also includes shared (or unshared) experiences.

Although cluster accounts are imperfect and controversial, they are useful frameworks to account for medical privacy issues, and they offer a better starting point than narrowing privacy to information, access, and/or consent. They are also invaluable for their conceptual clarity. Endorsing Allen's cluster model, Tom Beauchamp and James Childress write, "Definitions of privacy are too narrow if they focus entirely on limited access to *information* about a person" (2013, 312). Overly narrow or reductive conceptions of privacy disregard well-established and useful meanings of privacy and leave us unable to account for the full range of privacy needs and infringements. Cluster accounts thus put us in a better position to articulate medical privacy needs and the harms associated with privacy breaches.

15.3 The Value of Medical Privacy

Medical information has long been recognized as especially personal. Upon taking the Hippocratic Oath (c. 400 BCE), ancient Greek physicians vowed not to disclose what they saw and heard in practice ("Hippocratic Oath" 2002). The United Nations Universal Declaration of Human Rights (1948) identifies privacy as a fundamental human right (article 12). Medical privacy and confidentiality rules are recognized normative priorities in contemporary bioethics and medical practices (Beauchamp and Childress 2013, 312–321). Many people are selective about sharing medical information, even with medical providers and close loved ones (Allen 2021, pt. 1).

As such, it is one of few forms of information that enjoys legal protection. Medical information, including mental health information, reveals some of our deepest vulnerabilities, sensitivities, habits, traumas, personal decisions, and histories. It is not (usually) ethically loaded: medical conditions are largely unchosen, although habits and other decisions can play significant roles. Nonetheless, access to medical information introduces possibilities for stigma, distress, discrimination, and control. Little or no wrongdoing is reflected in such information, but we may still have something to hide.

Many commentators have argued that privacy is requisite to individuality, autonomy, relationality, growth, development, and freedom (Westin 1967; Reiman 1976; Benn 1984). Charles Fried (1968) and James Rachels (1975) frame privacy's value in terms of its ability to foster different relationships. The ability to selectively conceal some personal information makes it possible to have different types of relationships with varying levels of intimacy. For example, disclosure of certain personal medical details would be inappropriate in professional contexts but expected in medical or familial contexts.

Privacy is crucial for human flourishing and psychological well-being (Véliz 2024, 108). Medical privacy provides space for us to care for our health, consider our options, make medical decisions, recover (or fail to recover) from illnesses, give birth, miscarry, and die—all without unwanted interference. It allows a sense of safety and respite when we are most vulnerable. From this perspective, privacy is invaluable to health and wellness, both individually and collectively.

15.4 Informational Privacy and Surveillance

Surveillance capitalism poses significant threats to informational and decisional privacy in particular. As noted earlier, informational privacy is a state in which personal information remains unaccessed by unauthorized parties. It is closely associated with confidentiality, the handling of sensitive information to prevent unauthorized access or disclosure, particularly in a medical context (DeCew 2000; Beauchamp and Childress 2013; Allen 2021). Unauthorized access to medical information would qualify as a privacy infringement, but disclosure of shared private information by a trusted party is a breach of confidentiality (Beauchamp and Childress 2013, 316–317). Given the complexity of contemporary data ecosystems, Neil Richards and Jonathan King argue that privacy no longer refers to secrecy, but instead "the rules we have to govern information flows," with confidentiality as "a kind of privacy that is based on trust" (2014, 409, 413). Because personal information can remain confidential, privacy requires rules that protect shared information (426–432). For example, confidentiality laws such as HIPAA help protect patient information in medical settings, albeit with significant limitations (Tanner 2017).

Informational privacy "is disturbed when data, facts, or conversations that a person wishes to [keep] secret or anonymize are nonetheless acquired or disclosed," and it can be undermined in multiple ways (Allen 2011, 4). Surveillance refers to data collection through observation, monitoring, and recording of activities and personal information (Solove 2008, 106–112; see also Lyon 2007, 14). It is undertaken for a variety of purposes, including public health, law enforcement, "influence, management, protection or direction" (Lyon 2007, 14). It is not a new phenomenon, and it is not always unethical, but digital technologies facilitate unprecedented levels of intrusive health surveillance.

Most websites, apps, and devices use tracking technologies to collect vast troves of personal data, including medical data, with few legal obligations. Personal medical data can be collected and inferred from internet histories, online symptom checkers, health apps, messages, and social media activity, among other sources (Glenn and Monteith 2014, 2). A 2022 study found that thirty-three out of a hundred hospitals used a Meta pixel, a tracking tool that shares identified data with Meta (Facebook). The tool shared appointment scheduling data for twenty-six million appointments, including medications, conditions, and demographic information (Feathers et al. 2022). A 2023 study found that nine out of eleven major online pharmacies had third-party trackers, "including a Google Analytics tool and advertising technologies" (Gollan 2023). At the time of writing, LinkedIn, Meta, and three healthcare websites are being sued for collecting sensitive health information and using it for targeted advertising without obtaining consent (Alder 2024).

In addition to web activity, health apps and devices collect personal information such as vital signs, sleep patterns, and physical activity. Additional medical information is collected through payment and purchase histories, including medical bills, medications, and over-the-counter products, all of which can reveal medical conditions and decisions (Glenn and Monteith 2014, 2). Location history is routinely surveilled via mobile devices, and it can reveal visits to mental health professionals, rehabilitation facilities, reproductive healthcare clinics, and other specific providers (2).

Although it can have benefits, health surveillance can be ethically problematic. Where it is covert, Stanley Benn writes, surveillance is dishonest; it "deliberately deceives a person about [their] world" and thereby undermines their autonomy (1984, 230). Where it is overt, surveillance can cause emotional discomfort and distress, even leading some to "self-censorship and inhibition" (Solove 2008, 108). Jonathon Penney writes that a chilling effect occurs "when a person, deterred by fear of some legal punishment or privacy harm, engages in self-censorship," resulting in avoidance of lawful activities and forms of speech; in Penney's view, it pushes people in the direction of social conformity (2022, 1454). Because of its chilling effects, surveillance can function as "a tool of social control" (Solove 2008, 108).

Studies have shown a decrease in health app usage and web access as a result of mass surveillance, particularly after the *Dobbs* decision (Basavaraj et al. 2024) and the Snowden revelations (Penney 2022; Murray et al. 2024). After the *Dobbs* decision overturned *Roe v. Wade* in the United States, many people stopped using reproductive health apps, particularly in states where abortion was banned or restricted (Gross 2024). Naveen Basavaraj et al. found that after the *Dobbs* decision was leaked, there was a 9.6% reduction in weekly health app sessions and "a 31% reduction in the average time spent on health apps," especially among women (2024, 5). Medical tracking tools and information sources have incredible power to improve the quality of our lives and health, but we "pay" for access with our data. Because we cannot foresee all the possible future uses of our information—insurance rates, healthcare coverage, and employment can all potentially be impacted by health data—online self-censorship may be a reasonable and practical form of self-protection.

15.5 Information Processing: Aggregation, Secondary Use, and Exclusion

Informational privacy losses do not end with data collection, but may also occur through data processing and handling. Information processing refers to the analysis and usage of data collected. It includes *aggregation*, the compilation of data points from various sources; *secondary use*, the nonconsensual usage of data for additional purposes; and *exclusion*, the data subject's inability to access or modify personal data (Solove 2008, 104).

Aggregation refers to the process of compiling data points from public and private sources to build a larger profile. It is one of the central purposes and most promising features of big data, given its ability to reveal patterns, trends, and correlations that would be invisible with smaller datasets (Thorpe and Gray 2015, 171). Aggregated data can be vastly more revealing once compiled, but as Solove writes, this has significant privacy implications:

> A piece of information here or there is not very telling, but when combined, bits and pieces of data begin to form a portrait of a person. … Aggregated information can reveal new facts about a person that she did not expect would be known about her when the original, isolated data was collected. (2008, 118)

Aggregating information has always been possible, but data analytics tools available today enable data aggregation at an unprecedented scale. Aggregation can be harmful when it reveals highly personal information, and it can exacerbate the power differential inherent to information collection (118–119). For banks, insurance companies, and employers, access to a wider range of background information allows for more informed decision-making. This can improve productivity, but it expands possibilities for inaccuracies and omissions, loss of employment, insurance denial, and other concrete harms (O'Neill 2017; Véliz 2019, 2024). Aggregation may also facilitate the offloading of human decision-making onto algorithms, which can be highly efficient but can also lead to inaccurate, unfair, or biased decisions and can exacerbate inequalities (O'Neill 2017).

Because personal data are financially valuable, data aggregation is a highly lucrative practice, and the data broker industry has proliferated in recent decades. It is currently a multi-billion-dollar industry. Thousands of data brokers aggregate, analyze, and commodify personal data in the form of "prediction products," manufactured and sold in "a new kind of marketplace for behavioral predictions" called "behavioral futures markets" (Zuboff 2019, 8). These "prediction products" include consumer lists and other marketing tools. Some "segments" or lists available for purchase include "Anxiety Sufferers" and "Consumers with Clinical Depression" (Harwell 2023). In 2013, one pharmaceutical marketing company sold lists of "rape sufferers," HIV/AIDS patients, and domestic violence victims (Dwoskin 2013). Data brokers operate within and beyond HIPAA-protected contexts, as medical charting platforms and pharmacies legally sell de-identified patient data for research and commercial purposes (Tanner 2017). Their customers include businesses, political campaigns, and governments, including foreign adversaries (Arango 2023).

Data brokers erode privacy by indefinitely increasing the number of parties with unauthorized access to information, and, through aggregation, the quantity and sensitivity of information. Additional layers of privacy are lost as data are used for secondary (and tertiary) purposes without consent. According to Solove, secondary use is a privacy issue under the heading of information processing. It amounts to "a dignitary [harm] that emerges from denying people control over the future use of their data" (Solove 2008, 132). Secondary use tends to operate in tandem with exclusion, which refers to the inability to access, amend, or delete personal data (134). Some laws, such as the General Data Protection Regulation (GDPR) in the European Union and HIPAA and the Privacy Act of 1974 in the United States, offer partial restrictions on exclusion and secondary use. Outside of these contexts, data subjects are excluded from secondary data uses, with little recourse. Data subjects have minimal ability to access or modify personal data, let alone choose how personal information is used or with whom it is shared. This leaves people vulnerable to abuses and "divests people of control over their lives in a substantial way" (135).

One especially intrusive secondary use is predictive modeling. Combined with data aggregation, this form of modeling draws on aggregated data and advanced scientific research to make predictions and infer sensitive and predictive information that people do not volunteer. Genetic information is especially predictive (Laurie 2002; Allen 2021), but other health information can also reliably predict future needs and responses. Likewise, health conditions, pregnancies, and emotional states can be inferred from seemingly innocuous data such as purchase histories (Duhigg 2012). These inferences "may have the same consequences for an individual as if the information came from an electronic medical record" (Glenn and Monteith 2014, 4).

Even if predictive inferences are inaccurate, they can result in privacy losses. In addition to the attention and analysis on which inferences are based, the process of using advanced science to infer sensitive information is a process of obtaining unauthorized access to that information. Like deepfakes, which violate victims' privacy by making statistical inferences based on existing information and by drawing additional attention to the victim (Véliz 2024, 95), health inferences use detailed personal information to predict likely medical conditions the person did not consent to share. Both involve advanced statistical analysis to sketch sensitive personal information in detail and often with some degree of accuracy. "To respect people's privacy, there are some inferences that we shouldn't make if we can avoid it" (Véliz 2024, 95–96).

Another privacy-intrusive secondary use of aggregated data occurs through personalized content and targeted advertising. Personalized content is the algorithmic prioritization of individually tailored content in order to maximize time spent, advertising revenue, and data collection. Prioritized content tends to include click-bait and emotionally engaging content, including content that provokes anger or fear. Targeted advertisements based on demographic information, personal interests, and medical data can influence actions and worldviews. Some advertisements are precisely targeted to arrive at highly vulnerable moments, including during pregnancy (Duhigg 2012).

Although medical targeted advertising can be well-intentioned and sometimes helpful, it undermines privacy in several ways. First, privacy losses are integral to targeted advertising. These practices incentivize commodification and secondary use, and they permit an indefinite number of parties to access sensitive data. Medically sensitive targeted advertisements based on personal health information, collected or inferred, are especially invasive and can have devastating consequences. For example, Grindr, a gay dating app, is facing a class action lawsuit in the UK for allegedly sharing medical information without consent. Some data subjects received targeted advertisements for HIV therapies in multiple feeds after sharing their status with potential partners. As one anonymous man said, "I'm not ashamed of my status, but I didn't expect Grindr to go and sell it on like a piece of meat. It's not their business. It's my life" (Booth 2024). The comparison to "a piece of meat" suggests that the experience of health data commodification and targeting is not just embarrassing but also dehumanizing.

Second, by implying personal medical status, targeted advertisements can reveal health information to friends and family. For the anonymous man quoted above, a friend or colleague could have learned of his HIV-positive status by looking over his shoulder; because the advertisements were displayed in multiple feeds, his status could have been revealed by advertisements shown on other platforms. In another well-known example, Target used purchase patterns to infer that a teenager was pregnant before her father learned of the pregnancy, and Target sent precisely timed coupons and advertisements based on these inferences (Duhigg 2012). Rather than giving people the opportunity to make these disclosures for themselves, targeted advertisements risk disclosing sensitive health information nonconsensually. These revelations can cause distress and impact relationships.

Third, by attempting to influence medical decisions, targeted medical advertising may amount to decisional interference. As Zuboff argues, prediction products try not only to commodify our data but to influence our behaviors "toward profitable outcomes" such as platform engagement and purchases (2019, 8). Although personalized content can help people access relevant information and products, it can also negatively influence their medical decision-making. People may be exposed to misinformation and harmful, overpriced, or privacy-intrusive medical treatments in their most vulnerable moments, and they may suffer concrete harms as a result.

In recent years, data brokers have sold lists of people who visited reproductive healthcare clinics based on precise location histories. Anti-abortion organizations have purchased these lists and delivered targeted advertisements to people who had recently visited these clinics. At least one advertisement pushed misinformation: "Took the first pill at the clinic? It may not be too late to save your pregnancy," referring to a dangerous and medically unsupported practice of attempting to reverse a medication abortion (Tau and Haggin 2023).

Medical targeted advertisements violate the right to privacy in both decisional and informational forms. By accessing sensitive information without consent, they violate the right to informational medical privacy. By attempting to interfere with medical decision-making, they violate the right to decisional privacy. By advertising dangerous treatments, they also threaten public safety and expose people to harmful misinformation.

15.6 Anonymity and Identification

Identification connects de-identified data or other anonymous "informational baggage" to a specific person (Solove 2008, 124). Some examples include identity verification for account access and use of genetic material at a crime scene. Anonymity is valuable in biomedical research and public health surveillance (Allen 2021). Identification is a risk for medical records because de-identified medical records can be re-identified with relative ease (Tanner 2017). One study found that "99.98% of Americans would be correctly re-identified in any dataset using 15 demographic attributes" (Rocher et al. 2019, 1).

Identification is a risk for any anonymized or pseudonymized data, or for any publicly visible online account. Because it can serve as a tool of social control (Solove 2008, 125), identification is a legal risk in regions with restrictions on reproductive and gender-affirming healthcare. Online support forums and social media sites can help people facing various medical conditions, and some forums allow people to seek medical support pseudonymously. In these contexts, people may share information they do not feel comfortable sharing with family or friends. However, some medical and mental health support forums do not permit modification or deletion of posts or comments, further exposing data subjects to identification risks. One study found that YouTube comments containing personal medical information from multiple sclerosis patients remained visible after account deletion (Fernandez-Luque et al. 2009). Although people are responsible for their online disclosures, people in distress sometimes share extremely personal, stigmatizing information without awareness or consideration of the privacy risks. Such a lapse of judgment should not leave anyone at permanent risk of identification. Better disclosures and options, including the ability to delete posts and accounts, would help people to mitigate these risks.

15.7 Insecurity and Information Dissemination

In addition to the above information processing practices, privacy is further threatened through inadequate security practices. Insecurity refers to cybersecurity failures and poor data handling practices, including "glitches, security lapses, abuses, and illicit uses of personal information," potentially resulting in data breaches and other disclosures (Solove 2008, 127). Insecurity can result from inadequate or outdated security practices, device theft or loss, or "fraudulent or accidental access to data" (Allen 2021, pt. 1.3). Although hackers can sometimes overcome the most stringent of security systems, data stewards have a responsibility to take adequate preventative measures and to remediate the effects of breaches (Goodman 2015).

The view that insecurity is a privacy loss is controversial. Some commentators distinguish unrealized risks from harms or wrongs (Goodman 2015, 48), and they differentiate inaccessible, unaccessed, and accessed information (Véliz 2024, 76). Under this view, the right to privacy might be violated if data have been collected nonconsensually, but the privacy loss itself does not occur unless the information is accessed by another person (Véliz 2024, 85). Additionally, because insecurity is a matter of risks rather than their realization, it is difficult to determine the appropriate redress for victims (Allen 2021).

In my view, insecurity does qualify as a privacy infringement. When insecurity is a form of negligence, it demonstrates a lack of respect for private information and therefore a lack of respect for data subjects, whether or not a breach occurs. As Kenneth Goodman argues, information stewards have an obligation to minimize security risks (2015, 48). By collecting personal information, particularly medical information, they assume a moral responsibility to protect data from unauthorized access. Failing to take appropriate security measures when entrusted with this significant responsibility can also yield the same harms as intentional disclosure.

Solove identifies several privacy harms associated with information dissemination, which occurs when personal information is made available to unauthorized parties. This includes, but is not limited to, *disclosure,* which refers to "the revelation of truthful information about a person"; *exposure*, which "involves revealing another's nudity, grief, or bodily functions"; and *increased accessibility*, which makes personal data easier to access (Solove 2008, 142–143). Information dissemination can cause multiple harms, including stigma, discrimination, distress, identity theft, financial losses, employment and insurance denials, and even stalking and murder (142–143).[4] Exposure leaves us vulnerable by revealing especially personal "information about our bodies and health," aspects of our humanity that we conceal as a social practice and as a matter of dignity (148).

Medical information dissemination is a recognized harm (Biegelman 2009). Insecurity and resulting disclosures amount to informational privacy losses, with consequent harms for victims. And data breaches have become a routine occurrence. Between 2009 and 2023, 5,887 medical data breaches involving over five hundred individual medical records per breach occurred (Alder 2025). In 2024, a UnitedHealth data breach compromised the personal data of over one hundred million people—the largest health data breach in history so far (Reuters 2024). Recourse for victims is incommensurate to the risks and harms incurred. Data stewards undertake a responsibility to mitigate and remediate these risks and harms, but the frequency

---

[4] A man murdered a woman after purchasing her data from Docusearch, Inc., which resulted in a lawsuit against the company (*Remsburg v. Docusearch, Inc.*) (Solove 2008, 143).

of data breaches and lack of meaningful recourse for victims indicate that many data stewards do not undertake these responsibilities with the appropriate level of caution or respect for privacy.

15.8 Decisional Privacy and Decisional Interference

The right to decisional privacy is a right to be free from unauthorized interventions in personal decisions, including medical, sexual, reproductive, childrearing, and end-of-life decisions (Inness 1992; DeCew 1997; Solove 2008; Borgmann 2010; Allen 2011, 2021; Beauchamp and Childress 2013). These highly personal decisions are beyond the appropriate purview of governments and corporations. The right to decisional privacy protects our most personal decision-making processes from access and intervention by these and other unauthorized parties. It is distinct from, but closely related to, informational, physical, and associational privacy.

Decisional privacy is a controversial concept legally and philosophically. Some thinkers argue that decisional privacy is reducible to autonomy or liberty, and it is better explained as such (e.g., Thomson 1975; Parent 1983; Ursin 2008; Véliz 2019, 2024). However, this reduction is a mistake. Decisional privacy is a recognized and meaningful concept in philosophy, law, medicine, and public life. Allen defends the concept by noting its long history: "The decisional use of privacy has bona fide conceptual roots in Greek and Roman antiquity's public/private distinction, marking a boundary between affairs of politics and government (*res publicae*) and affairs of the household (*re privatae*)" (2021, pt. 5). While the line between public and private is variable and permeable, it can still be meaningfully drawn, and there is practical value in circumscribing a private space that is shielded from unauthorized access, which simultaneously limits informational, sensorial, and decisional access.

Decisional privacy has historically served as a legal premise in favor of protecting some personal medical decisions, especially regarding contraception and abortion. Although the US Constitution does not explicitly mention privacy, the Supreme Court in *Griswold v. Connecticut* (381 US 479 [1965]), which established the right of married couples to access contraception, found that the Constitution contained "penumbras" protecting the right to privacy, understood in decisional terms (14). *Eisenstadt v. Baird* (405 US 438 [1972]), which established the right of unmarried individuals to access contraception, defined the right to privacy as "the right of the individual, married or single, to be free from unwarranted governmental intrusion into matters so fundamentally affecting a person as the decision whether to bear or beget a child" (21). In *Roe v. Wade* (410 US 113 [1973]), the Court found that the right to privacy included the right to terminate a pregnancy (118). All these rulings relied on an understanding of a constitutional right to make personal medical, familial, sexual, and reproductive decisions without governmental interference. Although these cases and their justifications are controversial, they recognized and articulated meaningful decisional aspects of the right to privacy.

Restrictions on personal medical choices are forms of decisional interference. They legitimize governmental access to, and interference in, decisions typically made among patients, medical professionals, and loved ones. As such, these restrictions legitimize governmental access to personal medical information, private spaces, communications, and other aspects of our lives. Sensitive personal decisions and information thereby become accessible to government agents and other parties, including, potentially, the general public.

In this sense, the right to decisional privacy protects informational privacy. It protects medically relevant information, including health conditions and options chosen. For example, the surveillance required to enforce contraceptive bans was a motivating justification for the ruling in *Griswold v. Connecticut*, where the Justices argued that allowing the police to search the "sacred precincts of marital bedrooms" would be "repulsive to the notions of privacy surrounding the marriage relationship" (17).

The searches that transpire today are not simply or primarily physical. Police have little need to obtain a warrant or physically search homes when they can simply purchase it from data brokers. They can legally do so without a warrant in the United States under the third-party doctrine, which states that information shared with a third party is no longer covered by Fourth Amendment protections. Reproductive health data may be obtained from online activity and communications, health apps, location history, and other sources, with few restrictions (e.g., the Electronic Communications Privacy Act [1986]). A 2022 study found that 99% of abortion clinic websites had third-party data transfers and 69% used third-party cookies (Friedman et al. 2022). After the *Dobbs* decision, Google promised to delete location data after people visited "particularly personal" medical facilities, such as psychiatric and reproductive health providers (Fitzpatrick 2023), but subsequent studies have shown that these location histories persist (Bhuiyan 2022, 2024). Fortunately, some companies, including Google, require a warrant before sharing data with law enforcement. They received 87,000 search warrants in 2021 (Gollan 2023).

Surveillance technologies enable states to prosecute people who obtained, provided, or assisted illegal abortions. For example, in 2015, an Indiana woman who had a medication abortion was charged with "feticide" based on text messages, web searches, and email history. In 2017, a Mississippi woman who delivered a stillborn baby at home was charged with "killing her infant child" after police found that she had searched for medication abortion online (Zakrzewski et al. 2022). In 2022, a Nebraska teenager and her mother were prosecuted on multiple charges based on Facebook messages showing that the mother had assisted with a medication abortion. These high-profile examples emerge from a larger pattern: "Over the last two decades, at least 61 investigations have been initiated against pregnant women or individuals who aided them in self-managed abortions" (Dewan and Frenkel 2022).

In addition to directly limiting personal medical options and enforcing these limitations, the surveillance required for enforcement violates decisional privacy by wielding a panoptic power over people. Health surveillance has chilling effects on expression, information access, bodily autonomy, and medical decision-making. The fear of legal repercussions, combined with the constancy of surveillance, is likely to alter decisions for at least some people. These chilling effects, as I discussed above, already extend to health apps and platforms, but the surveillance is sweeping and extends far beyond health-related domains.

The combination of surveillance and decisional interference amounts to a complex of harms. As Jolynn Dellinger and Stephanie Pell argue, privacy losses for persons seeking abortions may include "invasion[s] of the body" in the form of mandatory medical exams; "limitation[s] on decision-making, or law enforcement access to profoundly personal data," with consequent harms, including legal repercussions; and "emotional trauma, distress, anxiety, physical discomfort or injury, loss of custody, financial loss, reputational damage, or stigma" (2024, 91–92). The consequences of these privacy losses may permanently impact quality of life and may limit future opportunities. In medical emergencies, these restrictions sometimes result in mortalities.

Importantly, privacy violations and harms are not equally distributed. Under reproductive healthcare bans, governmental surveillance and decisional interference disproportionately target marginalized groups, particularly people of color and LGBTQIA+ people (Dellinger and Pell 2024, 92). These bans, and the surveillance architecture used to enforce them, exacerbate social inequalities and leave marginalized populations especially vulnerable to privacy violations and associated harms. Minimizing the collection, storage, accessibility, and sale of reproductive health data would mitigate these privacy violations. As one privacy researcher concluded, "The best way to protect people who are seeking abortions is to stop collecting the data entirely" (Bhuiyan 2022).

15.9 Privacy and Consent

Most commentators acknowledge that information can be shared consensually and that the resulting reduction in privacy does not violate people's rights (Véliz 2024). In order for consent to obtain, however, it must be voluntary and informed. Consent for data usage is allegedly obtained through the privacy policies offered by websites, platforms, and devices, but this consent is neither fully informed nor fully voluntary. It is "murky" at best (Solove 2024).

First, assuming the condition of competence is met, informed consent is undermined by the length, difficulty, and vagueness of most privacy policies. The average privacy policy ranges from 1,000 to 1,700 words in length, with some as long as 25,000 words. On average, privacy policies require a reading level between grades twelve and fifteen (Ermakova et al. 2015; Fabian et al. 2017), even though 37% of Americans have a high school diploma or less (US Census Bureau 2023). Over the past twenty years, the average policy length has doubled, and the difficulty level has increased by a full grade level (Amos et al. 2021). In addition to their length and difficulty, privacy policies are not always forthcoming about their tracking technologies and data sharing practices (Ermakova et al. 2015; Amos et al. 2021). If not omitted entirely, these details are usually cloaked in vagueness. Policies stipulate that data may be shared with third parties, but they do not specify which data, with whom the information will be shared, or for what purposes. Even those who take the time to read privacy policies are not provided with a clear view of the terms to which they are agreeing. Without full disclosure and understanding, meaningful consent is impossible.

Second, the consent obtained is not always fully voluntary. In a medical setting, patients have no choice but to accept the policies of the provider's chosen platform, and many of these have a history of data breaches. Outside the scope of HIPAA protections, voluntary consent is further undermined. Someone who is struggling with severe or emergent medical symptoms may seek information online, and they may accept intrusive privacy policies under some degree of duress. Consent in these cases is constrained by the health needs people seek to meet through technology. In these cases, it cannot be fully voluntary.

Even where symptoms do not constitute a crisis, the internet is a vital resource for health information. It is unreasonable to expect people to forego medical information and tools in order to maintain control over personal health information. Access to health technologies and information should not require that we share our sensitive health information with an indefinite number of unknown, unaccountable third parties and accept whatever intrusive secondary and tertiary uses they choose. Given the sensitivity of medical information, the risks of data commodification, and the value of privacy, this is an asymmetrical, extortive, and exploitative trade. Under these circumstances, it is not possible to meet the basic conditions of voluntary informed consent, and the right to privacy is violated even when consent to a privacy policy seems to be obtained.

15.10 The Limits of Privacy

From a public health standpoint, an absolute commitment to privacy would be ethically untenable. As most commentators acknowledge, privacy rights are not absolute, and violations may be justifiable for purposes of public health, safety, and medical research. Although privacy-protecting measures should be taken wherever possible, health surveillance is an invaluable tool to monitor public health threats and make interventions (Beauchamp and Childress 2013, 314–315). Workplace health protection programs such as the Occupational Safety and Health Administration (OSHA) and the National Institute for Occupational Safety and Health (NIOSH) rely on surveillance to protect workers, conduct research, improve workplace safety, and hold employers accountable (Occupational Safety and Health Administration 2020; National Institute for Occupational Safety and Health 2024). Exposure notification systems allow for automated contact tracing, anonymously notifying people of exposure based on Bluetooth logs of nearby phones (Ladyzhets 2021). Governmental and law enforcement agencies use surveillance technologies to monitor for criminal activity and security threats, for example, by monitoring for bioweapons and terrorist activity. Although mass surveillance programs violate privacy rights through warrantless bulk data collection, targeted surveillance in the interest of public protection can justify some privacy violations.[5] In short, lifesaving and health-protecting objectives do require some privacy losses, and it is not always possible or practical to achieve these goals with anonymous, de-identified, or consensually collected data (Beauchamp and Childress 2013, 314). As I will discuss below, guardrails are needed for these data uses, but they may be justifiable for targeted public safety protections.

Medical research is another important and promising use of big data. Researchers can make significant advances by surveilling medical and pharmacy records, genetic databases, wearable devices, web activity, social media trends, environmental sensors, and other sources (Mooney and Pejaver 2024). These sources can reveal correlations that are not evident in clinical trials, at a larger scale and in real time. For these reasons, Bartha Knoppers and Adrian Thorogood argue in favor of a "right to science," a human right to benefit from advances in scientific research (2017, 53–57). In order to enjoy these benefits, they argue, improved data sharing is crucial; privacy and consent can inhibit these advancements (54). Considering the biomedical advancements that are possible through big data, the authors argue that obtaining "individual specific consent" poses logistical difficulties to the point that it "is simply no longer feasible" (156).

Public health and biomedical research objectives are laudable, and the concept of a right to science is compelling, so long as the public actually benefits and abuses are prevented. However, privacy harms and risks are legitimate liabilities that should not be minimized too quickly. Beauchamp and Childress offer criteria for justifiable medical privacy violations while protecting privacy and mitigating harms. They recommend considering the scope and severity of harm prevented and benefits achieved, likelihood of achieving the goal, necessity of privacy infringements, and presence of security measures to mitigate harms (2013, 316–322). Data stewards must make judgments about the preventability and foreseeability of harms and benefits, risks to patients (and data subjects) caused by breaches of confidentiality, and legal implications. Privacy and confidentiality infringements that are likely to

---

[5] One interesting example is the Golden State Killer, who was convicted in 2020 after investigators used a public genealogy website to match his DNA with a distant relative. In the process, police investigated a number of innocent people who were unaware that their genetic information was accessible to law enforcement (Wickenheiser 2019, 115). This investigation was controversial but arguably justifiable in the interests of justice and public safety. It was a targeted search for a specific, known violent offender, conducted on a public website. Although innocent people did lose some privacy, they voluntarily posted their genetic information, and public safety and justice outweigh those privacy claims.

Another interesting case was the recent identification of a suspect in the Idaho State killings. In this case, the FBI relied on genetic databases that were not available to the public and whose members had not consented to police access. Although the pursuit of justice and the protection of public safety do support data access, the police did not obtain a warrant, and they may have violated a Justice Department policy against law enforcement access to DNA databases without explicit consent (Baker 2025). This case highlights the power of big data to protect the public, but also the importance of requiring warrants and providing all information needed for people to give informed consent.

prevent major harm or death are justifiable, and measures should be taken to prevent abuse wherever possible (316–322).

15.11 Mitigating Abuses

Surveillance technologies empower governments and corporations to monitor and influence our actions, thoughts, and decisions at an unprecedented scale. We cannot safely assume that these powers will never be abused. For these reasons, Ferguson argues that, to protect ourselves, we must begin with the "tyrant test," which assumes that technologies will be abused:

> Because surveillance technology offers government a new power to monitor and control citizens, the response must check that power. The question is how, and the answer is to assume the worst. Power will be abused, and constraints must work backwards from that cynical starting point. The tyrant lens assumes that governmental power, including police power, must be checked (and checked again) because the government will misuse it against the less powerful. (2021, 262)

Because the potential for tyranny cannot be understated, Ferguson offers the tyrant test as an approach to checking the powers of governmental surveillance. Rather than simply trusting government agents not to abuse their power (the "trust lens"), banning police usage of surveillance technology entirely (the "trap lens"), or relying exclusively on technological solutions (the "technocratic lens"), Ferguson argues for a "tyrant lens" that permits mass surveillance technologies so long as sufficient legal and technological safeguards exist to check a hypothetical tyrant (2021, 270–283). Passing the tyrant test requires a robust system of "structural checks on power" with "legal and political oversight" to regulate deployment of surveillance technologies (271). New surveillance technologies would require democratic approval, and "liberty from surveillance would be the norm" (272). Authorities would be required to obtain limited, targeted warrants, or "super warrants," in order to access to sensitive data (272–277). Audits and accountability procedures would be implemented (273), and rights-based checks would provide recourse for privacy violations (277–278). Such an approach would limit data access and use but not necessarily data collection itself (276), although "certain types of searches would be prohibited" (283).[6] These guardrails would protect the public from privacy violations and power abuses by restricting access while still permitting some data collection for targeted purposes. Democratic processes would ensure that the uses of surveillance reflected the will of the people, and systems of checks and balances would mitigate the potential for abuses while still allowing some surveillance for public health and safety.

---

[6] Ferguson notes that there is early historical precedent for such a ban in English court cases *Wilkes v. Wood* (1763) and *Entick v. Carrington* (1765), which found that unpublished writings, including politically controversial or dissenting views, ought to be protected from government surveillance (2021, 285). In these early cases, even lawful searches and seizures were found to have tyrannical potential. Although these precedents are largely ignored today, Ferguson suggests that they are worth reconsidering.

Although the tyrant test is a useful framework, it might not successfully protect us from a hypothetical tyrant. The possibilities for insecurity, corruption, and collusion can never be fully eliminated. Risks of disclosure and abuse are inherent to surveillance systems, and the only way to eliminate these risks is to minimize data collection. Legal and technical safeguards are crucial and should be more widespread, but confidentiality-based protections will always carry risks. For this reason, Nicolas Terry argues that reducing data collection is the only way to protect ourselves from data abuses and harms (2013, 19). This would require "a true collection-regulating privacy model" rather than "a confidentiality model" such as HIPAA (19). Confidential information can always be breached, and justifications for access can expand over time. Only information that is not collected is safe from possibilities of disclosure or abuse. Just as there are some spaces in which non-consensual surveillance would be unwarranted and inappropriate, there are some types of information that are, except under narrow circumstances, too sensitive to be non-consensually collected or commodified.

Applied to private corporations, the tyrant test may turn out to support Zuboff's conclusion that we ought to reject the for-profit trade in personal data entirely, just as we previously banned child labor (2019, 343). Data brokers, corporations, and other entities that do not need medical information should be restricted or prohibited from collecting, inferring, aggregating, or selling health-related data without obtaining explicit voluntary informed consent. Where medically sensitive data collection cannot be minimized without compromising research, public health, or technological functions (e.g., fitness devices), better legal and technical safeguards should be implemented. Companies that must collect and store health data should be bound by confidentiality rules stricter than HIPAA. Their data responsibilities should parallel those of physicians, with revocation of licenses for abuses (Véliz 2019, 9). Stringent security measures should be legally required and ethically normalized, with regular audits and updates, and companies should be meaningfully held accountable for data breaches. Targeting based on medical information, location history, and other especially sensitive information should be restricted. Measures such as encryption, limited access, local storage, de-identification, and data deletion should be the default wherever possible. Some data should still be accessible for medical research and public health protection, but legal safeguards and ethical norms should mandate de-identification and other privacy-protecting measures, and access should be limited to authorized parties for specific purposes.

People need and deserve robust data privacy rights to protect us from abuses, and we should have recourse when our rights are violated. We should have the right to meaningfully consent to all data collection and usage, and the ability to opt out wherever possible. Although obtaining consent for each data use might be burdensome, this could be addressed by complex consent models such as tiered approaches that allow data subjects to specify boundaries (Mittelstadt and Floridi 2016) and "dynamic consent" models that permit broad or narrow consent and modifications (Kaye et al. 2015). Data subjects should be free to access, modify, move, and delete their data at will. Privacy policies should be legible, transparent, and specific, and clear summaries should be readily available. These and other consent models could protect medical privacy while allowing the public to benefit from advances in medical research. Although these measures may be imperfect and challenging to implement, they would be a vast improvement over the status quo.

15.12 Conclusion

The right to medical privacy is an ancient ethical principle and a basic human need. It is multifaceted and plural; as such, it needs complex protections. The right to informational medical privacy allows us to choose what medical information to share (or withhold), when, and with whom. Physical and associational privacy rights carve space for us to undergo medically challenging experiences without unwanted access or interactions. Decisional privacy rights protect autonomous personal medical decision-making and, with it, private information, from outside interference and access. These rights protect our health, well-being, autonomy, relationships, and other vital aspects of our lives.

Contemporary data commodification practices have reduced medical privacy almost to a vanishing point. By collecting, processing, and commodifying sensitive personal data without meaningful consent, corporations violate the right to medical privacy and expose people to significant risks and harms, including data breaches and decisional interference. Because we are excluded from secondary and tertiary uses of our information, we are unable to make corrections or anticipate possible future data abuses. Where governments are provided with warrantless access to health information, people are exposed to further privacy losses and possibilities for social control. The permanence of data and pervasiveness of data sharing exacerbate these privacy losses indefinitely. We now live with the ongoing risk and reality that our most sensitive data can be, and for some people, already has been, breached and used against us. Because we cannot foresee all possible future uses of our data, and because most corporate privacy policies are not sufficiently forthcoming about their data practices, we cannot meaningfully consent to the privacy losses to which we are routinely subjected.

Access to medical information and tools that allow us to flourish in contemporary society currently require that we subject ourselves to intrusive surveillance and share invaluable personal medical information with an indefinite number of unelected, unaccountable parties for unknown future uses. It is extortive to demand that people trade our privacy and, with it, portions of our autonomy and well-being, for access to technologies that are functionally required for modern life. We should be able to access websites and drive our vehicles without being reduced to "products" available for purchase by advertisers, political groups, and other parties. Protecting our privacy should not require that we relinquish the benefits of technologies or withdraw from participation in modern life. The risks of breach and abuse are too high, and existing safeguards and public benefits are, for the most part, too minimal, for this to be a fair or consensual exchange.

Big data can have many beneficial applications, including biomedical research and public health. Because rights are not absolute, some limited privacy infringements are justifiable in the presence of voluntary informed consent, and for significant and likely public health protections, so long as guardrails are in place to prevent abuses. However, most commercial data commodification practices provide minimal or no public benefit and occur without voluntary, informed consent. They reduce invaluable aspects of our lives to commodities in order to generate profits and power. We are told that these practices are inevitable and economically necessary, but these risky and degrading practices are not necessary for profitability. We can reject them, just as we have already rejected child labor, dangerous working conditions, and other unethical business practices (Zuboff 2019, 343).

Contemporary surveillance practices expose significant gaps in existing privacy laws and norms. The value and sensitivity of medical information, and the damaging consequences of disclosure, indicate a need for heightened privacy measures and a significant reduction in the data collected and commodified. Robust protections and data privacy rights are needed, especially for vulnerable and marginalized populations. Existing medical privacy laws provide some protections within limited contexts, but stronger measures are needed to protect us from present and future data abuses.

References

Alder, Steve. 2024. "LinkedIn, Meta, and Healthcare Companies Sued for Using Tracking Tools." *HIPAA Journal*. November 7. https://www.hipaajournal.com/linkedin-meta-healthcare-companies-sued-tracking-tools/.

Alder, Steve. 2025. "Healthcare Data Breach Statistics." *HIPAA Journal*. Last modified January 20, 2025. https://www.hipaajournal.com/healthcare-data-breach-statistics/.

Allen, Anita. 2011. *Unpopular Privacy: What Must We Hide?* Oxford: Oxford University Press.

Allen, Anita. 2021. "Privacy and Medicine." *Stanford Encyclopedia of Philosophy* (Spring 2021 Edition). Edited by Edward N. Zalta. https://plato.stanford.edu/archives/spr2021/entries/privacy-medicine/.

Amos, Ryan, Gunes Acar, Eli Lucherini, Mihir Kshirsagar, Arvind Narayanan, and Jonathan Mayer. 2021. "Privacy Policies over Time: Curation and Analysis of a Million-Document Dataset." In *Proceedings of the Web Conference 2021*, edited by Jure Leskovec, Marko Grobelnik, Marc Najork, Jie Tang, and Leila Zia, 2165–2176. Ljubljana: ACM. https://doi.org/10.1145/3442381.3450048.

Arango, Steven. 2023. "Data Brokers: A Benefit or Peril to U.S. National Security?" *Ohio State Technology Law Journal* 20. https://ssrn.com/abstract=4490939.

Aristotle. 1998. *Politics*. Translated by C. D. C. Reeve. Indianapolis: Hackett.

Baker, Mike. 2025. "To Identify Suspect in Idaho Killings, F.B.I. Used Restricted Consumer DNA Data." *New York Times*. February 25. https://www.nytimes.com/2025/02/25/us/idaho-murders-bryan-kohberger-dna.html.

Basavaraj, Naveen, Uttara M. Ananthakrishnan, and Catherine E. Tucker. 2024. "The Chilling Effect of Dobbs: A Study of Mobile Health Apps Usage." MIT Sloan Research Paper No. 7156-24. https://doi.org/10.2139/ssrn.4924919.

Beauchamp, Tom L., and James F. Childress. 2013. *Principles of Biomedical Ethics*. 7th ed. New York: Oxford University Press.

Benn, Stanley I. 1984. "Privacy, Freedom, and Respect for Persons." In *Philosophical Dimensions of Privacy*, edited by Ferdinand David Schoeman, 223–244. Cambridge: Cambridge University Press. https://doi.org/10.1017/CBO9780511625138.009.

Bhuiyan, Johana. 2022. "Googling Abortion? Your Details Aren't as Private as You Think." *Guardian.* November 29. https://www.theguardian.com/world/2022/nov/29/abortion-rights-us-google-roe-dobbs.

Bhuiyan, Johana. 2024. "Google Promised to Delete Location Data on Abortion Clinic Visits. It Didn't, Study Says." *Guardian.* January 17. https://www.theguardian.com/technology/2024/jan/16/google-keeps-location-history-data-abortion-clinics-despite-delete-pledge.

Biegelman, Martin T. 2009. *Identity Theft Handbook: Detection, Prevention, and Security.* Hoboken, NJ: Wiley.

Booth, Robert. 2024. "Grindr Accused of Treating Gay Man's Medical Data Like 'Piece of Meat.'" *Guardian.* May 26. https://www.theguardian.com/uk-news/article/2024/may/26/grindr-accused-of-treating-gay-man-medical-data-like-piece-of-meat.

Borgmann, Caitlin E. 2010. "Abortion, the Undue Burden Standard, and the Evisceration of Women's Privacy." *William & Mary Journal of Race, Gender, and Social Justice* 16 (2): 291–325. https://scholarship.law.wm.edu/wmjowl/vol16/iss2/3.

Caltrider, Jen, Misha Rykov, and Zoë MacDonald. 2023. "It's Official: Cars Are the Worst Product Category We Have Ever Reviewed for Privacy." **Privacy Not Included*. Mozilla Foundation. September 6. https://foundation.mozilla.org/en/privacynotincluded/articles/its-official-cars-are-the-worst-product-category-we-have-ever-reviewed-for-privacy/.

Cooley, Thomas McIntyre. 1888. *A Treatise on the Law of Torts, or, The Wrongs Which Arise Independent of Contract.* 2nd ed. Chicago: Callaghan.

DeCew, Judith Wagner. 1997. *In Pursuit of Privacy: Law, Ethics, and the Rise of Technology.* Ithaca, NY: Cornell University Press.

DeCew, Judith Wagner. 2000. "The Priority of Privacy for Medical Information." *Social Philosophy and Policy* 17 (2) (Summer): 213–234. https://doi.org/10.1017/S026505250000217X.

Dellinger, Jolynn, and Stephanie K. Pell. 2024. "Bodies of Evidence: The Criminalization of Abortion and Surveillance of Women in a Post-Dobbs World." *Duke Journal of Constitutional Law & Public Policy* 19: 1–108. https://scholarship.law.duke.edu/djclpp/vol19/iss1/1.

Dewan, Shaila, and Sheera Frenkel. 2022. "A Mother, a Daughter and an Unusual Abortion Prosecution in Nebraska." *New York Times.* August 18. https://www.nytimes.com/2022/08/18/us/abortion-prosecution-nebraska.html.

Duhigg, Charles. 2012. "How Companies Learn Your Secrets." *New York Times.* February 16. https://www.nytimes.com/2012/02/19/magazine/shopping-habits.html.

Dwoskin, Elizabeth. 2013. "Data Broker Removes Rape-Victims List after Journal Inquiry." *Wall Street Journal.* December 19. https://www.wsj.com/articles/BL-DGB-31536.

Ermakova, Tatiana, Benjamin Fabian, and Eleonora Babina. 2015. "Readability of Privacy Policies of Healthcare Websites." *Wirtschaftsinformatik Proceedings 2015*: 1085–1099. https://aisel.aisnet.org/wi2015/73.

Fabian, Benjamin, Tatiana Ermakova, and Tino Lentz. 2017. "Large-Scale Readability Analysis of Privacy Policies." In *WI '17: Proceedings of the International Conference on Web Intelligence*, 18–25. New York: Association for Computing Machinery. https://doi.org/10.1145/3106426.3106427.

Feathers, Todd, Simon Fondrie-Teitler, Angie Waller, and Surya Mattu. 2022. "Facebook Is Receiving Sensitive Medical Information from Hospital Websites." *Markup.* June 16. https://themarkup.org/pixel-hunt/2022/06/16/facebook-is-receiving-sensitive-medical-information-from-hospital-websites.

Fernandez-Luque, Luis, Najeed Elahi, and Francisco J. Grajales III. 2009. "An Analysis of Personal Medical Information Disclosed in YouTube Videos Created by Patients with Multiple Sclerosis." In *Medical Informatics in a United and Healthy Europe*, edited by Klaus-Peter Adlassnig, Bernd Blobel, John Mantas, and Izet Masic, 292–296. Amsterdam: IOS Press. https://doi.org/10.3233/978-1-60750-044-5-292.

Ferguson, Andrew Guthrie. 2021. "Surveillance and the Tyrant Test." *Georgetown Law Journal* 110 (2): 205–290. https://www.law.georgetown.edu/georgetown-law-journal/in-print/volume-110/volume-110-issue-2-december-2021/surveillance-and-the-tyrant-test/.

Fitzpatrick, Jen. 2023. "Protecting People's Privacy on Health Topics." *Google: The Keyword*. May 12. https://blog.google/technology/safety-security/protecting-peoples-privacy-on-health-topics/.

Fried, Charles. 1968. "Privacy." *Yale Law Journal* 77 (3) (January): 475–493. https://doi.org/10.2307/794941.

Friedman, Ari B., Lujo Bauer, Rachel Gonzales, and Matthew S. McCoy. 2022. "Prevalence of Third-Party Tracking on Abortion Clinic Web Pages." *JAMA Internal Medicine* 182 (11) (September 8): 1221–1222. https://doi.org/10.1001/jamainternmed.2022.4208.

Glenn, Tasha, and Scott Monteith. 2014. "Privacy in the Digital World: Medical and Health Data Outside of HIPAA Protections." *Current Psychiatry Reports* 16 (11) (November): article no. 494. https://doi.org/10.1007/s11920-014-0494-4.

Gollan, Jennifer. 2023. "Websites Selling Abortion Pills Are Sharing Sensitive Data with Google." *ProPublica*. January 18. https://www.propublica.org/article/websites-selling-abortion-pills-share-sensitive-data-with-google.

Goodman, Kenneth. 2015. *Ethics, Medicine, and Information Technology: Intelligent Machines and the Transformation of Health Care*. Cambridge: Cambridge University Press.

Gross, Paige. 2024. "Data Privacy after Dobbs: Is Period Tracking Safe?" *Stateline*. July 26. https://stateline.org/2024/07/26/data-privacy-after-dobbs-is-period-tracking-safe/.

Harwell, Drew. 2023. "Now for Sale: Data on Your Mental Health." *Washington Post*. February 13. https://www.washingtonpost.com/technology/2023/02/13/mental-health-data-brokers/.

"Hippocratic Oath." 2002. Translated by Michael North. National Library of Medicine, National Institutes of Health. https://www.nlm.nih.gov/hmd/greek/greek_oath.html.

Inness, Julie. 1992. *Privacy, Intimacy, and Isolation*. Oxford: Oxford University Press.

Kaye, Jane, Edgar A. Whitley, David Lund, Michael Morrison, Harriet Teare, and Karen Melham. 2015. "Dynamic Consent: A Patient Interface for Twenty-First Century Research Networks." *European Journal of Human Genetics* 23 (2) (February): 141–146. https://doi.org/10.1038/ejhg.2014.71.

Knoppers, Bartha Maria, and Adrian Mark Thorogood. 2017. "Ethics and Big Data in Health." *Current Opinion in Systems Biology* 4 (August): 53–57. https://doi.org/10.1016/j.coisb.2017.07.001.

Laurie, Graeme T. 2002. *Genetic Privacy: A Challenge to Medico-Legal Norms*. Cambridge: Cambridge University Press.

Ladyzhets, Betsy. 2021. "We Investigated Whether Digital Contact Tracing Actually Worked in the US." *MIT Technology Review*. June 16. https://www.technologyreview.com/2021/06/16/1026255/us-digital-contact-tracing-exposure-notification-analysis/.

Lyon, David. 2007. *Surveillance Studies: An Overview*. Cambridge: Polity.

Michael, Katina, and Roger Clarke. 2013. "Location and Tracking of Mobile Devices: Überveillance Stalks the Streets." *Computer Law & Security Review* 29 (3) (June): 216–228. https://doi.org/10.1016/j.clsr.2013.03.004.

Mittelstadt, Brent Daniel, and Luciano Floridi. 2016. "The Ethics of Big Data: Current and Foreseeable Issues in Biomedical Contexts." *Science and Engineering Ethics* 22 (2) (April): 303–341. https://doi.org/10.1007/s11948-015-9652-2.

Mooney, Stephen J., and Vikas Pejaver. 2024. "Big Data in Public Health: Terminology, Machine Learning, and Privacy." *Annual Review of Public Health* 39: 95–112. https://doi.org/10.1146/annurev-publhealth-040617-014208.

Murray, Daragh, Pete Fussey, Kuda Hove, Wairagala Wakabi, Paul Kimumwe, Otto Saki, and Amy Stevens. 2024. "The Chilling Effects of Surveillance and Human Rights: Insights from Qualitative Research in Uganda and Zimbabwe." *Journal of Human Rights Practice* 16 (1) (February): 397–412. https://doi.org/10.1093/jhuman/huad020.

National Institute for Occupational Safety and Health. 2024. "Surveillance Program." US Centers for Disease Control and Prevention. March 8. https://www.cdc.gov/niosh/research-programs/portfolio/surveillance.html.

Occupational Safety and Health Administration. 2020. "Rules of Agency Practice and Procedure Concerning OSHA Access to Employee Medical Records." US Department of Labor. https://www.osha.gov/laws-regs/regulations/standardnumber/1913/1913.10.

O'Neil, Cathy. 2017. *Weapons of Math Destruction: How Big Data Increases Inequality and Threatens Democracy.* New York: Crown.

Parent, W. A. 1983. "Privacy, Morality, and the Law." *Philosophy & Public Affairs* 12 (4) (Autumn): 269–288. https://www.jstor.org/stable/2265374,

Penney, Jonathon W. 2022. "Understanding Chilling Effects." *Minnesota Law Review* 106 (3): 1451–1530. https://minnesotalawreview.org/wp-content/uploads/2022/04/6-Penney_Web.pdf.

Rachels, James. 1975. "Why Privacy Is Important." *Philosophy & Public Affairs* 4 (4) (Summer): 323–333. https://www.jstor.org/stable/2265077.

Reiman, Jeffrey. 1976. "Privacy, Intimacy, and Personhood." *Philosophy & Public Affairs* 6 (1) (Autumn): 26–44. https://www.jstor.org/stable/2265060.

Reuters. 2024. "Hack at UnitedHealth's Tech Unit Impacted 100 Mln People, US Health Dept Says." *Reuters.* October 25. https://www.reuters.com/technology/cybersecurity/hack-unitedhealths-tech-unit-impacted-100-mln-people-2024-10-24/.

Richards, Neil M., and Jonathan H. King. 2014. "Big Data Ethics." *Wake Forest Law Review* 49 (2): 393–432. file:///C:/Users/philo/Downloads/ssrn-2384174.pdf.

Rocher, Luc, Julien M. Hendrickx, and Yves-Alexandre De Montjoye. 2019. "Estimating the Success of Re-Identifications in Incomplete Datasets Using Generative Models." *Nature Communications* 10: article no. 3069. https://doi.org/10.1038/s41467-019-10933-3.

Solove, Daniel J. 2008. *Understanding Privacy.* Cambridge, MA: Harvard University Press.

Solove, Daniel J. 2024. "Murky Consent: An Approach to the Fictions of Consent in Privacy Law." *Boston University Law Review* 104 (2) (March): 593–639. https://www.bu.edu/bulawreview/files/2024/04/SOLOVE.pdf.

Tanner, Adam. 2017. *Our Bodies, Our Data: How Companies Make Billions Selling Our Medical Records.* Boston: Beacon Press.

Tau, Byron, and Patience Haggin. 2023. "Antiabortion Group Used Cellphone Data to Target Ads to Planned Parenthood Visitors." *Wall Street Journal.* May 18. https://www.wsj.com/articles/antiabortion-group-used-cellphone-data-to-target-ads-to-planned-parenthood-visitors-446c1212.

Terry, Nicolas. 2013. "Protecting Patient Privacy in the Age of Big Data." *SSRN Electronic Journal.* Robert H. McKinney School of Law Legal Studies Research Paper No. 2013–04. https://doi.org/10.2139/ssrn.2153269.

Thomson, Judith Jarvis. 1975. "The Right to Privacy." *Philosophy & Public Affairs* 4 (4) (Summer): 295–314. https://www.jstor.org/stable/2265075.

Thorpe, Jane Hyatt, and Elizabeth Alexandra Gray. 2015. "Big Data and Public Health: Navigating Privacy Laws to Maximize Potential." *Public Health Reports* 130 (2) (March–April): 171–175. https://doi.org/10.1177/003335491513000211.

Ursin, Lars Øystein. 2008. "Biobank Research and the Right to Privacy." *Theoretical Medicine and Bioethics* 29 (4) (August): 267–285. https://doi.org/10.1007/s11017-008-9079-8.

US Census Bureau. 2023. "Census Bureau Releases New Educational Attainment Data." Press release no. CB23-TPS.21. February 16. https://www.census.gov/newsroom/press-releases/2023/educational-attainment-data.html.

Véliz, Carissa. 2019. "Medical Privacy and Big Data: A Further Reason in Favour of Public Universal Health-Care Coverage." In *Philosophical Foundations of Medical Law*, edited by Andelka M. Phillips, Thana C. de Campos, and Jonathan Herring, 306–319. Oxford: Oxford University Press.

Véliz, Carissa. 2024. *The Ethics of Privacy and Surveillance.* Oxford: Oxford University Press.

Warren, Samuel D., and Louis D. Brandeis. 1890. "The Right to Privacy." *Harvard Law Review* 4 (5) (December 15): 193–220. https://doi.org/10.2307/1321160.

Westin, Alan F. 1967. *Privacy and Freedom*. New York: Atheneum.
Wickenheiser, Ray A. 2019. "Forensic Genealogy, Bioethics and the Golden State Killer Case." *Forensic Science International: Synergy* 1: 114–125. https://doi.org/10.1016/j.fsisyn.2019.07.003.
Wittgenstein, Ludwig. 1958. *Philosophical Investigations*. Translated by G. E. M. Anscombe. New York: Prentice Hall.
Zakrzewski, Cat, Pranshu Verma, and Claire Parker. 2022. "Texts, Web Searches about Abortion Have Been Used to Prosecute Women." *Washington Post*. July 3. https://www.washingtonpost.com/technology/2022/07/03/abortion-data-privacy-prosecution/.
Zuboff, Shoshana. 2019. *The Age of Surveillance Capitalism: The Fight for a Human Future at the New Frontier of Power*. New York: PublicAffairs.

Lauren Nuckols is a Senior Lecturer in Philosophy at Central Washington University, USA. Her research is focused on American pragmatism and ethics, with an emphasis on environmental ethics and ethics of technology. More specifically, she works on the relationship between ethics and aesthetics, and its implications for environmental, technological, and human rights issues. She holds a PhD in Philosophy from The Pennsylvania State University.

Chapter 16
Preserving Autonomy, Promoting Health: A Defense of Digital Nudging in Healthcare

Matthew C. Altman

Abstract Behavioral economics has challenged the notion that people act rationally in maximizing their personal utility. Instead, people systematically misuse heuristics in ways that lead to poor outcomes, even when judged against their own conceptions of the good. Changing the context in which people choose can use those cognitive habits to promote what people themselves value. Nudges have been proposed and used in many areas of healthcare, including clinical and public health spaces. Critics object that nudges may not work and that they fail to respect individual autonomy. However, if nudges are subject to public scrutiny, they are not coercive or manipulative. And behavioral science can get us to a better understanding of people's true preferences, assisted by digital technology, to minimize the chance that choice architects will intervene in the wrong ways. Libertarian paternalism thus avoids the pitfalls of traditional medical paternalism by both respecting patient autonomy and promoting outcomes that patients themselves value.

Keywords Nudges · Paternalism · Patient autonomy · Behavioral economics · Digital technology

16.1 Introduction

People often make bad decisions when it comes to their health. If we care about their well-being but also want to respect their freedom, what should we do? Mandates and incentives often fail on both counts, as do traditional forms of medical paternalism, since they force decisions onto people and may be mistaken about what matters most to them. By contrast, well-designed nudges preserve freedom of choice while improving overall outcomes, even when judged against people's own conceptions of the good. In this chapter, I defend libertarian paternalism against both deontological and consequentialist objections. If nudges are subject to public scrutiny, they are

M. C. Altman (✉)
Central Washington University, Ellensburg, USA
e-mail: matthew.altman@cwu.edu

M. C. Altman and D. Schwan (eds.), *Ethics and Medical Technology*, The International Library of Bioethics 113, https://doi.org/10.1007/978-3-031-94690-5_16

not coercive or manipulative. And behavioral science can get us to a better understanding of people's true preferences, assisted by digital technology, to increase the chance that choice architects will intervene in the right ways. Thus, when properly implemented, nudges are a promising and morally permissible method of healthcare intervention.

16.2 Behavioral Economics

According to neoclassical economic theory, the free market drives innovation and increases productivity through competition. When people act out of self-interest, both buyers and sellers benefit, as if their actions were coordinated by an invisible hand that has the common good as its aim. However, the assumption that individuals act rationally in maximizing their personal utility has been called into question by psychologists and social scientists (for brief histories, see White 2013, 24–32; Halpern 2019, 13–58; Truc 2022). The field of study known as behavioral economics or behavioral science has revealed why we often perform erroneous cost-benefit analyses.

In their seminal article "Judgment under Uncertainty" (1974), Amos Tversky and Daniel Kahneman identify three heuristics, or mental shortcuts, that allow people to draw conclusions and make decisions quickly but that often lead us astray:

- Representativeness heuristic: People judge the likelihood of A being in category B by how much A is like their image or stereotype of B.
- Availability heuristic: People judge the likelihood of an event, including risks and benefits, based on how easily examples of that event can be brought to mind.
- Anchoring and adjustment: People make judgments by beginning from an initial idea or value and then adjusting, which anchors the judgment to the starting point.

In addition to these three heuristics, behavioral scientists have identified many other shortcuts, biases, and cognitive habits, including:

- Serial position effect: We more easily remember the first item (primacy effect) and the last item (recency effect) in a series, and we privilege those (Ebbinghaus 1885).
- Planning fallacy: We are unrealistically optimistic about how long it will take to complete a task (Kahneman and Tversky 1977).
- Loss aversion: We feel up to twice as bad when we lose something as we feel good when we gain the same thing (Tversky and Kahneman 1992).
- Status quo/present bias: We tend to prefer the current state of affairs, so we resist change (Samuelson and Zeckhauser 1988).
- Take-the-best heuristic: When presented with two options with many characteristics, we often focus on one characteristic that we use to compare the two, and we choose based solely on that (Gigerenzer and Goldstein 1996).

- Recognition heuristic: When we are unfamiliar with most of the alternatives, we tend to choose the one that we recognize because we perceive it to be more valuable (Goldstein and Gigerenzer 1999).

This is only a selection of heuristics that have been proposed by researchers on cognition and human behavior (see Gigerenzer and Todd 1999; Gilovich et al. 2002). And they are not mutually exclusive; often they overlap and support one another. For example, when we set out an initial timeline in planning a project, we tend to continue thinking in terms of that timeline even when deadlines are missed—in other words, anchoring supports the planning fallacy. Loss aversion and status quo bias together cause inertia because we want to maintain our present holdings, which are more vivid in the mind because of the recency effect.

Sometimes we think through our decisions carefully and rationally, and sometimes we use mental shortcuts, either appropriately or inappropriately. Behavioral economists explain this dichotomy in terms of two different ways of thinking, two cognitive systems, or two psychological functions. Keith Stanovich and Richard West (2000) call these System 1 and System 2, and Richard Thaler and Cass Sunstein (2008) call them the Automatic System and the Reflective System (see Stanovich and West 2000, Table 3 [p. 659] for a list of how different researchers refer to the two systems). According to the dual-process theory of mind, System 1 is driven by emotions, instincts, and habits; it acts unconsciously, associatively, and automatically in response to stimuli. System 2 is logical, analytical, and self-conscious; it acts deliberately and slowly, appealing to explicit rules to solve complex problems. Neurologically, System 1 tends to be associated with the limbic system, which emerged with the first mammals, while System 2 tends to be associated with the neocortex, which is evolutionarily recent and distinctively human (De Neys and Goel 2011).

In light of these discoveries, behavioral economists have fundamentally transformed how we understand decision-making. Neoclassical economists are right that people try to maximize personal utility, and in normal situations—"in contexts in which they have experience, good information, and prompt feedback"—heuristics usually serve them well (Thaler and Sunstein 2008, 9; see also Sunstein 2014b, 11). Heuristics reduce cognitive burden by focusing choosers on what tends to be most important. But in unusual or complex situations—when results are unpredictable, calculations of probable outcomes are difficult, or the consequences of a decision will not be felt for years—people often make choices that do not advance their personal welfare. Thus, people have bounded rationality, meaning that they do the best they can under suboptimal conditions, with limited information, limited time, and limited cognitive resources.

Stressors on human cognition that disrupt rational decision-making are prevalent in the healthcare context. Clinicians, public health officials, and patients often must decide quickly in situations of high stress and high cognitive load, which makes the use of heuristics more likely. For example, patients usually have to make treatment decisions when outcomes are uncertain and with limited understanding of the complex information that clinicians give them. And their choices are often clouded by emotional responses (such as denial) or psychological illnesses (such as depression)—what Terrence Ackerman (1982) calls, respectively, cognitive constraints and psychological constraints—that interfere with their ability to understand the current situation, weigh risks and benefits, and decide how to act in accordance with their values.

16.3 Ends Paternalism versus Means Paternalism

Traditionally, public and private organizations have tried to shape human behavior through mandates/bans and incentives/disincentives. Even when these are meant to prevent people from making unhealthy choices, they grate against our commitment to individual freedom. According to John Stuart Mill's harm principle, "the only purpose for which power can be rightfully exercised over any member of a civilized community, against his will, is to prevent harm to others" (1978, 9). He gives several arguments to justify noninterference when it comes to self-regarding behavior, what he calls "liberty of pursuits": individuals are in the best position to know what is right for them, they develop fuller characters by shaping their own lives rather than conforming, and people can learn from others' ways of living (Mill 1978, 53–71). Mill concludes that paternalism—restricting or managing other people's actions for their own good—is problematic because it imposes a commonly accepted conception of the good life on people to whom it may not apply: "The strongest of all the arguments against the interference of the public with purely personal conduct is that, when it does interfere, the odds are that it interferes wrongly and in the wrong place" (81).

In the healthcare arena, this is the main line of argument against medical paternalism and for patient autonomy. As Alan Goldman (1980) points out, clinicians are experts in diagnosis and treatment, but they are not experts in what their patients value. Clinicians are trained to treat health and continued life as the highest priority, but patients may make different tradeoffs. For example, a patient with a terminal illness may want medical aid in dying to avoid the loss of autonomy or dignity at the end of life rather than living as long as possible.

Mill and Goldman conclude that people are better able to achieve what they value when they are left to their own devices. However, this depends on two assumptions: individuals are the best judges of what is important to them, and they generally act in accordance with those values. The first claim is probably true. If individuals have privileged knowledge of what they want, then forcing my own conception of the good onto them—what Sunstein calls ends paternalism (2014b, 19)—does not respect their autonomy or maximize well-being. However, the second assumption, that people generally do what they must to achieve their ends, is belied by the findings of behavioral economics, which has shown that people do not always do what is best for themselves, even when measured against their own values. Unlike ends paternalism, which forces a conception of the good onto someone, means paternalism attempts to counteract the errors caused by System 1 and empower System 2 such that people are more likely to make choices that "*will promote their own ends, as they themselves understand them*" (Sunstein 2014b, 19).

16.4 The Variety of Nudges

Supporters of means paternalism disagree about the kinds of interventions that are justified, with Sarah Conly (2013) and Julian Le Grand and Bill New (2015) arguing for more coercive interventions, tending toward what is called hard paternalism, and Thaler and Sunstein (2008) and David Halpern (2019) arguing for nudges, the behavioral tools of soft paternalism. Both approaches try to get people to maximize what they value, but hard paternalism imposes higher, "material costs"—incentives such as fines or punishments, or mandates such as bans on products—while soft paternalism imposes less onerous, "psychic costs," such as having to redirect one's attention (Sunstein 2014b, 55–61).

Because of our heuristics and biases, the way our environment is set up affects how we act. On the whole, people at cafeterias eat healthier foods when they are placed early in the line. People tend to save more when contributions to a retirement plan are automatic unless they opt out. People are more likely to lose weight when they diet and exercise with other people. When changing the choice architecture—the context in which people make decisions—affects what some people do, but without coercing them, it results in a nudge. As Thaler and Sunstein define it, "a nudge … is any aspect of the choice architecture that alters people's behavior in a predictable way without forbidding any options or significantly changing the economic incentives" (2008, 6). By changing the choice architecture, we can make it so that (some) people's heuristics nudge them in a particular direction—ideally, toward the good as each of them defines it for themselves. Because people are free to opt out of what their biases incline them to do, but nudges are designed to influence people's choices to make them better off, Thaler and Sunstein call their position libertarian paternalism (2008, 4–6).

Nudges can take different forms to take advantage of different heuristics. Sunstein (2014a) lists ten of the most important kinds of nudges:

1. Default rules: A default rule determines what happens if a person decides not to choose. In most places, if a patient has not completed a proxy directive, the next of kin is the default surrogate decision-maker.
2. Simplification: The ideally rational chooser can determine the optimal choice regardless of complexity, but we cannot. In 2023, the US Centers for Medicare & Medicaid Services (CMS) adopted a marketplace rule requiring participating health insurance insurers to offer standardized plan design (SPD) options to consumers. This makes it easier to compare potential healthcare plans.
3. Uses of social norms: This is the bandwagon effect. If patients are told that most men and women over fifty get colonoscopies, they are more likely to get them.

4. Increases in ease and convenience: Scheduling someone for a follow-up medical appointment when they check out at the clinic is more likely to get them to return than if they are sent home with instructions to call the office.
5. Disclosure: People are less likely to notice or be motivated by hidden costs. Nutrition labels on food packaging may discourage the consumption of products with lots of added sugar.
6. Warnings: The US Food and Drug Administration (FDA) requires black box warnings on medications that may have serious side effects in order to decrease their use among at-risk populations.
7. Precommitment strategies: This is a broad category of strategies to increase the likelihood that someone will reach a goal—for example, agreeing to do something on a specific day and time (e.g., "I will go to the gym at 7:30 every morning before work"), limiting one's future options (e.g., not keeping ice cream in one's freezer), and so on.
8. Reminders: When people are forgetful or driven by inertia, reminders make something salient—for example, a morning text message reminding someone about a medical appointment later that day.
9. Eliciting implementation intentions: Asking someone what they are going to do makes them more likely to do it (e.g., "When are you planning to get your COVID vaccination booster?").
10. Informing people of the nature and consequences of their own past choices: If someone has never set money aside for a tax-exempt health savings account (HSA), telling them how much they would have saved last year may motivate them to start an HSA this year.

Although this is not an exhaustive list, it makes clear that there is a variety of nudges that draw on different heuristics.

16.5 Nudges in Healthcare

Nudges are ubiquitous across healthcare environments. First, the clinical space is full of nudges for providers, including warnings, reminders, and default stop dates for interventions; and many nudges have been proposed or trialed to change clinician behavior and promote patient health and safety (Nagtegaal et al. 2019; Last et al. 2021; Wolf et al. 2022). However, changing clinician behavior with nudges is different from other kinds of nudges. For one thing, although clinicians make mistakes as a result of inattention, haste, and the misuse of heuristics, there is no mismatch between what their impulsive and rational systems want (as there is with an addicted smoker, for example). Furthermore, nudging clinicians is not paternalistic because it promotes safe and effective care for patients, not the well-being of providers themselves. Thus, nudging clinicians tends to be uncontroversial because it reduces harm to others and does not get clinicians to do things that they, or even part of them, does not want to do.

More controversially, nudges are used to change individual and community health decisions. To address public health issues, many nudges have been proposed, trialed, or adopted to, for example, improve adult dietary behavior (Arno and Thomas 2016), encourage vaccination (Reñosa et al. 2021), and decrease alcohol and tobacco use (Sylvester and Gooch 2021). Nudges are also used to improve the health of individual patients in the clinical setting. For example, treatment options that providers offer to patients must meet the legal standard of care. Providers do not need to suggest things that a reasonably prudent person would not consider, such as herbal remedies for stage III breast cancer, thus defaulting to treatments that have been successful in clinical trials. As opposed to public health nudges, clinical nudges identify individual health preferences (ends) and appeal to patients' specific biases and desires (means). At Meritus Health in Maryland, for example, they ask each patient to complete a "What Matters Most" questionnaire in their MyChart account. Knowing what someone cares about helps to inform healing strategies. Since low mobility often correlates with poor health outcomes and higher mortality, Meritus got a portable putting green to motivate a golf-loving patient to get out of bed.

Digital technologies have the potential to improve the efficacy of nudges. For example, digital traces on social media can be used to predict personality traits, which can be used to tailor nudges to a particular person (Settanni et al. 2018; see also Chen and Patel 2020). As mobile technologies become capable of tracking individual health conditions, they have the potential to facilitate remote behavioral treatment—for example, having relaxation techniques pop up on a patient's phone when their blood pressure rises, or automatically scheduling a follow-up appointment if a treatment is not having the desired effect. A new app called WoeBot utilizes AI and natural language processing techniques to chat with users conversationally, to develop a picture of a user's mental state, and to deliver personalized interventions, drawing on cognitive behavioral therapy and other approaches.

16.6 Objections and Replies

A lot of choice architecture in everyday life nudges us toward unhealthy decisions, such as McDonald's using a red and yellow color scheme, the placement of candy bars at the grocery store checkout line, and the autoplay feature on YouTube. Should clinicians and public health officials use choice architecture to nudge patients and the broader public toward healthier options? Opponents of libertarian paternalism raise two kinds of objections: first, they say that nudges do not really make us better off, in either the short- or long-term; and second, they say that nudges violate people's freedom by manipulating them or otherwise forcing them to do what others (but not they themselves) think is best. Neither objection is compelling enough to rule out libertarian paternalism on either empirical or moral grounds. Nudges can be designed that both promote personal welfare and respect individual autonomy.

16.6.1 Consequentialist Objection #1: Nudges Are Ineffective or Misguided

Critics of nudges raise several empirical questions. For example, are nudges really effective at improving welfare individually and in the aggregate (Ploug 2019)? Will adopting nudges lead to a slippery slope toward ends paternalism and coercion (Rizzo and Whitman 2020, 349–397)? Are choice architects actually better than individuals themselves at moving them toward what they take to be good (White 2013, 61–80)? These kinds of questions are not objections per se; they are more like cautions. To be objections, we would have to assume that nudges are never effective, that there is no way to avoid the slippery slope, and that choice architects are always wrong. As Sunstein puts it, "In many contexts, the objections to paternalism depend on strong empirical assumptions, involving extreme optimism about private choosers and extreme pessimism about public officials, that do not always hold" (2014b, 22). The above questions cannot be settled a priori, only empirically. And there is no evidence to justify the pessimistic assumptions behind them.

As mentioned earlier, Mill's argument for liberty of pursuits depends on assumptions that have been called into question by behavioral science. Even if people can correctly identify what they value, that does not entail that they are well-equipped to achieve it. Because of people's bounded rationality, choice architects may be in a better position to guide other people's actions rightly, given what they themselves want, since choice architects can take the broad view, informed by System 2, rather than acting on impulse in the moment. In the clinical space, for example, medical professionals are in a good position to help patients with their affective forecasting (i.e., predicting how they will feel in the future). Patients are inclined to overestimate the negative impact of a disabling injury and to underestimate their ability to cope. A patient who is newly disabled has never experienced this before, but their clinician may know how other patients have responded and adapted to that condition. Also, a patient's temporary feelings may overwhelm them, but a clinician can help them recognize other elements of their lives that will continue to be valuable, such as interacting with family. The more that clinicians are aware of such affective forecasting errors, the better they are at countering them (Zamzow 2016).

If regulators or public health experts are wrong in what they are nudging us toward, there are plenty of checks. If a proposed nudge is publicized and debated (see below), and if people can easily choose options other than the default when the consequences are bad (or bad enough), then individual preferences are incorporated at both the policy and implementation stages. Furthermore, since behavioral economics is grounded in empirical observation—integrating economic principles with behavioral science—proponents of nudges only defend them if there is evidence that they work.

Consequentialist arguments against nudges are misguided, then, not because nudges are always good. They may be counterproductive, and choice architects may be corrupt or inept. There is some evidence that nudges are not as effective as they are purported to be (Hummel and Maedche 2019). However, proponents of nudges only accept them if the consequences are better than alternative arrangements. Although the effectiveness of nudges varies depending on the context and kinds of nudges used—a caveat that is hardly surprising—there is plenty of evidence that nudges can change behavior and improve outcomes (Arno and Thomas 2016; Mertens et al. 2021). The question is: can we empirically establish which nudges are effective, for whom, and under what circumstances?

Empirical science of any kind is always capable of improvement, and behavioral economics is a relatively new field. It began by discovering some of the ways that we diverge from the ideal chooser of neoclassical economics. It continues to identify cognitive heuristics, and it tries to show how we can change choice architecture to achieve better outcomes. This is a highly complex inquiry, challenging not only because of its interdisciplinarity but also because the effects of those common biases depend in part on the social contexts in which choices take place. However, all defenders of nudges want policymaking to be evidence-based, subject to cost-benefit analyses and guided by our best scientific knowledge, rather than appealing to moral intuition or public opinion (Sunstein 2019). The fact that nudge policies are open to empirical testing and replication makes them capable of continuous improvement. As Andreas Schmidt and Bart Engelen note, "That we regularly find ineffective nudges arguably indicates that the approach does reasonably well in separating effective from ineffective policies" (2020, 3).

The Behavioural Insights Team (BIT)—the UK's "Nudge Unit"—has outlined several ways to improve applied behavioral science research (Hallsworth 2023). For example, behavioral scientists should develop practical theories that show how universal explanations (e.g., about System 1 and System 2 thinking) relate to working hypotheses about specific biases and heuristics. BIT suggests resource rationality as an example, which "starts from the basis that people make rational use of their limited cognitive resources. Given that there is a cost to thinking, people will look for solutions that balance choice quality with effort" (17). Studies should include a wider range of contexts and participants, and meta-analyses and replications should be done to identify the most reliable nudges (16, 51–59; see also Szaszi et al. 2018). To increase effectiveness, interventions should be built into organizations' existing standard processes (Hallsworth 2023, 12–13, 29–34). As the field advances, following these and other proposals, the scientific grounding of behavioral economics will become more predictive, more instructive, and more useful.

16.6.2 Consequentialist Objection #2: Ends Are Moving Targets

A second, more serious but less frequently discussed consequentialist objection to libertarian paternalism is that someone's ends are in principle not identifiable because a person has no fixed values and inconsistent desires (Rizzo and Whitman 2020, 235–280). This is different from Mill's epistemic claim, which is an empirical generalization about the privileged perspective an individual has on their own true preferences. Rather, this objection is about the nature of end-setting for people who are not fully rational. If, for example, someone wants contradictory things—say, to lose weight and to enjoy the pleasures of eating decadent desserts—there may not be one end that the person "really" wants and that a choice architect can help them achieve. They may want both, even when having both simultaneously is impossible or their preferences fluctuate. As Tversky puts it,

> Individuals ... are not perfectly consistent in their choices. When faced with repeated choices between *x* and *y*, people often choose *x* in some instances and *y* in others. Furthermore, such inconsistencies are observed even in the absence of systematic changes in the decision maker's taste which might be due to learning or sequential effects. It seems, therefore, that the observed inconsistencies reflect inherent variability or momentary fluctuation in the evaluative process. (1969, 31)

Contrary to the transitivity of preferences, someone may prefer *a* to *b*, *b* to *c*, and *c* to *a*, and not simply because of inconsistency but because of ordering preferences (the serial position effect) and other heuristics. Thus, Tversky says, "preference should be defined in a probabilistic fashion" (1969, 31).

Under the circumstances, it seems that ends paternalism is unavoidable. A choice architect may assume that the person's System 1 wants to eat lots of sweets and System 2 wants to achieve a healthy weight, even though they may want both, or their order of preferences may switch. In the clinical context, patients' preferences may be tied to specific treatment options rather than holding abstract principles that apply consistently across treatments (Ploug 2019, 65). Thus, according to this objection, choice architects inevitably impose goals onto people that they do not consistently hold, and any choice architecture "interferes wrongly and in the wrong place" (Mill 1978, 81).

There are two reasons why this consequentialist objection to libertarian paternalism is not damning. First, there is no way to avoid choice architecture entirely. Critics of libertarian paternalism often assume that one can either have or not have choice architecture, as if people's choices could be untouched by the right setup, or that we could avoid responsibility by leaving it up to chance. In principle, however, there is no way to arrange things such that all people's choices, even when they are thoughtlessly driven by heuristics, are completely unaffected. For example, when a decision must be made but someone does not or cannot choose for themselves, there must be a default option:

> Default options are frequently unavoidable. Oncologists must decide what to do if a patient without an advanced directive has a cardiac arrest, emergency medicine physicians must have a policy for how to care for uninsured patients who require urgent attention, and cardiologists must decide the order in which they will present medical and surgical treatment options to patients with valvular heart disease. When default options are unavoidable, it makes little sense to consider whether setting them is unethical. Instead, we must ask which one of the many possible default options is most justifiable. (Halpern et al. 2007, 1342; see also Thaler and Sunstein 2008, 10, 85, 240-241; Sunstein 2014b, 118-122, 151)

If we need to have defaults, then we must make decisions about choice architecture, which is going to impact some people's decisions. As Thaler and Sunstein say, defaults do not "come from nature or from the sky" (2008, 241).

Mark White seems to think that mandated choice—forcing someone to choose rather than having a default—is the only way to remain neutral and respect personal autonomy (2013, 100). However, someone has to decide whether to mandate choice and how to phrase and order the options—both of which inevitably impact some people's decisions. Patients are influenced when a clinician tells them the preferred treatment of experts in the field (default rule), the option most patients choose (use of social norms), and the greater risks that come with alternative treatments (warnings). How much patients like and trust a clinician impacts how likely they are to follow the clinician's recommendation (affect heuristic), so the person who explains the options also impacts patients' choices. Furthermore, requiring mandated choice is paternalistic because it deprives people of the option of choosing not to choose (Sunstein 2014b, 95; 2016). Especially when people have little information about or understanding of the options, they generally prefer to have a default (Thaler and Sunstein 2008, 88–89). If we want to allow them not to choose when that is their preference, then there must be a default rule. This is not an unusual circumstance in the medical context, where patients often defer to the opinion of their medical practitioner rather than deciding for themselves.

Because choice architecture is ubiquitous, the question is not whether we ought to shape people's choices but which interventions are best given what we know, most reliable under the circumstances, or most warranted by the evidence. With regard to means—that is, which nudges to use—we must follow the most rigorous behavioral science. To follow Mill's injunction and respect people's individual ends—to be means paternalists rather than ends paternalists—the best we can do is probabilistic inferences about people's true preferences.

Despite White's insistence that "*only a person can know his or her true interests*" (2013, 62), there are several ways to increase the probability that we are not imposing our own ends onto others. Clinicians often begin with self-reporting from patients, such as the "What Matters Most" questionnaire at Meritus Health. Knowledge about what a particular patient wants—or what they think they want—helps to guide clinical interactions. For example, if an older patient indicates that running for exercise is important to them, clinicians should not repeatedly raise concerns about arthritis in the knees or pressure the patient to take up swimming. Engelen says that doctors can infer their patients' preferences reliably because they have known them for years or even decades (which is perhaps an outdated notion given the recent prevalence of team-based healthcare models) (2019, 52). For public health interventions, ends can be revealed through surveys and deliberative polls (52).

Clinicians also need to engage in open and honest dialogue with their patients about what they want, their habits, and how the two become disjoined. Clinicians often think that they empower patients by giving them objective information about their conditions and options, letting them choose treatments, and then carrying out their wishes. This model of the patient-physician relationship ignores the issues raised by behavioral science. Having ongoing, mutually respectful, and honest dialogue about what a patient wants and the obstacles to achieving it is more likely to reveal what matters to them (Emanuel and Emanuel 1992). It also helps the clinician to resist their own cognitive habits, such as generalizing about a patient based on their age, race, or ailment, which may be misplaced in particular cases (Capron and Spruijt-Metz 2016, 239).

Of course, in the current healthcare environment, physicians (especially harried residents) hardly have the time, skills, and inclination to dig down to their patients' true preferences. Luckily, technological advancements can help choice architects to overcome epistemic and other limitations when it comes to discerning people's values. All of us have digital traces (also called digital footprints or digital records) that reveal our choices and behaviors in real time, as a result of self-tracking devices such as Fitbit and mobile technologies such as GPS-enabled smartphones (Estrin 2014). Health-related data can be collected through social media activity, online search engine activity, and ecological momentary assessments (where users answer prompts on their smartphones to provide snapshots of their daily lives), all of which can be linked and analyzed with AI algorithms (Tucaković et al. 2021, 38). These serve as digital markers of healthy and risky behaviors, as well as physical and mental health. Technology companies are also developing mobile health information and sensing technologies (mHealth) that can be used not only for point-of-care diagnostics and portable imaging but also for monitoring treatment adherence and assessing the efficacy of treatments (Kumar et al. 2013; see also Marsch 2021). As Alexander Capron and Donna Spruijt-Metz note, the existence of voluminous "small data" about individual persons has the potential to reveal their true preferences more accurately than either self-reporting or clinician-patient interactions:

> "Small data" about the patient, competently analyzed and accessible on an ongoing basis, will help some [physicians] by showing what patients like to do (work, travel, garden, hike, read books, attend concerts, etc.) and even when and with whom (spouses, children, grandchildren, friends, co-workers, strangers, etc.). Such data can also provide clues about how patients' well-being and activities are affected by changes in health or by different medical interventions, and about how various features of the environment also affect patients' behavior, choices, and health status. They are more detailed and more reliable than what patients or family members typically report to physicians during office visits since they are free of the errors of memory and selective reporting that color normal narratives. (2016, 238)

In short, there are many ways to identify patients' true preferences so that they can be respected and furthered by choice architects. The dramatic improvement of AI and the expansion of digital technologies will make such identifications even more accurate.

Although such technologies raise privacy concerns, these can be reduced if clinicians explain how the information will be used and patients consent to be monitored. Research has shown that, in general, people are willing to share their data with clinicians and researchers in pursuit of health-related insights (Seltzer et al. 2019). If such data is used for medical purposes, it may also be protected by privacy laws such as HIPAA in a way that other big and small data—much of it owned by private companies—is not.

Before moving on, I want to be clear about what my responses to these consequentialist objections have and have not demonstrated. Obviously, the science regarding human cognition and decision-making is not settled. There is some controversy about whether the psychological discoveries underlying nudge theory accurately capture how people make difficult decisions, including accusations that some of the science suffers from greater or lesser degrees of conclusion-jumping. The point of this section is not to definitively establish the truth of libertarian paternalism, let alone the justifiability of any specific interventions. However, we have enough evidence to know that simply leaving people to their own devices does not result in optimal outcomes, even according to their own conceptions of the good. And instituting some kind of choice architecture is inevitable. Under the circumstances, what should we do? Choice architects are informed by empirical research on human cognition, and they are open to continuous improvement in a way that other approaches are not. Therefore, the previous arguments (in 16.6.1 and 16.6.2) mitigate consequentialist concerns that choice architects cannot effectively nudge decision-makers to choose rightly, as they would themselves if they reliably did what they needed to do to get what they want.

16.6.3 Deontological Objection #1: Nudges Are Manipulative

Some critics oppose nudges on principle, regardless of the consequences. The first and most common deontological objection is that libertarian paternalism is manipulative, erodes freedom, and does not respect subjectivity. If people are being unknowingly steered in one direction, then they are not consenting to the behavior and are thus being instrumentalized to achieve some outcome, even if it is for their own benefit.

This kind of objection paints all nudges with too broad a brush. The kind of nudge matters. Jeremy Waldron objects to nudges because they bypass his conscious reasoning: "I wish … that I could be made a better chooser rather than having someone on high take advantage (even for my own benefit) of my current thoughtlessness and my shabby intuitions" (2014, 23). However, some nudges—called Type 2 nudges—directly engage System 2, a person's thoughtful, deliberative capacities. These include disclosures, warnings, and reminders. How does texting someone about a doctor's appointment or informing someone that smoking causes cancer undermine a person's agency?

Furthermore, precommitment strategies undertaken by someone to change their own behavior could hardly be construed as manipulative. If I install the McDonald's app on my phone for ease of ordering but later find that I eat more fast food as a result, my uninstalling the app, thus making it harder for me to get the food that the impulsive part of me wants, is an act of agency. Involving someone else does not change the moral equation either. If patients agree to have their behavior monitored through mobile technologies and they agree to the nudges for the purpose of achieving their own freely adopted ends, then there is nothing objectionably paternalistic about such interventions. For example, using GPS on a recovering alcoholic's cell phone, their healthcare practitioner and their sponsor could be notified when they are near or at a bar that they used to frequent (Johnson et al. 2011). In the person's clearer moments, when guided by System 2, they could agree to this. One can imagine their clinician calling to remind them of the health effects of chronic drinking or their sponsor texting them pictures of their family. If such communications prevented the recovering alcoholic from impulsively deciding to start drinking again, it would not make the person less free.

Critics of nudges claim that such strategies are impositions on people's agency because they are not internally motivated to behave differently—in this case, to resist the impulse to drink alcohol. Typically, an alcoholic reaches out to their sponsor for support. Is getting a phone call from the sponsor, arranged in advance but unbidden in the moment, an intrusion on the person's agency? To answer in the affirmative, we have to assume a unified agency. However, one may experience contradictory motivations—in this case, to drink and not to drink—often simultaneously. The phone call is an imposition on System 1 but not System 2, as evidenced in this case by the fact that, when the recovering alcoholic is with their sponsor, they request the phone call. The temporal lag between the request and the call does not make it less the alcoholic's own doing. If the person defies the nudge—in this case, going into the bar anyway—all it says is that the incentive was not enough for System 2 to resist System 1, not that anyone infringed on their freedom.

Another way to understand this is that the sponsor and the clinician are trying to help bolster one of the recovering alcoholic's internal motivations, and specifically the more rational or reflective desire. Harry Frankfurt's (1998) distinction between first- and second-order desires makes this clearer: the person wants alcohol but does not want to want alcohol. Being free from interference to act on one's first-order desires is a kind of liberty in the sense that it is uncoerced, but insofar as nudges assist a person in acting according to their second-order desires, they are being helped to act autonomously. The person is able to do what their reflective self wants their impulsive self to want to do.

As noted earlier, choice architecture is unavoidable, but so are our intellectual habits. When we engage the world with our heuristics, they incline us in one direction or another, functioning as cognitive constraints (Ackerman 1982). The mere fact that heuristics are internal does not mean they are less coercive than the external conditions that also shape our behavior. Many critics of libertarian paternalism think that someone is free when we let them do what they want. But a person may want different, contradictory things. The question then is not whether we should let people do what they want but whether we should leave people at the mercy of System 1 or support System 2, both of which are part of them. To the extent that external choice architecture helps us to resist our impulses so we can better achieve the ends that we ourselves have chosen—means paternalism rather than ends paternalism—nudges support our freedom.

How should we feel about other Type 1 nudges such as default rules, which are not always explicit? Some critics worry that this is a form of domination, with choice architects working behind the scenes to control people's lives (Hausman and Welch 2010; Jones et al. 2011; Grüne-Yanoff 2012). Do nudges take advantage of a person's automatic processes in a way that treats them merely as a means to their own ends? Not necessarily. In a liberal democracy, the adoption of default rules by the government would be as subject to public scrutiny as any other law or regulation. In *Nudge*, Thaler and Sunstein endorse John Rawls's publicity principle: the government should only adopt policies, including paternalistic policies, that it is willing and able to defend to its own citizens (2008, 247–248). In *Why Nudge?* Sunstein goes beyond the willingness to defend and insists that nudges should actually go through a process of public vetting before implementation:

> Nothing should be hidden, and everything should be transparent. Soft paternalism, nudges, and any other behaviorally informed approaches, no less than hard paternalism, should be visible, scrutinized, and monitored. To the extent feasible, practices that embody soft determinism should be subject to public scrutiny in advance, often through notice-and-comment rule-making. (2014b, 147-148; see also Schmidt 2017; Engelen 2019, 52; Ivanković and Engelen 2019)

Often such reviews are done by people's elected representatives, such that the populace is indirectly consenting to them. But policymakers can also get people's input with surveys and public forums (Halpern 2019, 328–332). This process would mean that the people subjected to Type 1 nudges such as default rules would consent prior to being subjected to them. One cannot dominate oneself. Having public scrutiny of proposed nudges would also make the slippery slope less likely.

Under these circumstances, default rules come to resemble precommitment strategies: something that we consent to when we are thinking clearly and rationally, which we are then subjected to when we act carelessly and automatically. System 2 has given permission to nudge System 1. For example, as a matter of public policy, in the United States we have (historically) wanted to increase childhood vaccination rates. Parents do not need to make special appointments to vaccinate their children; during well-child visits to the clinic, providers are ready to administer vaccines on the recommended schedule—although parents can refuse. In all states, students must be vaccinated against specific communicable diseases as a condition of school attendance, or parents need to apply for exemptions. The easier it is to opt out—religious exemptions are always granted—the more people are allowed to decide for themselves. In Kantian terms, people are being treated as means to their own (and others') ends, but they are not treated *merely* as means, since they are consenting to the conditions under which they act—insofar as parents consent to the law and allow their children to be immunized (Kant 1996, 4:427–429). The fact that people generally approve of pro-self nudges, especially concerning health behavior, is evidence that most people consent to them, tacitly if not expressly (Hagman et al. 2015; Junghans et al. 2015; Reisch and Sunstein 2016).

Nudges are not coercive because, as Thaler and Sunstein say, "to count as a mere nudge, the intervention must be easy and cheap to avoid" (2008, 6). White claims that nudges "decide for me" or "ensure that I make 'better' choices" (2013, ix-x; see also Capron and Spruijt-Metz 2016, 234). However, unlike mandates or bans, nudges do not force anyone to do anything. People have all the options available to them that they would have without the nudge: less healthy foods are still available, just later in the cafeteria line. If one looks at the cafeteria line as a whole, it becomes clear that everything is there that was there prior to rearranging the order. As Yashar

Saghai (2013) puts it, nudges preserve the choice-set and are easily avoidable, so people's freedom of choice is preserved—this, despite the fact that some people's actual choices change depending on the choice architecture (see also Engelen 2019, 52).

16.6.4 Deontological Objection #2: Ends Paternalism Is Unavoidable

One worry about nudges, as voiced by White and others, is that choice architects must have a set conception of the good, and as Goldman points out, that may differ from what other people—the people who are being treated paternalistically—actually want. With the cafeteria line, choice architects assume that it is important for everyone to eat healthy, nutritious food. Everyone is then nudged to eat healthier. This is better when judged against the choice architects' set of values but not necessarily as the people who are being nudged define it for themselves. Not everyone wants the same healthy diet or wants to want the same healthy diet. Thus, choice architects cannot avoid ends paternalism.

To answer this objection, consider this: bans affect everyone, but whom do nudges affect? In the cafeteria, the people who really want to eat healthy food can do so and the people who really want to eat unhealthy food can do so. The people who eat more of whatever is placed early in the line are not motivated enough to incur the mild psychological cost of resisting what is more immediately available and waiting a few more seconds to fill their trays. It is hard to say that a conception of the good is imposed on them when their desire for unhealthy food is so unmotivating. To speak broadly, they want the unhealthy food, but do they *really* want it? If they succumb to the serial position effect, it must not be a true preference (of System 2) but only a shallow desire (of System 1), which the nudge helps them to resist.

Because of heuristics and biases, patients are sometimes not the best authority on the means to achieve their own ends. Means paternalism respects a person's choice of ends and helps them to choose what they want—or more precisely, what they want to want. Waldron's complaint—that he would like to be made a better chooser—may be more of a lament about what behavioral science has revealed about human decision-making than a criticism of nudges. If our choices were always guided by System 2, then nudges would be unnecessary. Indeed, nudges do not change the actions of the ideal rational chooser. However, given our bounded rationality, there is often a disconnect between what we want and the means that we choose to get there. Insofar as nudges help us achieve our own ends, they help us to act more rationally—that is, to align our actions and our goals. If we can accomplish this without nudges, that may be preferable (Engelen 2019, 54). It is good to educate and inform people. But there is no reason—certainly no empirically justified reason—to believe that, on the whole, people can reliably be made to be substantially better decision-makers about complicated things that they know very little about, such as healthcare, especially given the limited time and intellectual energy they have to make such important decisions. We need to evaluate the justifiability of nudges without appealing to mere intuitions about autonomy (a concept that is both vague and ambiguous) or unrealistic expectations about our own intellectual capabilities.

16.7 Conclusion

There are reasons not to force or coerce people to do what we think is best for them: autonomy has intrinsic value, and as Mill notes, we are liable to get things wrong, making people conform to someone else's conception of the good life. However, the idea that people will be better off if they are left to their own devices has been convincingly challenged by the behavioral science of the last fifty years. Furthermore, neutrality is not an option for public health officials, healthcare systems, and clinicians: the government has to establish vaccine policies, emergency department staff have to know whether to perform CPR on patients in cardiac arrest, and clinicians have to select and present treatment options in some order or other. Such decisions ought to be guided by libertarian paternalism, which both respects people's freedom and improves the welfare of those who rely too much on heuristics. Although nudges raise the specter of manipulation—a worry exacerbated by the addictive nature of many digital technologies and corporate ownership of personal data—being transparent about nudges achieves consent (either explicit or tacit), and if they are easily avoided, no one is being forced to do anything. Under these conditions, and being careful to respect privacy, digital technology can be used to develop individualized nudges, thus increasing the chances that they appropriately and effectively help people to satisfy their own true preferences. Libertarian paternalism is not the paternalism of the past. It allows government regulators, public health officials, and clinicians to act beneficently and to respect autonomy, even when we are inclined, against our own better judgment, to make unhealthy choices.[1]

References

Ackerman, Terrence F. 1982. "Why Doctors Should Intervene." *Hastings Center Report* 12 (4) (August): 14–17. https://doi.org/10.2307/3560762.

Arno, Anneliese, and Steve Thomas. 2016. "The Efficacy of Nudge Theory Strategies in Influencing Adult Dietary Behaviour: A Systematic Review and Meta-analysis." *BMC Public Health* 16 (676). https://doi.org/10.1186/s12889-016-3272-x.

Capron, Alexander M., and Donna Spruijt-Metz. 2016. "Behavioral Economics in the Physician-Patient Relationship: A Possible Role for Mobile Devices and Small Data." In *Nudging Health: Health Law and Behavioral Economics*, edited by I. Glenn Cohen, Holly Fernandez Lynch, and Christopher T. Robertson, 233–243. Baltimore: Johns Hopkins University Press.

[1] I am grateful to Cynthia D. Coe for providing helpful feedback on an early draft. Part of this chapter was presented at an annual meeting of the Association for Practical & Professional Ethics.

Chen, X. Shirley, and Mitesh S. Patel. 2020. "Digital Health Tools Offer New Opportunities for Personalized Care." *Harvard Business Review.* November 18. https://hbr.org/2020/11/digital-health-tools-offer-new-opportunities-for-personalized-care.
Conly, Sarah. 2013. *Against Autonomy: Justifying Coercive Paternalism.* Cambridge: Cambridge University Press.
De Neys, Wim, and Vinod Goel. 2011. "Heuristics and Biases in the Brain: Dual Neural Pathways for Decision Making." In *Neuroscience of Decision Making*, edited by Oshin Vartanian and David R. Mandel, 125–141. New York: Psychology Press. https://doi.org/10.4324/9780203835920.
Ebbinghaus, Hermann. 1885. *Über das Gedächtnis: Untersuchungen zur experimentellen Psychologie.* Leipzig: Duncker & Humber.
Emanuel, Ezekiel J., and Linda L. Emanuel. 1992. "Four Models of the Physician-Patient Relationship." *JAMA: Journal of the American Medical Association* 267 (16) (April 22–29): 2221–2226. https://doi.org/10.1001/jama.1992.03480160079038.
Engelen, Bart. 2019. "Ethical Criteria for Health-Promoting Nudges: A Case-by-Case Analysis." *American Journal of Bioethics* 19 (5) (May): 48–59. https://doi.org/10.1080/15265161.2019.1588411.
Estrin, Deborah. 2014. "Small Data, Where N = Me." *Communications of the ACM* 57 (4) (April): 32–34. https://doi.org/10.1145/2580944.
Frankfurt, Harry G. 1998. *The Importance of What We Care About: Philosophical Essays.* Cambridge: Cambridge University Press.
Gigerenzer, Gerd, and Daniel G. Goldstein. 1996. "Reasoning the Fast and Frugal Way: Models of Bounded Rationality." *Psychological Review* 103 (4) (October): 650–669. https://doi.org/10.1037/0033-295x.103.4.650.
Gigerenzer, Gerd, and Peter M. Todd, eds. 1999. *Simple Heuristics That Make Us Smart.* Oxford: Oxford University Press.
Gilovich, Thomas, Dale Griffin, and Daniel Kahneman, eds. 2002. *Heuristics and Biases: The Psychology of Intuitive Judgment.* Cambridge: Cambridge University Press.
Goldman, Alan H. 1980. "Refutation of Medical Paternalism." In *The Moral Foundations of Professional Ethics*, 173–195. Totowa, NJ: Rowman & Littlefield.
Goldstein, Daniel G., and Gerd Gigerenzer. 1999. "The Recognition Heuristic: How Ignorance Makes Us Smart." In *Simple Heuristics That Make Us Smart*, edited by Gerd Gigerenzer and Peter M. Todd, 37–58. Oxford: Oxford University Press.
Grüne-Yanoff, Till. 2012. "Old Wine in New Casks: Libertarian Paternalism Still Violates Liberal Principles." *Social Choice and Welfare* 38 (4) (April): 635–645. https://doi.org/10.1007/s00355-011-0636-0.
Hagman, William, David Andersson, Daniel Västfjäll, and Gustav Tinghög. 2015. "Public Views on Policies Involving Nudges." *Review of Philosophy and Psychology* 6 (3) (September): 439–453. https://doi.org/10.1007/s13164-015-0263-2.
Hallsworth, Michael. 2023. *A Manifesto for Applying Behavioral Science.* Behavioural Insights Team. March 20. https://www.bi.team/publications/a-manifesto-for-applying-behavioral-science/.
Halpern, David. 2019. *Inside the Nudge Unit: How Small Changes Can Make a Big Difference.* New updated ed. London: Penguin.
Halpern, Scott D., Peter A. Ubel, and David A. Asch. 2007. "Harnessing the Power of Default Options to Improve Health Care." *New England Journal of Medicine* 357 (13) (September 27): 1340–1344. https://doi.org/10.1056/NEJMsb071595.
Hausman, Daniel M., and Brynn Welch. 2010. "Debate: To Nudge or Not to Nudge." *Journal of Political Philosophy* 18 (1) (March): 123–136. https://doi.org/10.1111/j.1467-9760.2009.00351.x.
Hummel, Dennis, and Alexander Maedche. 2019. "How Effective Is Nudging? A Quantitative Review on the Effect Sizes and Limits of Empirical Nudging Studies." *Journal of Behavioral and Experimental Economics* 80 (June): 47–58. https://doi.org/10.1016/j.socec.2019.03.005.

Ivanković, Viktor, and Bart Engelen. 2019. "Nudging, Transparency, and Watchfulness." *Social Theory and Practice* 45 (1) (January): 43–74. https://doi.org/10.5840/soctheorpract20191751.

Jones, Rhys, Jessica Pykett, and Mark Whitehead. 2011. "Governing Temptation: Changing Behaviour in an Age of Libertarian Paternalism." *Progress in Human Geography* 35 (4) (August): 483–501. https://doi.org/10.1177/0309132510385741.

Junghans, Astrid F., Tracy T. L. Cheung, and Denise D. T. De Ridder. 2015. "Under Consumers' Scrutiny—an Investigation into Consumers' Attitudes and Concerns about Nudging in the Realm of Health Behavior." *BMC Public Health* 15 (336). https://doi.org/10.1186/s12889-015-1691-8.

Kahneman, Daniel, and Amos Tversky. 1977. "Intuitive Prediction: Biases and Corrective Procedures." Decision Research Technical Report PTR-1042–77–6. Eugene, OR: Decision Research. https://apps.dtic.mil/sti/pdfs/ADA047747.pdf.

Kant, Immanuel. 1996. *Groundwork of the Metaphysics of Morals*. In *Practical Philosophy*, translated and edited by Mary J. Gregor, 41–108. Cambridge: Cambridge University Press.

Kumar, Santosh, Wendy J. Nilsen, Amy Abernethy, Audie Atienza, Kevin Patrick, Misha Pavel, et al. 2013. "Mobile Health Technology Evaluation: The mHealth Evidence Workshop." *American Journal of Preventive Medicine* 45 (2) (August): 228–236. https://doi.org/10.1016/j.amepre.2013.03.017.

Last, Briana S., Alison M. Buttenheim, Carter E. Timon, Nandita Mitra, and Rinad S. Beidas. 2021. "Systematic Review of Clinician-Directed Nudges in Healthcare Contexts." *BMJ Open* 11 (7) (July): e048801. https://doi.org/10.1136/bmjopen-2021-048801.

Le Grand, Julian, and Bill New. 2015. *Government Paternalism: Nanny State or Helpful Friend?* Princeton, NJ: Princeton University Press.

Marsch, Lisa A. 2021. "Digital Health Data-Driven Approaches to Understand Human Behavior." *Neuropsychopharmacology* 46 (1) (January): 191–196. https://doi.org/10.1038/s41386-020-0761-5.

Mertens, Stephanie, Mario Herberz, Ulf J. J. Hahnel, and Tobias Brosch. 2021. "The Effectiveness of Nudging: A Meta-analysis of Choice Architecture Interventions across Behavioral Domains." *PNAS* 119 (1) (December 30): e2107346118. https://doi.org/10.1073/pnas.2107346118.

Mill, John Stuart. 1978. *On Liberty*. Edited by Elizabeth Rapaport. Indianapolis: Hackett.

Nagtegaal, Rosanna, Lars Tummers, Mirko Noordegraaf, and Victor Bekkers. 2019. "Nudging Healthcare Professionals towards Evidence-Based Medicine: A Systematic Scoping Review." *Journal of Behavioral Public Administration* 2 (2): 1–20. https://doi.org/10.30636/jbpa.22.71.

Ploug, Thomas. 2019. "Easy Resistible, Means-Paternalist Nudging in the Clinical Context Is an Untenable Proposal." *American Journal of Bioethics* 19 (5) (May): 48–59. https://doi.org/10.1080/15265161.2019.1588421.

Reisch, Lucia A., and Cass R. Sunstein. 2016. "Do Europeans Like Nudges?" *Judgment and Decision Making* 11 (4) (July): 310–325. https://doi.org/10.1017/S1930297500003740.

Reñosa, Mark Donald C., Jeniffer Landicho, Jonas Wachinger, Sarah L. Dalglish, Kate Bärnighausen, Till Bärnighausen, and Shannon A. McMahon. 2021. "Nudging toward Vaccination: A Systematic Review." *BMJ Global Health* 6 (9) (September): e006237. https://doi.org/10.1136/bmjgh-2021-006237.

Rizzo, Mario J., and Glen Whitman. 2020. *Escaping Paternalism: Rationality, Behavioral Economics, and Public Policy*. Cambridge: Cambridge University Press.

Saghai, Yashar. 2013. "Salvaging the Concept of Nudge." *Journal of Medical Ethics* 39 (8) (August): 487–493. https://doi.org/10.1136/medethics-2012-100727.

Samuelson, William, and Richard Zeckhauser. 1988. "Status Quo Bias in Decision Making." *Journal of Risk and Uncertainty* 1 (1) (March): 7–59. https://doi.org/10.1007/BF00055564.

Schmidt, Andreas T. 2017. "The Power to Nudge." *American Political Science Review* 111 (2) (May): 404–417. https://doi.org/10.1017/S0003055417000028.

Schmidt, Andreas T., and Bart Engelen. 2020. "The Ethics of Nudging: An Overview." *Philosophy Compass* 15 (4) (April): e12658. https://doi.org/10.1111/phc3.12658.

Seltzer, Emily, Jesse Goldshear, Sharath Chandra Guntuku, Dave Grande, David A. Asch, Elissa V. Klinger, and Raina M. Merchant. 2019. “Patients’ Willingness to Share Digital Health and Non-health Data for Research: A Cross-Sectional Study.” *BMC Medical Informatics and Decision Making* 19 (157). https://doi.org/10.1186/s12911-019-0886-9.

Settanni, Michele, Danny Azucar, and Davide Marengo. 2018. “Predicting Individual Characteristics from Digital Traces on Social Media: A Meta-analysis.” *Cyberpsychology, Behavior, and Social Networking* 21 (4) (April): 217–228. https://doi.org/10.1089/cyber.2017.0384.

Stanovich, Keith E., and Richard F. West. 2000. “Individual Differences in Reasoning: Implications for the Rationality Debate?” *Behavioral and Brain Sciences* 23 (5) (October): 645–726. https://doi.org/10.1017/S0140525X00003435.

Sunstein, Cass R. 2014a. “Nudging: A Very Short Guide.” *Journal of Consumer Policy* 37 (4) (December): 583–588. https://doi.org/10.1007/s10603-014-9273-1.

Sunstein, Cass R. 2014b. *Why Nudge? The Politics of Libertarian Paternalism*. New Haven, CT: Yale University Press.

Sunstein, Cass R. 2016. Foreword to *Nudging Health: Health Law and Behavioral Economics*, edited by I. Glenn Cohen, Holly Fernandez Lynch, and Christopher T. Robertson, xi–xxvii. Baltimore: Johns Hopkins University Press.

Sunstein, Cass R. 2019. *The Cost-Benefit Revolution*. Cambridge, MA: MIT Press.

Sylvester, Benjamin, and Stephen Gooch. 2021. “A Realist Review of Nudge Interventions to Decrease Alcohol and Tobacco Use.” Defence Research and Development Canada, Scientific Report, DRDC-RDDC-2021-R136. September. https://cradpdf.drdc-rddc.gc.ca/PDFS/unc367/p813561_A1b.pdf.

Szaszi, Barnabas, Anna Palinkas, Bence Palfi, Aba Szollosi, and Balazs Aczel. 2018. “A Systematic Scoping Review of the Choice Architecture Movement: Toward Understanding When and Why Nudges Work.” *Behavioral Decision Making* 31 (3) (July): 355–366. https://doi.org/10.1002/bdm.2035.

Thaler, Richard H., and Cass R. Sunstein. 2008. *Nudge: Improving Decisions About Health, Wealth, and Happiness*. New Haven, CT: Yale University Press.

Truc, Alexandre. 2022. “Forty Years of Behavioral Economics.” *European Journal of the History of Economic Thought* 29 (3): 393–437. https://doi.org/10.1080/09672567.2021.1993295.

Tucaković, Lana, Nemanja Nikolić, and Ljubiša Bojić. 2021. “How Digital Data Are Used in the Domain of Health: A Short Review of Current Knowledge.” In *Proceedings of the PaKSoM 3rd Virtual International Conference: Path to a Knowledge Society—Managing Risks and Innovation*, edited by M. Stanković and V. Nikolić, 37–41. Niš, Serbia: Complex System Research Centre and Serbia Mathematical Institute of the Serbian Academy of Sciences and Arts.

Tversky, Amos. 1969. “Intransitivity of Preferences.” *Psychological Review* 76 (1) (January): 31–48. https://doi.org/10.1037/h0026750.

Tversky, Amos, and Daniel Kahneman. 1974. “Judgment under Uncertainty: Heuristics and Biases.” *Science* 185 (4157) (September 27): 1124–1131. https://doi.org/10.1126/science.185.4157.1124.

Tversky, Amos, and Daniel Kahneman. 1992. “Advances in Prospect Theory: Cumulative Representation of Uncertainty.” *Journal of Risk and Uncertainty* 5 (4) (October): 297–323. https://doi.org/10.1007/BF00122574.

Waldron, Jeremy. 2014. “It’s All for Your Own Good.” Review of *Why Nudge? The Politics of Libertarian Paternalism* and *Conspiracy Theories and Other Dangerous Ideas*, by Cass R. Sunstein. *New York Review of Books* (October 9): 21–23. https://www.nybooks.com/articles/2014/10/09/cass-sunstein-its-all-your-own-good/.

White, Mark D. 2013. *The Manipulation of Choice: Ethics and Libertarian Paternalism*. New York: Palgrave Macmillan.

Wolf, Axel, Anita Sant’Anna, and Andreas Vilhelmsson. 2022. “Using Nudges to Promote Clinical Decision Making of Healthcare Professionals: A Scoping Review.” *Preventive Medicine* 164 (November): article no. 107320. https://doi.org/10.1016/j.ypmed.2022.107320.

Zamzow, Jennifer L. 2016. "Affective Forecasting in Medical Decision-Making: What Do Physicians Owe Their Patients?" In *Nudging Health: Health Law and Behavioral Economics*, edited by I. Glenn Cohen, Holly Fernandez Lynch, and Christopher T. Robertson, 222–232. Baltimore: Johns Hopkins University Press.

Matthew C. Altman is Chair and Professor of Philosophy at Central Washington University, USA. His research focuses on applied ethics, the history of philosophy, and the philosophy of law. Altman has published on such diverse topics as restorative justice, performance-enhancing drugs, mass incarceration, suicide, the problem of other minds, mandatory ultrasound laws, same-sex marriage, and the state of academic philosophy. He is the author, co-author, or editor of nine books, including *The Hackett Introduction to Medical Ethics* (with Cynthia D. Coe, 2025) and *A Theory of Legal Punishment* (2021).

Chapter 17
Conclusion: Technology, Values, and the Critical Role of Bioethics

David Schwan and Matthew C. Altman

Abstract This Conclusion identifies three lessons that follow from the chapters in the book. First, we ought to identify and critically reflect on the ideological assumptions that are embodied in new technologies. Second, we ought to design or redesign technologies with an awareness of their impact on people and how the effects vary depending on local circumstances. Third, we ought to draw on bioethics as we develop new medical technologies so that we can challenge common assumptions and appeal to deeply held moral values to inform our decisions.

Keywords Ideology · Technological determinism · Technological universalism · Bioethics · Medical ethics

17.1 Introduction

It is often tempting to overstate the importance of the current historical moment. However, the medical technologies discussed in this contributed volume are, arguably, revolutionary. In the past decade, we have witnessed the rise of widely available gene therapies, the expansion of big data into predictive medicine and public health, and the rapid growth of AI-powered diagnostic and treatment tools. In addition to improving health outcomes, these technologies are reshaping the nature and norms of medicine itself. What lessons should a reader carry forward into this period of significant change?

D. Schwan (✉) · M. C. Altman
Central Washington University, Ellensburg, WA, USA
e-mail: david.schwan@cwu.edu

M. C. Altman
e-mail: matthew.altman@cwu.edu

M. C. Altman and D. Schwan (eds.), *Ethics and Medical Technology*, The International Library of Bioethics 113, https://doi.org/10.1007/978-3-031-94690-5_17

17.2 Technology Embodies and Reinforces Values

It is common knowledge that how we design and use technology is value-laden. But our tendency to adjust to new technological norms means that the ideological assumptions embodied in these tools are often obscured. One advantage of periods of rapid change is that at least some of these assumptions are foregrounded, giving us the opportunity to critically reflect on their status and value.

For example, consider medical diagnosis. For much of history, medical decision-making has centered on the clinician's education, practical training, and judgment, in the context of a relationship with patients in which their needs and values could be clarified and could guide treatment decisions. Yet in just a decade, some AI-driven diagnostic support systems are already able to outperform human diagnosticians. As impressive as these tools appear, they inherently privilege efficiency and predictive accuracy, framing medical concerns primarily as technical problems to solve. If effective medical diagnosis and treatment decisions also involve personal connection with patients or social practices that support the ongoing cultivation of interpretive human judgment, medical institutions should carefully consider whether these values are being displaced.

Electronic health records raise similar issues. While the development of EHRs continues to evolve, their design still frequently prioritizes coding for insurance claims, regulatory compliance, and redundant documentation to guard against potential lawsuits. Such systems reinforce the assumption that clinical encounters are primarily economic transactions between "providers" and "customers" rather than interpersonal relationships between clinicians and patients focused on health and well-being. In our view, clinicians are so frustrated with EHRs in part because of the values they privilege. Instead of being designed to foster better clinical communication, EHRs function as cumbersome billing and compliance checklists. Spending hours a day on these tasks is a constant reminder that modern medicine often is not primarily about patient care. For those who pursued medicine as a vocation because they want to help people, the practical dissonance they experience produces deep dissatisfaction and burnout.

Finally, consider some of the values embedded in telemedicine, remote monitoring technologies, and wearable health trackers. In their own ways, each emphasizes accessibility, convenience, and (in some cases) regular observation and data collection. Telemedicine has improved accessibility for many patients, but at the cost of direct personal interaction. Wearable devices, which have rapidly grown in popularity, convey the assumption that continuous self-monitoring and quantification of health is desirable, reduce patients' privacy by continuously recording their activity, and shift more responsibility for health management onto them. Furthermore, while there are clear benefits to tracking and utilizing personal health data, overemphasizing objective measures may displace more collaborative patient-clinician relationships grounded in dialogue and subjective experience.

The lesson here is that new and existing technologies are not neutral tools; they embody and reinforce underlying assumptions about medical practice, clinical judgment, and patient care. Periods of rapid transition can remind us of the contingency of our social structures and how they privilege some values over others. They also provide us with the collective opportunity to reassess how we organize our institutions and whether they promote what we consider to be essential to good medicine.

17.3 Resisting Technological Determinism and Universalism in Medicine

Given the value-laden nature of technology, we should be cautious about two downstream generalizations: that the development and deployment of new technologies are necessary for progress (technological determinism), and that technologies can be one-size-fits-all solutions to problems in medicine (technological universalism).

First, many of the innovations being utilized in medical contexts are not inevitable, particularly in their current forms. For example, EHRs could have been designed to facilitate ease of use and promote better health outcomes, with billing concerns a secondary function. Or consider the growing collection, use, and sale of health and genomic data outside of medical institutions and clinics. Given the deeply personal nature of this information and the potential for misuse, there may be good reason to prohibit organizations from collecting and storing this information without explicit consent rather than accepting the permissibility of data mining by default. It is important to recognize that what may seem like inevitable consequences of technological progress depend on choices we make, which should be interrogated by those whom the technology would impact. And we should scrutinize the intended purposes and collateral effects of new technologies early, since assumptions and standards tend to become fixed and entrenched over time, making later reforms more difficult.

Second, new technologies are often framed as universal solutions to many different problems, which risks overlooking social contexts and local variation. For example, staff may deploy AI companions or carebots in an eldercare facility in an effort to provide entertainment or even emotional support for residents. Deciding what is ethically appropriate involves answering practical and ethical questions about the specific facility, such as: How costly are these tools and will they replace care staff over time? Will they expand residents' options or will other activities and resources be reduced, effectively forcing them to engage with the carebots? In short, will carebots supplement their current human interactions or displace existing relationships? And how comfortable are residents with these kinds of tools? For those with robust social connections and tech literacy, such tools may be welcomed as an enjoyable and futuristic novelty. But the same tools offered in a place with greater social disconnection and lack of staffing may provoke serious offense or be interpreted as profoundly dystopian. Technology is implicated in social justice issues because it often enhances the lives of the privileged and further impoverishes the lives of the underprivileged. The permissibility of a new technology thus depends on the local cultural, social, and political dynamics that shape its impact.

17.4 The Role of Bioethics

Public discussion of emerging medical technologies regularly appeals to values such as autonomy, dignity, well-being, privacy, equity, transparency, and justice. With broad input from different stakeholders—including patients, clinicians, technology developers, and policymakers—a wide range of voices and experiences can be represented. However, open public discourse on emerging bioethical issues comes at a cost. Those without formal training in value theory may overlook conceptual distinctions or arguments that have been rigorously analyzed in the academic literature.

Bioethicists help to illuminate key concepts and carefully formulate what is stake in theoretical and practical disputes in medicine. Historically, they have clarified distinctions such as informed consent versus assent, privacy versus data security, pain versus harm, and genetic therapy versus genetic enhancement. By parsing such distinctions, unpacking their nuances, and drawing on historical arguments, bioethicists approach these ethical debates not merely as technical or abstract puzzles. Rather, they are opportunities to address fundamental questions about who we are, how we should relate to each other, and what kinds of social institutions best support human flourishing.

This book provides a snapshot of the current state of medical technology and its attendant ethical issues, and its contributors confront many such questions. Although they also try to anticipate the moral challenges posed by future technologies, they are not fortune-tellers; they cannot predict what revolutionary innovations will appear in the coming years. Nonetheless, the chapters of this book give us guidance about the sorts of questions to ask as we evaluate new or proposed medical technologies, such as:

- Does the technology enhance or restrict individual autonomy? Do benefits to the individual produce broader social harms? For example, even if small data allows us to improve our health through targeted interventions, will it erode personal privacy?
- What kinds of benefits and harms does the technology produce, and how do we weigh them against one another? For example, do EHRs improve communication among providers but sacrifice interpersonal engagement in the clinical setting?
- Does the technology change the physician's role from healer to something else, and is that good or bad? For example, will telehealth give patients in rural areas access to more medical specialties, or will it require patients to do a lot of self-diagnosis,

making doctors into little more than prescribers? Will caregivers at home have to take on tasks that would once have been done by trained professionals? Will care for elderly and disabled people become more the responsibility of family members, especially women?
- Does the technology reproduce existing biases or create new biases? Does it help to address injustices, produce new injustices, or both? For example, will new gene therapies provide improvement opportunities for the rich while making the poor into a biological underclass, or will costs decrease over time and provide more opportunities for everyone? Will individuals who opt out of enhancement face the social stigma of disability?
- Does the technology fundamentally change who we are and how we understand ourselves? Do the material benefits incur moral costs? For example, carebots may help overworked parents with their children, but what happens when children feel more of an emotional attachment to their carebots than their parents? Are personal, even romantic connections with AI companions simulacra of relationships, or can there be meaningful relationships between persons and nonpersons?
- Are there historical precedents that could help us anticipate the ethical implications of the technology or how to appropriately regulate its use? For example, critiques of early allocation schemes for penicillin or dialysis may help to inform the distribution of neurotechnologies. Will they be used to support medical decision-making for disabled people or to enhance the cognitive capabilities of the already well off?

Bioethicists prepare for coming uses of technology in medical practice not by knowing the future but by formulating the right questions to ask and articulating the values that ought to inform our answers.

Bioethicists also challenge common assumptions and practices when appropriate. Too often, decisions about whether to deploy new technologies are made by administrators or medical professionals who prioritize efficiency, profitability, legal compliance, or technical convenience over patient-centered values or concerns. Given the profound impact that new forms of AI, genomics, and applications of big data will have on medicine in the twenty-first century, decisions about whether to adopt them must involve more patient and caregiver voices in the deliberative process to promote safe, equitable, and just outcomes. In addition, if we want to ensure that the future of medical practice continues to preserve and promote the core values of human flourishing, dignity, and justice, bioethicists must play a crucial role.

David Schwan is a Senior Lecturer in the Department of Philosophy and Comparative Religion at Central Washington University, USA. In addition, he serves as the Director of the EthicsLab initiative at CWU. His research focuses on the intersection between applied ethics and moral psychology. He has published on empathy in medicine, the ethics of electronic health records, and medical scribes. His current research focuses on the ethics of advanced technology (AI/carebots) in medical care.

Matthew C. Altman is Chair and Professor of Philosophy at Central Washington University, USA. His research focuses on applied ethics, the history of philosophy, and the philosophy of law. Altman has published on such diverse topics as restorative justice, performance-enhancing drugs, mass incarceration, suicide, the problem of other minds, mandatory ultrasound laws, same-sex marriage, and the state of academic philosophy. He is the author, co-author, or editor of nine books, including *The Hackett Introduction to Medical Ethics* (with Cynthia D. Coe, 2025) and *A Theory of Legal Punishment* (2021).

GPSR Compliance
The European Union's (EU) General Product Safety Regulation (GPSR) is a set of rules that requires consumer products to be safe and our obligations to ensure this.

If you have any concerns about our products, you can contact us on

ProductSafety@springernature.com

In case Publisher is established outside the EU, the EU authorized representative is:

Springer Nature Customer Service Center GmbH
Europaplatz 3
69115 Heidelberg, Germany

www.ingramcontent.com/pod-product-compliance
Lightning Source LLC
Chambersburg PA
CBHW072122030825
30554CB00002B/11
* 9 7 8 3 0 3 1 9 4 6 8 9 9 *